Series on Mathematics Education Vol. **1**

How CHINESE

LEARN MATHEMATICS

Perspectives from Insid

Fan **uo**
Nanyang Technologica ngapore

Won i-Ying
The Chinese University of Ho ong, Hong Kong

Cai Jinfa
The University of Delaware, USA

Li Shiqi
East China Normal University, China

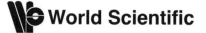

World Scientific

NEW JERSEY · LONDON · SINGAPORE · BEIJING · SHANGHAI · HONG KONG · TAIPEI · CHENNAI

Published by

World Scientific Publishing Co. Pte. Ltd.

5 Toh Tuck Link, Singapore 596224

USA office: 27 Warren Street, Suite 401-402, Hackensack, NJ 07601

UK office: 57 Shelton Street, Covent Garden, London WC2H 9HE

British Library Cataloguing-in-Publication Data
A catalogue record for this book is available from the British Library.

First published 2004
Reprinted 2006

ISBN   981-270-414-0 (pbk)

Printed in Singapore by B & JO Enterprise

Focusing on the Chinese Way of Learning Mathematics: An Introduction

The last decades have seen a mounting interest in Asian education amongst politicians, policy makers, educational researchers and practitioners around the world. In particular, being part of Asian education, Chinese education has attracted much attention. This growth of interest is clearly relevant to the widely acclaimed performance of Asian and particularly Chinese students that people have observed in large-scale international comparisons, such as those conducted in the International Assessment of Educational Progress (IAEP), the Third International Mathematics and Science Study (TIMSS), and the Programme for International Student Assessment (PISA) during this period. In those comparisons, mathematics as a school subject has been a focus because of its importance in children's school education and its comparability in contents being taught in different countries. Needless to say, many questions in this regard remain to be studied, or even identified.

This book intends to present a concerted effort in the study of Chinese mathematics education by a group of international researchers, both Chinese and non-Chinese, who we believe have insiders' experience, expertise, and more importantly a passion concerning Chinese mathematics education. The focus of the book is on how Chinese learn mathematics. Given the long history of Chinese culture, the rich practice of Chinese pedagogy, and the large population of Chinese learners, the value of studying on Chinese mathematics education to itself and beyond is easy to see.

The origin of the book can be traced back to the Ninth International Congress on Mathematical Education (ICME-9) held in Tokyo, Japan in 2000, during which a special event of the congress, *Forum of All Chinese Math Educators: Festive and Academic Gathering of Chinese Descendants and Other Interested Parties*, drew much interest from an unexpectedly large number of audience from Mainland China, Hong Kong, Singapore, Taiwan, Russia, Japan, and the United States, etc., in its two sessions[1]. With the momentum and encouragement we gained from the event and all the interested scholars and researchers including particularly the four advisors of this book, we started our journey of more than three years, from the initial discussion of the main theme and structure to the organization of peer-reviewing for all the contributions, and finally to the completion of the book.

This book consists of four sections. In **Section 1, "Overview and International Perspectives",** we start off in Chapter 1 with a comprehensive overview and synthesis by Fan and Zhu about the performance of Chinese students as revealed in large-scale international comparative studies in mathematics education conducted over the past few decades. The overview is followed by Wong, Han, and Lee's investigation of current mathematics curricula in 10 countries/regions in Chapter 2, providing readers with a broad background from an international and comparative perspective to understand the curriculum environment, under which Chinese students learn mathematics. In Chapter 3, Cai and Cifarelli provided an insightful review of smaller-scale and more specific cross-national comparative studies of the US and Chinese students and presented a profile of Chinese learners' mathematical thinking in problem solving and problem posing. In particular, they identified six characteristics of Chinese learners' mathematical thinking in problem solving. Following that, Wang and Murphy further led us in Chapter 4 into the Chinese classroom by analyzing discourse in a model Chinese mathematics classroom and developing the concept of coherence to describe the   most salient

---

[1] Also see "A Report on the Forum of All Chinese Math Educators at ICME-9", by L. Fan, D. Zhang, and L. Gu, 2000, *Bulletin of the International Commission on Mathematical Instruction. 49*, pp. 8-10.

features found in the classroom, that is, coherence in the instructional, psychological, and social dimensions. In Chapter 5, Li Jin in a more generic meaning proposed a Chinese cultural model of learning, based on her examination of Chinese learners' beliefs with respect to the learning purposes, processes, achievement standards, and affect by contrasting with the American ones. Meanwhile, Siu in Chapter 6 further opened up the cultural root of the Chinese mathematics learners by a uniquely "animated" reflection from a historical perspective on the official mathematics curriculum and the state examination system in ancient China. The chapter showed that study in mathematics in ancient China did not proceed in an examination-oriented, rote-based learning environment. In sum, by looking into the Chinese mathematics learners with different glass (telescopic, microscopic and longitudinal), we hope a general image of the Chinese mathematics learners is portrayed in Section 1.

Section 2, "Context and Teaching Materials", examines the social and pedagogical context and teaching materials particularly textbooks with the focus on how they affect the way Chinese students learn mathematics in classrooms, in schools, and in their own homes. In Chapter 7, Zhang, Li Shiqi, and Tang analyzed a once most coherent and visible principle for mathematics instruction in Mainland China, the "two basics" principle: "basic knowledge and basic skills", and discussed its both positive and negative influences on Chinese students' learning of mathematics. Bao in Chapter 8 evaluated the difficulty levels of new and old mathematics textbooks measured in five dimensions and provided us with an updated view of the mathematics curriculum in Mainland China. Also focusing on the mathematics textbooks, Fan, Chen, Zhu, Qiu, and Hu investigated in Chapter 9 the role of textbooks in the process of Chinese students' learning of mathematics through looking into how they are used by teachers and students within and beyond classrooms in two Chinese cities, Kuming and Fuzhou, providing readers with insights on how textbooks as main teaching materials shape the way of teaching and learning. Differently, Li Jianhua in Chapter 10 focused on a popular Chinese elementary school mathematics teacher manual in the topic of multi-digit multiplication, and illuminated a significant feature of the Chinese teachers' manual, that is, offering a thorough understanding of the student text and detailed suggestion for teachers' teaching. In Chapter 11, Huang Hsin Mei examined the effects of cram schools in Taiwan on children's mathematics learning. As the influence of non-formal mathematics education students received outside schools on their achievement particularly in Asia societies, such as Singapore, Hong Kong, Taiwan, Japan and Mainland China, have received growing attention in international mathematics education community[2], and yet they are still under-researched, this chapter opened a fresh and meaningful window for us to view mathematics instruction beyond the regular school settings.

Section 3, "**Pedagogy and Learning Processes**", focuses on the general pedagogy and learning processes in the Chinese mathematics classrooms. It begins with an analysis in Chapter 12 by Gu, Huang Rongjin, and Marton on how Chinese teachers promote effective mathematics learning even with large classes by teaching with variation, a characteristic they identified in Chinese mathematics classroom and a theory they have been working first independently then collaboratively on mathematics pedagogy. Still with the perspective of variations, Huang Rongjin and Leung in Chapter 13 further looked into the Hong Kong and Shanghai classroom, and their findings challenged the very idea of the so-called paradox of Chinese learners. Similarly taking a Shanghai classroom as a focal point of investigation, Lopez-Real, Mok, Leung, and Marton revealed in Chapter 14 that although one might be able to identify a "pattern" of teaching that characterizes a teacher's approach, it is dangerous to attempt to look for a national "script" of mathematics lessons. Consistently, Ma, Zhao, and Tuo further in Chapter 15 alerted us to the diversity within the perceived communality of the so-called "Chinese" mathematics classrooms by showing a vast difference in teachers and their preparation and implementation of teaching in rural and urban regions in Northeast China. In Chapter 16, Li Jun examined the learning results of using both theoretical and experimental

---

[2] For example, see the Discussion Document of ICMI Study 13, "Mathematics education in different cultural traditions: A comparative study of East Asia and the West", retrievable at its official website at http://www.inf.fu-berlin.de/icmics (as of 15 May 2004).

approaches in teaching a specific topic of mathematics curriculum, probability, on Chinese students, and hence revealed the advantages and disadvantages of both approaches. Using date collected from mathematics classrooms in Jiangsu Province of China, An in Chapter 17 identified and discussed a unique characteristic of Chinese mathematics teaching and learning: using the learning-questioning and learning-reviewing instructional model to enhance students' understanding of mathematics concepts and reinforce mathematics proficiency. Finally, Xu in Chapter 18 reported a study on the effects of using different representations in problem solving activities on Chinese children's learning of mathematics, and concluded that by means of different representations the Chinese children could exhibit their different preferred cognitive structures, which signals a challenge for teachers to change their conception about teaching and learning.

Section 4, "Inspiration and Future Directions", presents the last two chapters of the book. In Chapter 19, Wong firstly provided a comprehensive review on the trend of CHC (Confucian Heritage Culture) studies over the past fifteen years, and then examined the three Chinese traditions of calligraphy, martial art, and seal carving, and their implications for our understanding the learning of mathematics, and thus finally provided his perception of the "CHC script" concerning our main theme. In Chapter 20, Cai, Lin, and Fan offered a summary of research-based evidences that characterize how Chinese learn mathematics around the following four key issues: (1) Are Chinese learners really higher achievers in mathematics? (2) Does the teaching of Chinese learners necessarily lead to rote learning? (3) How is the intended curriculum structured to support teaching and learning? and (4) How do Chinese families support students' learning? Furthermore, for each of these questions, they discussed needed directions to better understand Chinese learners and their learning of mathematics, and thus closed the whole book.

This book could not have been completed without many people's help, support, and cooperation. As editors, first we would like to thank our advisors, Zhang Dianzhou of East China Normal University, Lee Peng Yee of the National Institute of Education (NIE) of Nanyang Technological University, Lin Fou-Lai of National Taiwan Normal

University, and Gu Lingyuan of Shanghai Academy of Educational Sciences for their invaluable advices, support, and encouragement. Three editorial meetings were held in the National Institute of Education of Singapore in May 2002, East China Normal University and Shanghai Academy of Educational Sciences in October 2002, and Shenzhen University in January 2004, and we are grateful to these institutions for their various support and/or sponsorships; besides, we owe a special thanks to Kang Wu of Shenzhen University for organizing the last editorial meeting. We also wish to thank Ren Zizhao of the National Education Examinations Center of China, Bao Jiansheng of Soochow University, Zhang Jianyue of People's Education Press of Beijing, Lionel Pereira-Mendoza of NIE, and Tso Tai-Yih of National Taiwan Normal University for various support and help they gave us at different stages. In addition, our editorial assistants, Zhu Yan, and Yeo Shu Mei of NIE, offered a great amount of editorial and technical support especially during the last stage of the completion of the book, and we truly appreciate their important assistance. Finally, we must not forget all the authors; without their effort and contribution, we could never have done our work as editors.

It is clear to us that, in many senses, this book only represents a starting point in our understanding the phenomenon and exploring the value of mathematics education involving Chinese students, and there is much to do further along this direction. In this connection, we hope the book can contribute meaningfully in the long way to the advancement of research in Chinese mathematics education, and hence more broadly in the international mathematics education.

Fan Lianghuo
Wong Ngai-Ying
Cai Jinfa
Li Shiqi

May 2004

Contents

Section 3 Pedagogy and Learning Processes

Section 4   Inspiration and Future Directions

Section 1

OVERVIEW AND
INTERNATIONAL PERSPECTIVES

Chapter 1

How Have Chinese Students Performed in Mathematics? A Perspective from Large-Scale International Mathematics Comparisons

FAN Lianghuo   ZHU Yan

This chapter primarily aims to provide readers with an overview and synthesis of the performance of Chinese students, mainly from Mainland China, Hong Kong, and Taiwan, as revealed in large-scale international comparative studies in mathematics education conducted over the past few decades. Overall, the results from those international comparisons consistently indicated that Chinese students were among the top performers, though evidences also suggested that Chinese learners were relatively weak in some mathematics areas. Attention is also paid to the interpretations and issues raised by researchers concerning those international comparisons and Chinese students' performance from various perspectives.

Key words: Chinese students, mathematics performance, large-scale international comparisons

1 Introduction

Over the past few decades, a considerable number of influential large-scale international comparative studies have been conducted in mathematics education, centering on measuring students' mathematical achievements in different countries. The results from those studies have provided a most important benchmark for comparing students' performance across different countries. As Medrich and Griffith (1992) pointed out, those studies were the most completely executed large-scale international surveys in the education domain. Therefore, it is quite understandable that they have attracted much attention from researchers, policy makers, educators, and the general public who have an interest or a stake in mathematics education in different countries.

Chinese students, including those from Mainland China, Hong Kong, and Taiwan, participated in most of the large-scale international studies, including those organized by the International Association for the Evaluation of Educational Achievement (IEA), Educational Testing Service (ETS), and the Organization for Economic Cooperation and Development (OECD). This chapter is mainly intended to provide readers with an overview and synthesis of the performance of Chinese students in those prominent international comparisons, though attention is also paid to the interpretations and issues raised by researchers concerning those international comparisons and Chinese students' performance.

Before we proceed, we should point out that although this chapter will naturally mention, to different degrees, the large-scale international comparative studies concerned, it is not intended to present a comprehensive review of those studies. Readers who are interested to know more about those studies should refer to relevant publications, which are often well-circulated and easily accessible through online resources.

2 The IEA Studies

According to Husén (1996), the idea of measuring the performance of different educational systems by testing the achievement of large samples of students was first suggested at the end of the 1950s (also see Husén & Tuijnman, 1994). In this sense, the International Association for Evaluation of Educational Achievement (IEA) was believed to be the first organization conducting large-scale international surveys in education (Robitaille & Travers, 1992). Since its inception in 1958, the IEA has conducted more than 20 large-scale comparative studies in student achievement, and five of them were in the subject of mathematics.

In 1959, the IEA began to organize its first cross-national comparison in mathematics, the First International Mathematics Study (FIMS), which was carried out from 1961 to 1967. The FIMS was believed to be an experiment in international studies on mathematics achievement (Travers & Weinzweig, 1999). Twelve countries participated in that study, mainly consisting of industrialized Western European countries, but no Chinese students from Mainland China, Hong Kong, and Taiwan were involved.

In 1976, the IEA embarked on conducting its second mathematics study the Second International Mathematics Study (SIMS). The number of participating countries increased to twenty and more than 5000 students from 130 classes in Hong Kong attended this study. Two age levels were involved in the study, that is, 13-year-old students (Population A) and students in the final grade of secondary education (Population B). At each age level, students' performance was measured and reported separately for different mathematics areas, as shown in Table 1 (Robitaille & Garden, 1989a).

Table 1
Breakdown of the SIMS Item Pool for Population A and Population B

Population A	Population B
• Arithmetic (29%)	• Sets, relations, functions (5%)
• Algebra (19%)	• Number systems (13%)
• Geometry (25%)	• Algebra (19%)
• Measurement (15%)	• Geometry (19%)
• Descriptive statistics (11%)	• Analysis (34%)
	• Probability and statistics (5%)
	• Others (5%)

At the Population A level, Hong Kong students' overall performance ranked eighth, whereas Japanese students were the first. Regarding each particular mathematics area, the SIMS found that Hong Kong students ranked eighth in arithmetic, tenth in both algebra and geometry, seventh in measurement, and fourteenth in statistics. At this age level, Japanese students received the highest average scores in all the subtests but measurement test, on which Hungary students performed the best. Figure 1 shows the mean percent correct achieved by the best performers and Hong Kong students on the five mathematics areas as well as the corresponding international mean percent correct.

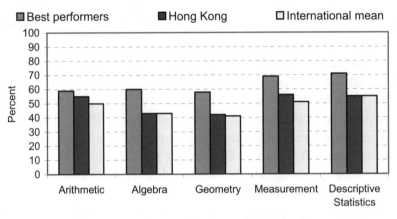

Figure 1. Students' achievements: Population A

Source. "The IEA Study of Mathematics II: Contexts and Outcomes of School Mathematics", by Robitaille and Garden, 1989a.

In order for the readers to see more specifically what were tested in the study, Table 2 shows some sample items from the five mathematics areas along with a summary of the results, including the average percentage of all the students, the average percentage of Hong Kong students, and the range of percentages of all the students who answered correctly, on each of the items.

Table 2
Percent Correct for Sample Items at the Population A Level

Item No.	Stem	Int'l mean (%)	H. K. mean (%)	Range (%)
142	Arithmetic <table><tr><td>x</td><td>3</td><td>6</td><td>P</td></tr><tr><td>y</td><td>7</td><td>Q</td><td>35</td></tr></table> The table above shows the values of x and y, where x is proportional to y. What are the values of P and Q?	22	24	50 (JPN) to 6 (LUX)
151	Algebra If $5x + 4 = 4x - 31$, then x is equal to	26	24	58 (JPN) to 9 (SWA)

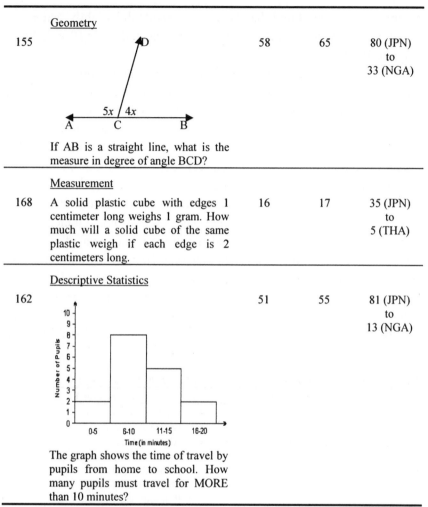

155	Geometry If AB is a straight line, what is the measure in degree of angle BCD?	58	65	80 (JPN) to 33 (NGA)
168	Measurement A solid plastic cube with edges 1 centimeter long weighs 1 gram. How much will a solid cube of the same plastic weigh if each edge is 2 centimeters long.	16	17	35 (JPN) to 5 (THA)
162	Descriptive Statistics The graph shows the time of travel by pupils from home to school. How many pupils must travel for MORE than 10 minutes?	51	55	81 (JPN) to 13 (NGA)

Note. JPN: Japan; LUX: Luxembourg; SWA: Swaziland; NGA: Nigeria; THA: Thailand.
Source. "Second International Mathematics Study", by Robitaille and Garden, 1989b.

At the final grade of secondary school, students from Hong Kong obtained the highest scores on almost all the subtests. In particular, the percent correct in each major subtest by the Hong Kong students was 80% in "sets, relations and functions", 78% in "number systems" and "algebra", 65% in "geometry", 71% in "elementary functions and calculus", and 73% in "probability and statistics". However, within algebra test, it was found that Japanese students did slightly better than Hong Kong students on "equations and inequalities" (Robitaille & Garden, 1989a).

Compared to the first two IEA studies, many more countries/regions participated in its third study, the Third International Mathematics and Science Study (TIMSS), which was believed to be "the largest international assessment that has been conducted to date in the field of education" (Beaton & Robitaille, 1999, p.31). Moreover, because of its success, it turned out to be retrospectively the first in a four-year cycle of assessment of trends in students' mathematics achievement[1].

The TIMSS study was conducted at three age levels: 9-year-olds (Grades 3 and 4 in most countries/regions), 13-year-olds (Grades 7 and 8 in most countries/regions), and students in their final year of secondary education. Students from East Asia including Hong Kong and Singapore participated in the test for the first two age but not the last age levels.

Similar to the SIMS, the TIMSS attempted to measure students' achievement in different areas with mathematics (see Table 3). The results showed that East Asian students took overall the first four places

Table 3
Mathematics Content Areas Involved in the TIMSS Tests by Grade Levels

Primary School Years	Middle School Years
• Whole numbers (25%)	• Fractions and number sense (34%)
• Fractions and proportionality (21%)	• Geometry (15%)
• Measurement, estimation, and number sense (20%)	• Algebra (18%)
• Data representation, analysis, and probability (12%)	• Data representation, analysis, and probability (14%)
• Geometry (14%)	• Measurement (12%)
• Patterns, relations, and functions (10%)	• Proportionality (7%)

Source. "Mathematics Achievement in the Middle School Years: IEA's Third International Mathematics and Science Study", by Beaton et al., 1996; "Mathematics Achievement in the Primary School Years: IEA's Third International Mathematics and Science Study", by Mullis, Martin, Beaton, et al., 1997.

---

[1] TIMSS has later been renamed Trends in International Mathematics and Science Study.

in mathematics for both young age levels: Singapore[2], Korea, Japan, and Hong Kong.

There are totally 102 items in the mathematics test at the primary school level (Mullis, Martin, Beaton, et al., 1997). The average percent correct by Hong Kong third graders on the items was 59%. The corresponding percent obtained by Korean students (first place) was 67%, while the international average percent correct was 47%. Regarding different mathematics content areas, the results showed that Hong Kong students ranked second on "geometry" items, third on "measurement, estimation, and number sense" items, and fourth on all the other items. Similar results were found for the fourth graders. Overall, Hong Kong close to 9000 primary participants ranked fourth. On each subtest, those students ranked first on "geometry" items, second on "fractions and proportionality" items, and fourth on the others. Table 4 shows some sample items from the six mathematics content areas along with a summary of students' performance on each of them.

Table 4
Percent Correct for Sample Items at the Primary School Level

Sample Items	Third Grade		Fourth Grade	
	Int'l mean (%)	H. K. mean (%)	Int'l mean (%)	H. K. mean (%)
Whole numbers				
25 × 18 is more than 24 × 18. How much more?	30	35 (5th)	45	63 (3rd)
Fractions and proportionality				
Mario uses 5 tomatoes to make half a liter of tomato sauce. How much sauce can he make from 15 tomatoes?	42	61 (1st)	53	73 (1st)

[2] Given that Singapore is a typical multi-ethnic country with the majority of population being Chinese (77%), attention is also paid to Singaporean students' performance in this Chapter.

Measurement, estimation, and number sense A thin wire 20 centimeters long is formed into a rectangle. If the width of this rectangle is 4 centimeters, what is its length?	21	20 (21st)	23	29 (5th)
Data representation, analysis, and probability The graph shows the number of cartons of milk sold each day of a week at a school. How many cartons of milk did the school sell on Monday?	19	23 (7th)	37	38 (12th)
Geometry This picture shows a cube with one edge marked. How many edges does the cube have altogether? 	35	53 (2nd)	42	72 (1st)
Patterns, relations, and functions These numbers are part of a pattern. 50, 46, 42, 38, 34, … What do you have to do to get the next number?	41	43 (10th)	57	65 (10th)

Note. From Table 4 to Table 8, the ordinal numbers in the brackets represent the ranking of Chinese students concerned on the particular test item in all the participating countries. *Source.* "Mathematics Achievement in the Primary School Years: IEA's Third International Mathematics and Science Study", by Mullis, Martin, Beaton, et al., 1997.

At the middle school year level, Hong Kong students also ranked fourth, whereas both seventh and eighth graders from Singapore became the best performers. On the 151 test items at this school level, the average percent correct obtained by Hong Kong seventh graders was 65% and that by eighth graders was 70%, and the corresponding percent by Singaporean students was 73% and 79%, while the international average percent correct was 49% and 55%, respectively. Moreover, the TIMSS revealed that in the defined six major mathematics content areas, Hong Kong close to 7000 participants were relatively weak on "measurement" and "proportionality" items. Some sample items and students' corresponding performance are given in Table 5.

Table 5
Percent Correct for Sample Items at the Middle School Level

Sample Items	Seventh Grade		Eighth Grade	
	Int'l mean (%)	H. K. mean (%)	Int'l mean (%)	H. K. mean (%)
Fractions and number sense				
If the price of a can of beans is raised from 60 cents to 75 cents, what is the percent increase in the price?	23	47 (2nd)	28	54 (2nd)
Geometry				
What is the ratio of the length of a side of a square to its perimeter?	50	63 (7th)	56	71 (5th)
Algebra				
If $3(x + 5) = 30$, then $x =$	62	87 (2nd)	72	92 (2nd)
Data representation, analysis, and probability				
Each of the six faces of a certain cube is painted either red or blue. When the cube is tossed, the probability of the cube landing with a red face up is $\frac{2}{3}$. How many faces are red?	41	70 (3rd)	47	72 (3rd)

Measurement

| Which of these angles has a measure closest to 30°? | 62 | 69 (14th) | 64 | 68 (16th) |

A.   B.

C.   D.

Proportionality

| Peter bought 70 items and Sue bought 90 items. Each item cost the same and the items cost \$800 altogether. How much did Sue pay? | 32 | 52 (6th) | 38 | 62 (4th) |

Source. "Mathematics Achievement in the Middle School Years: IEA's Third International Mathematics and Science Study", by Beaton et al., 1996.

Although student mathematics achievement in the TIMSS was measured primarily through written tests, participating countries also had an opportunity to administer a performance assessment, which consisted of a set of practical tasks. The performance assessment was available for administration to a sub-sample of both fourth and eighth graders that completed the written tests. At the eighth grade level, there were 19 education systems participating in the mathematics performance assessment and among them Singapore was the only Asian country[3]. However, at the fourth grade level, students from nine education systems including Hong Kong participated in the performance assessment. The performance assessment is the largest international one of its kind that has bee conducted so far.

At each grade level, the study set a total of five mathematics performance tasks. Table 6 shows the overall results for both Singapore and Hong Kong students.

---

[3] Hong Kong also participated in the eighth grade performance assessment, but it failed to meet the sampling criteria, hence the results were excluded in the official report.

Table 6
Average Percentage Scores on Performance Assessment Tasks in the TIMSS

Tasks	Fourth Grade			Eighth Grade		
	Best performers (%)	Hong Kong (%)	Int'l ave. (%)	Best performers (%)	Singapore (%)	Int'l ave. (%)
Dice	54 (AUS)	48 (2nd)	42	84 (SIN)	84 (1st)	73
Calculator	50 (HKG)	50 (1st)	40	66 (ROM)	60 (4th)	54
Folding and cutting	63 (SLO)	40 (3rd)	38	84 (ROM)	80 (3rd)	69
Around bend	57 (HKG)	57 (1st)	44	67 (NTH)	63 (3rd)	54
Packaging	34 (IRA)	15 (5th)	17	65 (SIN)	65 (1st)	44
Overall	44 (SLO)	39 (5th)	36	71 (SIN)	71 (1st)	59

Note. 1. AUS: Australia; SIN: Singapore; HKG: Hong Kong; ROM: Romania; SLO: Slovenia; NTH: Netherlands; IRA: Iran, Islamic Republic. 2. The overall score is the average of percentage scores across tasks, including one combination task (i.e., Plasticine) with all tasks being weighted equally.
Source. "Performance Assessment in IEA's Third International Mathematics and Science Study", by Harmon et al., 1997.

During 1997-2001, a replication of the TIMSS, known as TIMSS-Repeat (TIMSS-R), was conducted. It measured progress in the eighth grade mathematics in thirty-eight countries/regions. About 5000 students from Hong Kong and 6000 from Taipei participated in the study. In the TIMSS-R, the mathematics test was also designed to enable reporting by various content areas, including *fractions and number sense, measurement, data representation, analysis, and probability, geometry,* and *algebra.* Consistent to the TIMSS, the TIMSS-R found that East Asian students (i.e., Singapore, Korea, Chinese Taipei, Hong Kong, and Japan) again achieved highest scores in overall mathematics assessment as well as in each of the major content areas. Table 7 shows Chinese Taipei and Hong Kong students' overall performance in the TIMSS-R.

Table 7
Chinese Students' Mathematics Performance in the TIMSS-R

	Best performers	Chinese Taipei	Hong Kong
Fractions and number sense	608 (SIN)	576 (3rd)	579 (2nd)
Measurement	599 (SIN)	566 (4th)	567 (3rd)
Data representation, analysis, and probability	576 (KOR)	559 (3rd)	547 (5th)
Geometry	575 (JPN)	557 (4th)	556 (5th)
Algebra	586 (TAP)	586 (1st)	569 (5th)
Overall	604 (SIN)	585 (3rd)	582 (4th)

Note. SIN: Singapore; KOR: Korea; JPN: Japan; TAP: Chinese Taipei.
Source. "TIMSS 1999 International Mathematics Report: Findings From IEA's Repeat of the Third International Mathematics and Science at the Eighth Grade", by Mullis, Martin, Gonzalez, et al., 2000. The international average for each content area as well as for the overall performance was scaled to be 487.

Among the 38 participating educational systems, 26 systems, including Hong Kong, took part in both TIMSS studies, which provided a unique opportunity to investigate the change in mathematics achievement over the four years in an international context. The comparison of students' performance between the two time periods reveals that the average mathematics achievement across the 26 countries increased slightly, from a scale score of 519 in 1995 to 521 in 1999 (Mullis, Martin, Gonzalez, et al., 2000). The greatest increase was received in Latvia (Latvian-Speaking Schools) with an increase of 17 scale-score points. The next highest increase, 13 scale-score points, occurred in Hong Kong, which was much higher than the other three Asian regions (Korea: 4, Japan: -4, Singapore: -7). Moreover, it was found that Hong Kong students got slight improvement in all individual mathematics content areas ranging from 1% in *measurement* and *algebra* to 4% in *data representation, analysis, and probability* (Leung, Yung, & Tso, 2002).

3 The ETS Studies

Claiming to be the largest private educational testing and measurement organization, the Educational Testing Service (ETS) has for a long time been active in educational testing in the United States and taken charge of the National Assessment of Educational Progress (NAEP) program since 1983 (Robitaille & Travers, 1992). In 1988 and 1990/91, the ETS further carried out two large-scale international studies entitled *International Assessment of Educational Progress* (IAEP). The purpose of IAEP was to collect and report data on what students know and can do, on educational and cultural factors associated with achievement, and on students' attitudes (Mead, 1995).

In the first study (IAEP1), 13-year-old students from the United States and five other countries were assessed in their mathematics and science achievement, but no Chinese students were involved.

More than a dozen countries/regions participated in the second study (IAEP2) and students at two age levels (9-year-old and 13-year-old) were assessed. About 1650 Students from Mainland China participated in the 13-year-old test, while about the same number of students from Taiwan attended each of the two age level tests. It is worth noting that, among the IEA and ETS international comparisons, the IAEP2 is the only one involving students from Mainland China, and the participants were selected from only 17 provinces and 3 municipal cities, representing 38% of the total age-eligible children (Lapointe, Mead, & Askew, 1992).

The mathematics achievement tests in the IAEP2 lasted one hour at both age levels and covered five content areas: *Numbers and operations, Measurement, Geometry, Data analysis, statistics, and probability*, and *Algebra and functions*. At the 9-year-old level, students from Taiwan ranked third among the 14 educational systems, while Korean students performed best. At the elder level, students from Mainland China were the top performers. However, as shown in Table 8, Chinese students were relatively weak in *Data analysis, statistics, and probability*.

Table 8
Chinese Students' Performance (Percent Correct) in IAEP studies

	9-year-old			13-year-old			
	Best performers (%)	Taiwan (%)	Int'l ave. (%)	Best performers (%)	Mainland China (%)	Taiwan (%)	Int'l ave. (%)
N.O.	74.6 (KOR)	67.1 (4th)	61.2	84.9 (CHI)	84.9 (1st)	74.7 (3rd)	61.0
Mea.	73.3 (ITA)	69.3 (7th)	67.2	71.4 (CHI)	71.3 (1st)	63.7 (2nd)	46.9
Geo.	75.4 (KOR)	69.2 (2nd)	63.9	80.2 (CHI)	80.2 (1st)	76.6 (4th)	62.2
D.S.P.	79.3 (KOR)	72.8 (3rd)	67.6	81.8 (SWI)	75.4 (10th)	81.2 (2nd)	69.1
A.F.	72.4 (HUN)	64.2 (5th)	61.8	82.4 (CHI)	82.4 (1st)	69.2 (5th)	54.2
Ove.	74.8 (KOR)	68.1 (3rd)	63.3	80.2 (CHI)	80.2 (1st)	72.7 (3rd)	58.3

Note. 1. N.O. = Number and operations; Mea. = Measurement; Geo. = Geometry; D.S.P. = Data analysis, statistics, and probability; A.F. = Algebra and functions; Ove. = Overall; 2. CHI: Mainland China; HUN: Hungary; KOR: Korea; ITA: Italy; SWI: Swaziland.
Source. "Learning Mathematics", by Lapointe, Mead, and Askew, 1992.

Moreover, the IAEP also investigated students' mathematics achievement in three process aspects, including *Conceptual understanding* (understanding of mathematical facts and concepts), *Procedural knowledge* (application of knowledge and concepts in solving routine problems using procedures taught in the classroom), and *Problem solving* (application of several skills to a unique situation, which usually involved multiple steps) (Lapointe, Mead, & Askew, 1992). The results showed that at the 14-year-old age level, students from Mainland China ranked first in all the three aspects, whereas those from Taiwan also performed quite well, ranking either second or third. However, at the 9-year-old age level, the Chinese students did not do well on *Problem solving* tasks and their average percent correct (55.7) was lower than the international average (58.5), ranking tenth among the 14 educational systems.

4 The OECD Studies

The fact that the Organization for Economic Cooperation and Development (OECD), as a global organization, started in the early 1990s to organize large-scale international comparative studies reflects the value of such cross-national comparison. The OECD organized its first one called the International Adult Literacy Surveys (IALS) between 1994 and 1998. Later, it initiated another new system of international assessment, Programme for International Student Assessment (PISA), which is a three-yearly survey of the knowledge and skills of 15-year-olds in reading, mathematical, and scientific literacy. In each survey, two-thirds of testing time will be devoted to one major literacy domain: reading in 2000, mathematics in 2003, and science in 2006.

Rather than focusing on school mathematics curriculum as it is often seen in other large-scale cross-national comparisons such as the TIMSS, PISA defined mathematical literacy broadly as the capacity to identify, understand and engage in mathematics as well as to make well-founded judgment about the role of mathematics plays in an individual's current and future private life, occupational life, social life with peers and relatives, and life as a constructive, concerned and reflective citizen (OECD, 2003). Accordingly, three broad dimensions were further identified in PISA for use in assessing students' mathematics literacy.

- *Mathematical content.* It was organized around two aspects: mathematical big ideas including chance, growth and change, dependency and relationships, and space and shape, and mathematical curricular strands including number, measurement, estimation, algebra, functions, geometry, probability, statistics, and discrete mathematics.
- *Mathematical processes.* PISA organized them into three classes, consisting of Competency Class 1: representation, definitions, and computations; Competency Class 2: connections and integrations for problem solving; and Competency Class 3: mathematisation, mathematical thinking, generalization and insight.
- *Mathematical situations and context.* The situations in which the PISA items were set were categorized as community;

educational; occupational, personal and scientific, to ensure the tasks were based on authentic contexts which can be likely found in the actual experiences and practices of students in a real-world setting.

A total of 4405 students from 140 schools in Hong Kong were randomly selected to participate in the mathematics assessment of PISA 2000, whose main focus was though on reading as indicated earlier. The results suggested that Hong Kong students were overall the best performers. They obtained a mean of 560 on mathematical literacy scale, which has a mean of 500 points and a standard deviation of 100 points, significantly higher than all the other 40 participating countries/regions except Japan (mean score: 557) and Korea (mean score: 547).

Furthermore, Hong Kong students performed substantially better than their international peers in all the three broad dimensions explained above and sub-areas under these dimensions. In content areas, the largest lead was seen in algebra and measurement but more moderate lead was observed in functions, geometry, and statistics. Table 9 presents part of the results.

Table 9

Comparison of Students' Average Scores of Hong Kong and OECD Countries/Regions on Some Dimensions and Sub-areas of the PISA Framework

	Hong Kong average (%)	OECD Average (%)
Mathematical curricular strands (Content)		
Algebra	55	28
Functions	62	55
Geometry	65	54
Measurement	56	41
Statistics	58	50
Mathematical processes (Competency Class)		
1: Representation, definitions, and computations	75	65
2: connections and integrations for problem solving	55	41
3: mathematisation, mathematical thinking, generalization and insight	27	14

Source. "The First HKPISA Report: Monitoring the Quality of Education in Hong Kong from an International Perspective", by HKPISA Center, 2003.

In addition, results showed that the differences in scores at different percentiles of students is quite uniform, suggesting students at different levels within Hong Kong are doing equally well in comparison with their international counterparts at corresponding levels (HKPISA Center, 2003).

5 Summary and Discussions

Table 10 presents a synthesis of Chinese students' performance and relevant information in all the above-mentioned international large-scale mathematics comparative studies.

From the results revealed in those large-scale international comparative studies, the most obvious conclusion that we can draw is that Chinese students, whether they are from Mainland China, Hong Kong, or Taiwan, were overall among the top performers by international standards. Meanwhile, under this general observation, it should be noted that evidences also suggested that Chinese learners were relatively weak in some mathematics areas, which was most evident in IAEP2, which showed that students from Mainland China were at the 10th place in the area of data analysis, statistics, and probability[4] while they were the best in all the other areas, and the performance of students from Taiwan were below the international average level in problem solving tasks.

It should be pointed out that Chinese students' outstanding academic performance in mathematics was also manifested in the International Mathematics Olympiads (see the appendix), and in particular, a large number of small-scale cross-national comparative studies conducted by individual researchers over the past two decades, most notably by Stigler, Stevenson, and their colleagues (e.g., Chen & Stevenson, 1995; Stevenson, Chen, & Lee, 1993; Stevenson & Stigler, 1992; Stigler, Lee, Lucker, & Stevenson, 1982; Stigler, Lee, & Stevenson, 1990). Those small-scale comparisons often provide us with more in-depth views and

---

[4] The reason seems to be related to the fact that data analysis, statistics, and probability were ignored in the school mathematics curriculum for a long time in Mainland China. The new reformed curriculum has explicitly included those topics (also see Li Jun, this volume), and it would be interesting to see how Chinese students will perform in this area in the future international comparisons.

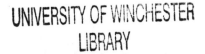

Table 10

Chinese Students' Performance in Large-scale International Mathematics Comparative Studies

International Study	No. of participating education systems	Age groups tested	Participation by Chinese students	Chinese students' performance (ranking)
FIMS (1961 – 1967)	11	13	None	NA
	12	17/18		
SIMS (1976 – 1989)	20	13	Hong Kong (5548 students, 125 schools)	8th
	15	17/18	Hong Kong (3294 students, 131 schools)	1st
IAEP1 (1988)	6	13	None	NA
IAEP2 (1990 – 1991)	13	9	China Taiwan (about 1650 students, 110 schools)	3rd
	20	13	Mainland China (about 1650 students, 110 schools)	1st
			China Taiwan (about 1650 students, 110 schools)	3rd
TIMSS (1991 – 1998)	26	9	Hong Kong (8807 students, 124 schools)	4th
	42	13	Hong Kong (6752 students, 86 schools)	4th
	24	17/18	None	NA
TIMSS-R (1997-2001)	38	13	Chinese Taipei (5772 students, 150 schools)	3rd
			Hong Kong (5179 students, 137 schools)	4th
PISA 2000 (2000 – 2002)	41	15	Hong Kong (4405 students, 140 schools)	1st
TIMSS 2003 (2000-2004)	27	9	Chinese Taipei (4661 students, 150 schools)	4th
			Hong Kong (4608 students, 150 schools)	2nd
	49	13	Chinese Taipei (5379 students, 150 schools)	4th
			Hong Kong (4972 students, 150 schools)	3rd
PISA 2003 (2002-2003)	42	15	Hong Kong (4478 students, 145 schools)	1st
			Macau (1250 students, 39 schools)	9th

Source. "Implementation of the TIMSS Sample Design", by Foy, 1996; "Implementation and the Sample Design", by Foy and Joncas, 1999; "Second International Mathematics Study", by Robitaille and Garden, 1989b; "Mathematics Achievement in Hong Kong Secondary Schools", by Brimer and Griffin, 1985; "The First HKPISA Report: Monitoring the Quality of Education in Hong Kong From an International Perspectiv", by HKPISA Center, 2003; "International Assessment of Educational Progress", by Mead, 1995; "Highlights from the Trends in International Mathematics and Science Study (TIMSS) 2003", by Gonzales et al., 2004; "PISA Learning for Tomorrow's World: First Results from PISA 2003", by Centre for Educational Research and Innovation, 2004; except for the durations of the IEA studies, which are retrieved March 15, 2004, from the IEA's official website at http://www.iea.nl/iea/hq

analysis on relevant issues. Nevertheless, to discuss in detail those small-scale studies is beyond the scope of this chapter.

On the other hand, the methodological issues of those large-scale international studies have recently received increasing attention from researchers (e.g., see Postlethwaite, 1999). In particular, different researchers have questioned the reliability and validity of the results obtained from those large-scale comparative studies and the generalizability of those from the small-scale ones (e.g., Bracey, 1993, 1996, 2000; Jaeger, 1992; Rotberg, 1990; Wang, 1996, 2001). Concerning the large-scale comparisons, researchers have argued that the majority of mathematics problems used in those studies were routine and traditional, which were hard to detect students' higher order thinking skills, for example, about 83% of the TIMSS items were multiple-choice questions for Population 2 students (International Association for the Evaluation of Education Achievement, 1996). Others have found that when more challenging tasks, such as open-ended problems, were used for comparisons, Chinese students did not demonstrate much superior performance in mathematics (e.g., Brenner, Herman, Ho, & Zimmer, 1999; Cai, 1998; also see Cai & Cifarelli, this volume).

Despite the criticisms and doubts about the past cross-national studies, many researchers in the international mathematics education community have tried to explore the possible reasons for Chinese students' outstanding performance in mathematics as revealed in the cross-national comparisons. They have interpreted such phenomenon from different perspectives and examined different factors that might affect students' learning in mathematics, including students' mother tongue (e.g., Fuson & Kwon, 1991; Geary, Bow-Thomas, Liu, & Siegler, 1996), societal expectation (e.g., Jiang & Eggleton, 1995; Stevenson et al., 1990), parental involvement (e.g., Stevenson & Stigler, 1992), social beliefs and cultural values (e.g., Stevenson, Chen, & Lee, 1993; Wong, 1998), learning behavior such as the amount of time spent on mathematics (e.g., Stevenson, Stigler, & Lee, 1986), curriculum and textbooks (e.g., Cai, Lo, & Watanabe, 2002; Zhu, 2003), among others. Although the available studies in this area have enhanced people's understanding concerning the way in which students learn mathematics in different countries and societies, it appears clear that we are at an explorative but not confirmative stage (also see Leung, 2002). There is still a long way for us to go to understand more precisely and definitely what contributed to the differences in students' achievements in mathematics, and how we can learn better from cross-national comparisons to further improve students' learning experiences in mathematics in different countries and educational systems.

Acknowledgements

The authors wish to thank Drs. Lionel Pereira-Mendoza, Chua Seng Kiat, Wong Ngai-Ying, and Frederick K. S. Leung for their various helps and suggestions in writing this chapter.

References

Beaton, A. E., Mullis, I. V. S., Martin, M. O., Gonzalez, E. J., Kelly, D. L., & Smith, T. A. (1996). *Mathematics achievement in the middle school year: IEA's Third International Mathematics and Science Study.* Chestnut Hill, MA: TIMSS International Study Centre, Boston College.

Beaton, A. E., & Robitaille, D. F. (1999). An overview of the Third International Mathematics and Science Study. In G. Kaiser, E. Luna, & I. Huntley (Eds.), *Studies in mathematics education series II: International comparisons in mathematics education* (pp. 30-47). London: Falmer Press.

Bracey, G. (1993). American students hold their own. *Educational Leadership, 50*(5), 66-67.

Bracey, G. (1996). International comparisons and the condition of American education. *Educational Researcher, 25*(1), 5-11.

Bracey, G. (2000). The TIMSS final year and report: A critique. *Educational Research, 29*(4), 4-10.

Brenner, M. E., Herman, S., Ho, H., & Zimmer, J. M. (1999). Cross-national comparison of representational competence. *Journal for Research in Mathematics Education, 30*(5), 541-557.

Brimer, A., & Griffin, P. (1985). *Mathematics achievement in Hong Kong secondary schools.* Hong Kong: Center of Asian Study, University of Hong Kong.

Cai, J. (1998). An investigation of U.S. and Chinese students' mathematical problem posing and problem solving. *Mathematics Education Research Journal, 10*(1), 37-50.

Cai, J., Lo, J. J., & Watanabe, T. (2002). Intended treatment of arithmetic average in U.S. and Asia school mathematics textbooks. *School Science and Mathematics, 102*(8), 1-13.

Centre for Educational Research and Innovation. (2004). *PISA learning for tomorrow's world: First results from PISA 2003*. Paris, France: Organization for Economic Co-operation and Development.

Chen, C., & Stevenson, H. W. (1995). Motivation and mathematics achievement: A comparative study of Asian American, Caucasian American, and East Asian high school students. *Child Development, 66*, 1215-1234.

Foy, P. (1996). Implementation of the TIMSS sample design. In M. O. Martin & D. L. Kelly (Eds.), *TIMSS technical report volume II: Implementation and analysis (primary and middle school years)* (pp. 21-45). Retrieved March 10, 2004, from http://isc.bc.edu/timss1995/TIMSSPDF/TR2chap2.pdf

Foy, P., & Joncas, M. (1999). Implementation and the sample design. In M. O. Martin, K. D. Gregory, & S. E. Stemler (Eds.), *TIMSS 1999 technical report* (pp. 155-168). Retrieved March 10, 2004, from http://isc.bc.edu/timss1999i/pdf/T99_TR_Chap09.pdf

Fuson, K. C., & Kwon, Y. (1991). Chinese-based regular and European irregular systems of number words: The disadvantages for English-speaking children. In K. Durkin & B. Shire (Eds.), *Language in mathematics education: Research and practice* (pp. 211-226). Milton Keynes, PA: Open University Press.

Harmon, M., Smith, T. A., Martin, M. O., Kelly, D. L., Beaton, A. E., Mullis, I. V. S., et al. (1997). *Performance assessment in IEA's Third International Mathematics and Science Study*. Retrieved March 1, 2004, from http://timss.bc.edu/timss1995/TIMSSPDF/PAreport.pdf

HKPISA Center (2003). The *HKPISA report: Monitoring the quality of education in Hong Kong from an international perspective*. Hong Kong: Author.

Husén, T. (1996). Lessons from the IEA studies. *International Journal of Educational Research, 25*(3), 207-218.

Husén, T., & Tuijnman, A. C. (1994). Monitoring standards in education: Why and how it came out. In A. C. Tuijnman & T. N. Postlethwaite (Eds.), *Monitoring standards in education: Paper in honor of John P. Keeves* (pp. 1-22). Oxford: Pergamon.

Geary, D. C., Bow-Thomas, C. C., Liu, F., & Siegler, R. S. (1996). Development of arithmetical competencies in Chinese and American children: Influence of age, language, and schooling. *Child Development, 67*(5), 2022-2044.

Gonzales, P., Guzman, J. C., Partelow, L., Pahlke, E., Jocelyn, L., Kastberg, et al. (2004). *Highlights from the Trends in International Mathematics and Science Study: TIMSS 2003*. Washington, DC: National Center for Education Statistics.

International Association for the Evaluation of Education Achievement. (1996). *TIMSS mathematics items: Released set for population 2 (seventh and eighth grades)*. Chestnut Hill, MA: Boston College.

Jaeger, R. M. (1992). Weak measurement serving presumptive policy. *Phi Delta Kappan, 74*(2), 118-128.

Jiang, Z., & Eggleton, R. (1995). A brief comparison of the U.S. and Chinese middle school mathematics programs. *School Science and Mathematics, 95*(4), 187-194.

Lapointe, A. E., Mead, N. A., & Askew, J. M. (1992). *Learning mathematics*. New Jersey: Educational Testing Service.

Leung, F. K. S. (2002). Behind the high achievement of East Asian students. *Educational Research and Evaluation. 8*(1), 87-108.

Leung, F. K. S., Yung, B. H. W., & Tso, A. S. F. (2002). *Secondary analysis of the TIMSS-R data for Hong Kong*. Hong Kong: Hong Kong IEA Center.

Mead, N. A. (1995). International Assessment of Educational Progress. In *International comparative studies in education: Descriptions of selected large-scale assessments and case studies* (pp. 48-57). Washington, DC: National Research Council. (ERIC Documents Reproduction Service No. ED383761)

Medrich, E. A., & Griffith, J. (1992). *International mathematics and science assessment: What have we learned?* National Center for Education Statistics Research and Development Report (NCES Publication No. 92-011). (ERIC Document Reproduction Service No. ED 342680)

Mullis, I. V. S., Martin, M. O., Beaton, A. E., Gonzalez, E. J., Kelly, D. L., & Smith, T. A. (1997). *Mathematics achievement in the primary school years: IEA's Third International Mathematics and Science Study*. Chestnut Hill, MA: TIMSS International Study Center, Boston College.

Mullis, I. V. S., Martin, M. O., Gonzalez, E. J., Gregory, K. D., Garden, R. A., O'Connor, et al. (2000). *TIMSS 1999 international mathematics report: Findings from IEA's repeat of the Third International Mathematics and Science Study at the eighth grade*. Chestnut Hill, MA: Boston College.

Organization of Economic Cooperation and Development (2003). *Literacy skills for the world of tomorrow: Further result from PISA 2000*. Retrieved March 1, 2004, from http://www1.oecd.org/publications/e-book/960301E.PDF

Postlethwaite, T. N. (1999). *International studies of educational achievement: Methodological issues*. Hong Kong: Comparative Education Research Centre, The University of Hong Kong.

Robitaille, D. F., & Garden, R. A. (Eds.) (1989a). *The IEA study of mathematics II: Contexts and outcomes of school mathematics*. New York: Pergamon Press.

Robitaille, D. F., & Garden, R. A. (Eds.) (1989b). *Second International Mathematics Study*. Stockholm: International Association for the Evaluation of Educational Achievement.

Robitaille, D. F., & Travers, K. J. (1992). International studies of achievement in mathematics. In D. A. Grouws (Ed.), *Handbook of research on mathematics and teaching* (pp. 687-709). New York: Macmillan.

Rotberg, I. C. (1990). I never promised you first place. *Phi Delta Kappan, 72*(4), 296-303.

Stevenson, H. W., Chen, C., & Lee, S. Y. (1993). Mathematics achievement of Chinese, Japanese, and American children: Ten years later. *Science, 259*(1), 53-58.

Stevenson, H. W., Lee, S. Y., Chen, C., Lummis, M., Stigler, J. W., Fan, L., et al. (1990). Mathematics achievement of children in China and the United States. *Child Development, 61*(4), 1053-1066.

Stevenson, H. W., & Stigler, J. W. (1992). *The learning gap: Why ours schools are failing and what we can learn from Japanese and Chinese education?* New York: Summit Books.

Stevenson, H. W., Stigler, J. W., & Lee, S. Y. (1986). Achievement in mathematics. In H. W. Stevenson, H. Azuma, & K. Hakuta (Eds.), *Children development and education in Japan* (pp. 201-218). New York: Freeman.

Stigler, J. W., Lee, S. Y., Lucker, G. W., & Stevenson, H. W. (1982). Curriculum and achievement in mathematics: A study of elementary school children in Japan, Taiwan and the United States. *Journal of Educational Psychology, 74*(3), 315-322.

Stigler, J. W., Lee, S. Y., & Stevenson, H. W. (1990). *Mathematical knowledge of Japanese, Chinese, and American elementary school children.* Reston, VA: National Council of Teachers of Mathematics.

Travers, K. J., & Weinzweig, A. I. (1999). The Second International Mathematics Study. In G. Kaiser, E. Luna, & I. Huntley (Eds.), *Studies in mathematics education series II: International comparisons in mathematics education* (pp. 19-29). London: Falmer Press.

Wang, J. (1996). Letter to the editor. *Journal for Research in Mathematics Education, 27*(5), 619-620.

Wang, J. (2001). TIMSS primary and middle school data: Some technical concerns. *Educational Researcher, 30*(6), 17-21.

Wong, N. Y. (1998). In search of the "CHC" leaner: Smarter, works harder or something more? In H. S. Park, Y. H. Choe, H. Shin, & S. H. Kim (Eds.), *Proceedings of the ICMI-East Asian Regional Conference on Mathematics Education I* (pp. 85-98). Chungbuk, Korea.

Zhu, Y. (2003). *Representations of problem solving in China, Singapore and US mathematics textbooks: A comparative study.* Unpublished doctoral dissertation, National Institute of Education, Nanyang Technological University, Singapore.

Appendix

Chinese Students' Performance in the International Mathematics Olympiads (1994-2004)

	No. of participating countries/regions	Mainland China (1985)	Hong Kong (1988)	Taiwan (1992)	Singapore (1988)
2004	85	1st	30th	6th	18th
2003	82	2nd	28th	16th	36th
2002	83	1st	24th	7th	30th
2001	87	1st	19th	9th	29th
2000	82	1st	28th	8th	37th
1999	81	1st	33rd	9th	36th
1998	76	NA	25th	5th	22nd
1997	82	1st	30th	14th	41st
1996	75	6th	27th	20th	25th
1995	73	1st	20th	12th	26th
1994	69	2nd	16th	12th	29th

Note. 1. All the results are retrieved from http://olympiads.win.tue.nl/imo/ as March 15, 2004 and http://www.imo2004/fimo as March 31, 2005. They are also available online in other IMO relevant websites. 2. The number in each bracket indicates the year for the first time of participation in the IMO. 3. All the students, except two, in the Singapore's teams participating in the IMOs from 1988 to 2004 were ethnically Chinese (Source: personal communication with Dr. Chua Seng Kiat, who led the Singapore IMO Teams in the 1990s).

Chapter 2

The Mathematics Curriculum:
Toward Globalization or Westernization?[1]

WONG Ngai-Ying   HAN Jiwei   LEE Peng Yee

The mathematics curricula of various educational regions have experienced their reform at the turn of the millennium. All these worldwide curriculum reforms precisely signify how great the challenge we have to face. We have to prepare our youngsters for an age in which the economy is globalized, the society is "knowledge-based", and information-rich. Previous analysis on the mathematics curricula showed that there had been a difference (now matter how small) in the approaches and pedagogical philosophies between "Western" and "Far Eastern" regions. The positions of their curricula were different too. However, in recent years, regions around the world seem to be meeting the same challenges and so the notions of accountability, valued-addedness, curriculum standardization, higher order abilities, ICT, life-long and life-wide learning have become world trends, which is common to both the "East" and the "West". In this chapter, the authors would first analyze and compare the mathematics curricula of major "Western" and "Far Eastern" regions. Their communalities and differences will then be drawn. The problems that arose from these trends will be discussed and possible solutions will be put forth.

Key words: curriculum, process ability, globalization, educational control

1 Introduction

The mathematics curricula of various educational regions in the world have experienced their reforms at the turn of the Millennium. While the

---

[1] The authors wish to thank Mrs. Siu Chan Fung Kit for translating part of the French mathematics Curriculum into English.

standard-based curriculum movement started off in the United States, along with the publication of *Curriculum and Evaluation Standards for School Mathematics* in 1989, the United Kingdom also had its first the national curriculum in the same year. In Australia, the *National Statement on Mathematics for Australian Schools* was published in 1990 and a new mathematics curriculum was published in New Zealand in 1992. Curriculum innovation also happened in continental Europe like France and Germany. The Netherlands had its new curriculum in 1998 too.

The same holds true in the other side of the globe. Educational and curriculum reform had been taken place in Mainland China, Taiwan and Hong Kong towards the end of the 20th century. Macau also published the first mathematics curriculum of its own after its reunion with China. Japan had its new mathematics curriculum in 2000, South Korea in 1998, Singapore in 1998 and again in 2000, Malaysia in 1993, which introduced the new concept of "Smart Schools" in 1998.

All these worldwide curriculum reforms, in particular in the subject of mathematics, clearly indicate how great the challenge we have to face. We have to prepare our youngsters for an age in which the economy is globalized, and the society is "knowledge-based" and information-rich. Previous analysis on the mathematics curricula showed that there had been a difference (no matter how small) in the approaches and pedagogical philosophies between "Western" and "Eastern" regions (N. Y. Wong & K. M. Wong, 1997). The positioning of their curricula was different too. However, in recent years, regions around the world seem to be facing the same challenges. As a result, the notions of accountability, valued-addedness, curriculum standardization, higher-order abilities, ICT (information and communication technology), life-long and life-wide learning have become world trends. They are now common emphases in the "East" and the "West" alike.

Before inspecting the curricula of various countries, we would like to have a look on the notion of curriculum itself. There are a lot of definitions of "curriculum" (D. Tanner & L. N. Tanner, 1980), each carrying a different perspective, or even conception, of it. While the International Association for the Evaluation of Educational Achievement (IEA) "intended – implemented – attained" curriculum is often used (Robitaille & Garden, 1989), Goodlad (1979) further identified the aspects of ideological, formal, perceived, operational, and experiential curricula (see also B. Clarke, D. Clarke, & Sullivan, 1996). Certainly one can get a holistic picture of what is happening in the classroom only by ethnographic observation of the implemented curriculum. In this chapter, though we can only focus on the intended curriculum as exhibited by the official curriculum documents, they can still reveal the general orientation of the curricula. One should also note that the curriculum could have different roles in different regions. Curriculum documents are more mandatory in some regions than in others. Some are meant to be a checklist of the attained curriculum (attainment targets, attainment standards, etc.); some are "code of practices" to be followed by teachers; some are programs of studies; some are curriculum frameworks for curriculum developers or textbook writers; and some are general principles and directions just for teachers' references (N. Y. Wong & K. M. Wong, 1997). In "Eastern" regions where public examinations often play a leading role, many of these documents originated from examination syllabi and thus more attention was paid on the regulations regarding examinations rather than on the teaching process in the presentation of the curriculum.

Naturally, like most other educational studies, a single investigation can only explore a few facets of the problem; however, we believe that the stated educational goals of curricula constitute essential parts of them. In this chapter, we will first provide a general picture by making a comparison of these goals, which will be subordinated by some of the specific objectives stated in the curricula. We hope that, by doing so, we can provide the readers with a broad backdrop to understand the curriculum environment, under which Chinese students learn mathematics, from an international and comparative perspective. Then, we will attempt to depict a world trend of the mathematics curriculum in the new Millennium. We will see in a moment the impact of such a trend on the Chinese mathematics curriculum and the possibility of blurring of local traditions in the wave of globalization.

2 "Western" Mathematics Curricula

2.1 *The United States*

School mathematics experienced tremendous change in the "Modern Mathematics" reform in the 1960s (Thwaites, 1972). In the United States, alongside with the "back-to-basic" movement in the 1970s, problem solving was identified as one of the most important basic skills as asserted in the position paper for basic mathematics in 1977 that "learning to solve problems is the principal reason for studying mathematics" (National Council of Supervisors of Mathematics, 1977, p. 2). Problem solving was thus put forth as the focus of school mathematics in the 1980s (National Council of Teachers of Mathematics [NCTM], 1980). With the decline of mathematical competence (National Commission on Excellence in Education, 1983), the necessity of setting up a national standard was put forth (see e.g., NCTM, 1989, pp. 45-56). Though there are different conceptions regarding "standards" (Raizen, McLeod, & Rowe, 1997), Robson and Latiolais (1999, 2000) identified the notions of content standards, curriculum standards, competency standards, and performance standards. In brief, they are benchmarks for or descriptions of contents of study, curricula, or students' performance. With such a movement, the *Curriculum and Evaluation Standards for School Mathematics* (commonly known as the NCTM standards) was published in 1989 (NCTM, 1989), which was said to be influenced by the California frameworks published regularly since the early 1960s (Raizen et al., 1997). The general goals for students were set in the NCTM standards "that students learn to value mathematics, become confident in their ability to do mathematics, become mathematical problem solvers, learn to communicate mathematically, and learn to reason mathematically" (NCTM, 1989, p. 5). We can see that these are in line with the "expanding goals" as stated in *Reshaping School Mathematics* (Mathematical Sciences Education Board, 1990) in which the practical, civic goal, professional and cultural goals were elaborated (p. 7).

Thirteen to fourteen standards were developed for Grades K–4, 5–8 and 9–12 (see Table 1).

Table 1

The Learning Dimensions in Various Regions before 1995

	U.S. (1989)			U.K. (1989)	Australia (1990)	New Zealand (1992)	Taiwan (1994)	Hong Kong (1992)
	K–4	5–8	9–12					
	- problem solving - communication - reasoning - connections	(as left)	(as left)	- using & applying math	- attitude & appreciation - math inquiry - choosing & using math	- reasoning & strategy		
	- estimation - number sense & numeration - whole number operation - whole number computation - fractions & decimal	- number & number relationships - number system & number theory - computation & estimation		- number	- number	- number	-concept of number	-number
		- algebra	(as left)	- algebra	- algebra	- algebra	- algebra	- algebra
	- geometry & spatial sense	- geometry	- synthetic geometry - algebraic geometry - trigonometry	- shape & space	- space	- space	- plane geometry - coordinate geometry	- shapes & space
	- measurement	(as left)			- measurement	- measurement	-	- measure
	- statistics & probability	(as left)	- statistics - probability - discrete math	- data handling	- chance and data	- measurement & data - chance & data	- data handling & probability	- data handling
	- patterns & relationships	(as left)	- functions - initial calculus - math structure					

Source. Extracted and translated from N. Y. Wong and K. M. Wong (1997).

The standard was attached with "focus" and "discussion." These standards describe more or less "students' action," or (learning) opportunities for students' actions.

After ten years of its publication, the NCTM standards underwent revision following extensive consultations. Finally, the NCTM (2000) published the *Principles and Standards for School Mathematics* in the new Millennium. The dimensions were sort of condensed into eleven standards of different grade levels (see Table 2). The learning stages were changed from "K–4, 5–8, 9–12" to "Pre-K–2, 3–5, 6–8, 9–12" too.

How Chinese Learn Mathematics: Perspectives From Insiders

Table 2
The Learning Dimensions in Various Regions after 1995

U.S. (2000)	U.K. (2000)	Victoria (2000)	China (2000)	Shanghai (2001)		Taiwan (1999)	Hong Kong (1999)		Macau	Japan (2000)		South Korea (2000)
				Primary	Secondary		Primary	Secondary		Elementary	Lower secondary	
- problem solving - reasoning & proof - communication - connections - representation	- reasoning & strategy	- reasoning & strategy	- practical & synthetic application			- connections					- Math & human activities - Mathematical considerations in society	
- number & operation	- number (become number & algebra starting from KS4)	- number	- number & algebra	- number & quantity	- number & number system	- number & quantity	- number	- number & algebra	- number & computation	- number & calculation	- number & algebraic expressions	- number & operation
- algebra	- algebra starting from KS4	- algebra		- pattern & algebra	- pattern, algebra & function	- algebra	- algebra					- Letters & expression
- geometry	- shape, space, & measures	- space	- shapes & space	- shape & space	- shape, space & geometry	- shapes & space	- shapes & space	- measure, shape & space	- shape & space			- geometric figures
- measurement	(see above)	- measurement & data					- measure		- quantity & measurement			- measurements
- data analysis & probability	- handling data (starting from KS2)	- chance and data	- statistics & probability	- data & statistics	- data, statistics & probability	- statistics & probability	- data handling	- data handling	- statistical charts		- elementary statistics	- Probability & statistics
				(see above)	(see above)							
											- fundamentals of mathematics	

Note. Though the mathematics curricula of Macau and South Korea were not described in the text, their learning dimensions were analyzed and are included in this table

In the new curriculum, the format of the standards was more or less the same. The *Number & Operations Standard* states that:

> Instructional programs from pre-kindergarten through grade 12 should enable all students to
> (a) understand numbers,
> (b) ways of representing numbers,
> (c) relationships among numbers, and number system;
> (d) understand meanings of operations and how they relate to one another; and
> (e) compute fluently and make reasonable estimates.
>
> (NCTM, 2000, p. 32; numbering added)

In line with the *Curriculum and Evaluation Standards for School Mathematics* published in 1989, California developed its own curriculum framework in 1992, in which "mathematical power" was stressed (California State Board of Education, 1992). The notion of "mathematical power" was elaborated in the beginning of the framework. It was conceptualized to include the dimensions of mathematical thinking, mathematical communication, mathematical ideas as well as mathematical tools and techniques. The issue of individual differences (including gender, race, class, and culture; California State Board of Education, 1992, pp. 44–46), tracking and grouping area were addressed (pp. 62–65). The standards could be seen as elaborations of the NCTM standards. For K–8, the strands of functions, algebra, geometry, statistics and probability, discrete mathematics, measurement, number, logic and language were found with the "underlying ideas" of "how many?", "how much?", "finding, making, and describing patterns," and "representing quantities and shapes." We can see that the process abilities were incorporated into the strands of contents. For 9–12, we have the strands of functions, algebra, geometry, statistics and probability, discrete mathematics, measurement, number, logic and language with the "underlying ideas" of "mathematical modeling", "variation", "algorithmic thinking", "mathematical argumentation", and "multiple representations". Teaching ideas (in the form of suggested units) were provided at different levels. The framework initiated the "California Math War" (Jackson, 1997a, 1997b) and finally California published its mathematics content standards (California State Board of Education, 1999).

Though some described the new California mathematics content standards as relatively conservative, the goals stated there still reflect an expanding goal of school mathematics (like the inclusion of interest and appreciation).

We can have a look at specific standards. For example, the standards of *Number Sense* in Grade 5 were: "interpret percents as a part of a number; find decimal and percent equivalent for common fractions and explain why they represent the same value; compare a given percent of a whole number" (California State Board of Education, 1999, p. 52). From this specific standard, we see that basically they are also descriptions of students' behaviors. When we compare them with the NCTM standards, they are more specific. The descriptions in NCTM standards were only put down in broad stroke.

2.2 *The United Kingdom*

The famous Cockcroft report (Cockcroft, 1982), which was meant to go for a holistic review of mathematical education in the United Kingdom, devoted an entire chapter on "why teach mathematics." The usefulness of mathematics was particularly stressed: "… This suggests that mathematics is in some way thought to be of especial importance. If we ask why this should be so, one of the reasons which is frequently given is that mathematics is 'useful'; it is clear, too, that this usefulness is in some way seen to be of a different kind from that of many other subjects in the curriculum" (Cockcroft, 1982, p. 1).

In the first National Curriculum in the United Kingdom published shortly afterwards (Department of Education and Sciences and the Welsh Office, 1989), learning targets (or "attainment targets" as originally called) were put into five dimensions laid out in four key stages. These dimensions included: *Using & Applying Mathematics, Number, Algebra, Shape & Space*, and *Data Handling* (see Table 1). In the 2000 revised National Curricula (Department for Education and Employment and Qualifications and Curriculum Authority, 2000), some "generic skills" were listed as general (non-mathematical) goals that one should aim to obtain through the learning of mathematics. They included spiritual, moral, social and cultural developments among the students. The key skills of communication, application of number, information technology, working with others, improving own learning and performance, problem solving, as well as other skills like thinking skills, financial capability, enterprise and entrepreneurial skills, and work-related learning were also elaborated (Department for Education and Employment and Qualifications and Curriculum Authority, 2000, pp. 8–9).

A brief comparison of the National Curricula issued in 1989, 1991, 1995, and 2000 to depict the trend of development is presented as follows.

The 1989 National Mathematics Curriculum was arranged in four key stages (corresponding to years 1–3, 2–6, 3–8, 4–10; the overlapping of years indicates the flexibility of arrangement) with 14 attainment targets: *Using & Applying Mathematics (I), Number (I), Number (II), Number (III), Number/Algebra, Algebra (I), Algebra (II), Measures, Using & Applying Mathematics (II), Shape & Space (I), Shape & Space (II), Handling Data (I), Handling Data (II), Handling Data (III)* (numbering added). There are 10 levels of performance within each attainment target. So, they are presented in the form of 14 charts (with one attainment target each), each presented in the three columns of "level", "statements of attainment" and "example".

Programs of study were also provided which move along the 10 levels but the dimensions were condensed into six, namely: *Using & Applying Mathematics, Number, Algebra, Measures, Shapes & Space,* and *Handling Data.* Obviously, the attainment targets are more or less description of students' expected performance and the programs of study are recommended teaching strategies, so to speak.

In the 1991 edition (Department for Education and the Welsh Office, 1991), attainment targets were then organized into 5 dimensions: *Using & Applying Mathematics, Number, Algebra, Shape & Space,* and *Handling Data.* Among them, all are content-related except possibly "using and applying mathematics," which was deemed so important in the Cockcroft report. The 10 levels of performance were maintained and the programs of study were merged into the statements of attainment, coming up with five charts, again with three columns. However, the "statements of attainment" came last, preceded with "level" and "programs of study". One may be aware of the shift from assessment to emphasizing the program of study.

Although learning targets in the mathematics curricula in the United States and the United Kingdom are more or less the same, those in the United Kingdom seems to be put down in more details and are more concrete and specific.

In the 1995 version, the division of the four key stages was changed to Year 1–2, 3–6, 7–9, and 10–11. In other words, the key stages correspond more closely, or rigidly, to school years, and overlapping of the years no longer exists. Programs of study include statements that are more or less teachers' action.

What follows are statements that begin with "Pupils should be taught to ..." and these statements fall into the categories of "understanding place value and extending the number system," "understanding and using relationship between numbers and developing methods of computation," and "solving numerical problems" (Department for Education and the Welsh Office, 1995, pp. 13–14). We see that, differing from the NCTM standards, process abilities were incorporated into content-based standards. In this version, attainment targets were separated from programs of study, and it seems that the "assessment component" is downplayed. More attention is paid on the program of learning, especially when one compare with earlier versions of the curriculum. Programs of study were presented first, with the following dimension in various key stages:

Key stage 1:	*Number; Shape, Space & Measures*
Key stage 2:	*Number; Shape, Space & Measures; Handling Data*
Key stage 3/4:	*Number & Algebra; Shape, Space & Measures; Handling Data.*

There were descriptions of further materials for Key Stage 4 too. The number of attainment levels was reduced to eight.

The 2000 National Curriculum framework basically resembles that of the 1995 version. Only the key stages were redefined by terminal year, namely: Key Stage1, till age 7; Key Stage2, till age 11; Key Stage3, till age 14. The original dimension *Using & Applying Mathematics* was merged into each dimension and the first learning target of *Number* becomes

Using & Applying Number. The same is true for all other dimensions (see Table 2).

The original four dimensions of *Using & Applying Mathematics*; *Number & Algebra*; *Shape, Space & Measures*; and *Handling Data* (with slight revisions) were retained in the attainment targets. The number of levels of attainment remained eight.

2.3 *Australia*

The first three chapters of the *National Statement on Mathematics for Australian Schools* (Australian Education Council, 1990) were devoted to the "importance of mathematics," "goals for school mathematics", and "enhancing mathematics learning." They are the philosophical position, curriculum goal, and teaching/learning approaches. In Chapter Two, the goals for school mathematics were spelt out as follows:

(a) Students should develop confidence and competence in dealing with commonly occurring situations.
(b) Students should develop positive attitudes towards their involvement in mathematics.
(c) Students should develop their capacity to use mathematics in solving problems individually and collaboratively.
(d) Students should learn to communicate mathematically.
(e) Students should learn techniques and tools which reflect modern mathematics.
(f) Students should experience the processes through which mathematics develops.

(Australian Education Council, 1990, p. 11)

Again, we can see clearly common features like affect, process ability, and information technology. In a decade later, Victoria revised its curriculum and standards framework (Board of Studies, 2000), which was originally published in 1988.

The learning outcome was arranged in six "levels" (or key stages if borrowing the jargon of the U.K. National Curriculum) and eight Key Learning Areas (The six levels are: end of preparatory year, end of Year 2, end of year 4, end of Year 6, end of Year 8, and end of Year 10. The eight

Key Learning Areas include: the arts, English, health and physical education, languages other than English, mathematics, science, studies of society and environment, and technology). The learning outcomes in mathematics were expressed by strands and sub-strands. The strands in the curriculum are *Space, Number, Measurement & data* (level 2), *Measurement* (from level 3), *Chance & Data* (from level 3), *Algebra* (from level 5), and *Reasoning & Strategies.*

The other component of the framework is a set of standards, with the pathways to VCE (Victorian Certificate Education), which serves as a bridge between learning and public examination. Obviously, the learning outcomes and the description of the expected student performances are very specific.

2.4 *Germany*

After the reunion of East and West Germany in 1991, each state of Germany had to reorganize its school system and to develop new curricula (Universität Würzburg, 2001). There are three types of schools in Germany: (1) Hauptschule, which provides a basis for subsequent vocational training; (2) Realschule, which equips young people for subsequent careers in positions located between the purely theoretical and the purely practical; and (3) Gymnasium, which equips students for intellectual activity and prepares them for higher/academic education (Schumann, 2002). The goals of mathematics teaching in the new curricula were stated below:

- mathematics as a theory and as a tool for solving problems in natural and social sciences, including modeling;
- experiences with fundamental ideas in mathematics like the idea of generalization, the need for proving, structural aspects, algorithms, the idea of infinity, and deterministic versus stochastic thinking;
- methods of getting insight like inductive and deductive reasoning, methods for proving, axiomatics, formalization, generalization/ specification, heuristic work;
- variation of argumentation levels and representation levels in

all fields and aspects of mathematics teaching; and
● historical aspects of mathematics.

(Schumann, 2002)

New orientations of the curriculum were also identified, including mathematization and modeling, cooperation between teachers of mathematics and other subjects, and mathematics as a history of ideas (Universität Würzburg, 2001).

The curriculum for mathematics in Germany is laid down in the form of syllabi for each state and for different types of schools. These syllabi advise teachers on aims, content, teaching approaches, and methods of assessment. The German Association for promoting mathematical & scientific studies (Deutscher Vereinzur Förderung des mathematischen und naturwisschnschaftliche Unterrichts) also put forth recommendations for erecting curricula for mathematics:

"In general, the Syllabi state that the general aims of mathematics education are to: provide fundamental knowledge and skills in important areas of mathematics; provide security in the techniques, algorithms, and concepts which are necessary for mastering everyday life in society; develop the ability to state facts mathematically and to interpret the contents of mathematical formulae; it should make possible the solving of non-mathematical or environmental phenomenon through mathematics; teach pupils to think critically and to question; give examples of mathematics as a cultural creation in its historical development and in its importance in the development of civilization; and provide terms, methods, and ways of thinking that are useful in other subject." (Schumann, 2002).

2.5 *France*

Let us conclude the descriptions of "Western" mathematics curricula by inspecting the case of France. There are three cycles in the French primary schools (l'Ecole primaire): Cycle 1 (Kindergarten: Age 2 to 6), Cycle 2 (Elementary school, the cycle of fundamental learning: Age 7 to 8), and Cycle 3 (Elementary school, the cycle of deepening learning: Age 9 to 10). There are also three cycles in junior secondary schools (collège), namely

Cycle 1 (Sixth Grade: Age11), Cycle 2 (Fifth Grade and Fourth Grade: Age 12 to 13), and Cycle 3 (Third Grade: Age 14). Again, three cycles are present in senior secondary schools (lycée): Second Grade (Age 15), First Grade (Age 16), and Terminal (Age 17) that lead to the national examination "Baccalauréat."

The French mathematics curriculum is revised about every ten years since the Modern Mathematic reform in 1974. The present secondary curriculum was implemented in 1996, proceeding grade by grade each year (Laborde, 2002).

The objectives of mathematics learning were stated for each grade. We will just focus on the sixth grade of junior secondary schools. One can refer to Ministère de l'éducation nationale, 2002 and 1999 for the curricula at Primary and senior secondary levels.

The general objectives are:

The teaching of mathematics in the sixth grade carries two aspects:
- it teaches to connect observations of real situations to representations: diagrams, tables, figures;
- it teaches also to connect these representations to a mathematical activity and to concepts.

This procedure makes it possible to build up mathematics from problems encountered in other disciplines and, in return, to utilize the mathematical knowledge in different fields.

It gives room to the activity of construction, realization of drawing, solution of problems, organization and treatment of data, of calculation … Students can thus learn the character that mathematics is a "tool".

It works toward the intellectual formation of the student, the formation of a citizen, and should particularly:
- develop the ability of reasoning: observation, analysis, deductive thinking;
- stimulate imagination, intuition;
- accustom the student to express clearly, both orally and in writing;
- strengthen the quality of working with order and care.

Thus, from the 6th grade onward, mathematics teaching develops the student's abilities in his own work and in his aptitude to search, to communicate and to justify his assertions.

(Translated from Ministère de l'éducation nationale, 2000, p.27)

Though they are only general guidelines and principles rather detailed descriptions of expected learning outcomes, the actual content as mentioned above were elaborated by the three columns of "notion", "expected student abilities" and "comments" (see, e.g. Laborde, 2002).

We see from the above that mathematics is positioned as a tool for students to understand the world around us and thus the connection (or even integration) between mathematics and other disciplines was emphasized.

As pointed out by Laborde (2002), there are some general orientations of the current curriculum. They are experimenting, modeling and formulating, interdisciplinary projects, mastering of mathematical techniques, and use of information technology.

3 "Far Eastern" Mathematics Curricula

3.1 *Mainland China*

China enforced its compulsory education in 1992. In the same year, the policy of allowing different teaching materials under a single national curriculum was implemented. In 1997, Shanghai and Zhejiang were allowed to have their own curricula (Leung, Lam, Mok, K. M. Wong, & N. Y. Wong, 1999; N. Y. Wong & K. M. Wong, 1997). The national curriculum (Basic Education Curriculum Material Development Centre [BECMDC], 2001) is under revision and the new national mathematics curriculum standard was released for consultation. Almost at the same time, Shanghai published the second edition of the mathematics curriculum in 2001.

The high regard of basic skills has long been a tradition of mathematics education in Mainland China. The "2 basics" (basic knowledge and basic skills) and the "3 abilities" (calculation, logical thinking, and spatial visualization) were explicitly stated as the overall goals in the 1992 curriculum, the origin of which can be dated back to the 1960s.

Six underlying principles in the development of mathematics curriculum material were stated in the new Basic Education Mathematics Curriculum, the focus of which were on the mathematics curriculum, mathematics itself, mathematics learning, mathematics activities, assessment, and information technology. For the first one, it was stated that:

> The mathematics curriculum in the free education stage puts its emphases on the basic, general and developmental nature of mathematics, to make mathematics counts for all students, in the hope of realizing:
> - everybody learn valuable mathematics;
> - everybody can acquire necessary mathematics;
> - different person can have different development in mathematics."
>
> (Translated from BECMDC, 2001, p.1)

Several principles of designing the curriculum were also stated. As for the principle about standards, it was mentioned that there were two types of learning targets. For those concerning "knowledge and skill," the levels of "knowing," "comprehending" and "grasping," "flexibly applying" were identified. This resembled very much the 1991 Shanghai curriculum (see below). Clearly, its origin is Bloom's taxonomy. And for those concerning "process," the levels of "acquaintance," "experience," and "exploration" were identified (BECMDC, 2001, pp. 3-4).

As for the principle about contents, the dimensions *Number Sense, Symbol Sense, Spatial Sense, Statistical Idea, Awareness of Application,* and *Deductive Ability* were further explained (BECMDC, 2001, pp. 4-5). Obviously, these principles are targeted to curriculum and textbook developers rather than frontline teachers. The overall objectives of the mathematics curriculums were also stated. These were spelt out in the dimensions of knowledge and skill, mathematical thinking, problem solving, and affect & attitude (BECMDC, 2001, pp. 6–7).

Like the mathematics curricula in many "Western" regions, the contents were arranged in several dimensions, key stages, and categories of mathematics abilities. There were four dimensions: *Number & Algebra,* *Shape & Space, Statistics & Probability,* and *Practical & Synthetic Application* (including the use of projects). These dimensions were allocated in three key stages (Year 1–3, Year 4–6, and Year 7–9), each with a specific objectives. The four categories of mathematics abilities included "knowledge and skill", "mathematics thinking", "problem solving", and "affect & attitude" (BECMDC, 2001, pp. 8–11).

The standards depict basically the expected student performance. For example, we have "able to use paper and pencil to multiple a 3-digit number with a two-digit number; divide a 3-digit number with a two-digit number" for *Number & Algebra* in the second key stage (Translated from BECMDC, 2001, p. 21).

The senior secondary mathematics curriculum, now under preparation, will basically go for a modular approach (Standards 2002 Writing Group, 2002).

Shanghai was selected in 1997 as the only city in China with the privilege of having its own curriculum as well as examination. In fact, the Shanghai mathematics curriculum had already been proposed earlier in 1991. The "requirements on teaching" (which were in fact sort of attainment levels) include cognitive, affective, and psychomotor domains. There are the levels of "knowing," "understanding," "comprehending," and "applying," which were then reconstructed as Levels 1–4 in the 2001 edition. Let us take the standard "Apprehensions of counting numbers less than 10 and addition & subtractions with them" in Primary 1 as an example. Curriculum requirements were laid down in the cognitive, affective and psychomotor domains.

The curriculum was revised in 2001 (Curriculum Reform Committee, 2001) though the National Curriculum was published earlier and was seen to be big leap forward.

The "basic–extension" curriculum structure was adopted and the dimension of *Number & Quantity*; *Pattern & Algebra*; *Shape & Space*; and *Data & Statistics* were found at the primary level, whereas *Pattern, Algebra & Function*; *Number & Number System*; *Shape, Space & Geometry*; and *Data, Statistics & Probability* were found at the secondary level.

3.2 *Taiwan*

After the martial law was lifted in Taiwan in 1987 and the "Period of Mobilization and Pacification" was ended in 1991, the mathematics curriculum was revised in the mid-1990s (N. Y. Wong & K. M. Wong, 1997). The general direction for change are "heading for the future, moving along with international trend, going for integration, seeking relevance in real life, going for humanization, and allowing flexibility". The mathematics curriculum has gone through another change to go for the policy of "1st – 9th Grades Curriculum Alignment." Previously, as in many other regions, primary and secondary curricula were designed and reviewed separately.

In the domain of mathematics, the educational goals are:

1. Acquisition of the concepts and relationships among number, quantities and shapes
2. Development of the mathematics caliber needed in daily life
3. Development of the abilities in formulating and solving mathematics problems
4. Development of the abilities in using mathematics as a tool for precise expression and communication
5. Development of the abilities in critical analysis in mathematics
6. Development of the abilities in mathematics appreciation.
   (Translated from Ministry of Education, Taiwan, 2001, p. 20)

The standards were then arranged in four key stages (Years 1–3, 4–5, 6–7, 8–9) and the learning dimensions of *Number & Quantity, Shape & Space, Statistics & Probability, Algebra,* and *Connections.* We can see that besides the last dimension, all others involve "content" rather than "process abilities." The standards are basically the expected student performances, as seen in the example of Standard "N-2-2" key stage 2: "[students are] able to extend addition, subtraction, multiplication and division to make sense in different tasks so as to apply to more real life situations and solve the problems involved; and [are] able to use calculating devices to do manipulations with large numbers" (Translated from Ministry of Education, Taiwan, 2001, p. 21). The "constructivist curriculum", which was introduced in 1994, initiated heated debate and after several revisions, the new mathematics curriculum was finally published towards the end of 2003, which can be regarded as another "back to basic" movement.

3.3 *Hong Kong*

Hong Kong has its first mathematics curriculum for primary schools in 1967, replacing its previous arithmetic curriculum. Innovations that originated from the Modern Mathematics reform were introduced into secondary school mathematics in 1964 and Nuffield mathematics was incorporated into the primary mathematics curriculum, which was later revised in 1973. With all the controversies that sprung out from Modern Mathematics, the primary and secondary school mathematics curricula were restructured in 1983 and 1985 respectively under the Curriculum Development Committee, which was established in 1973 (and later restructured into the Curriculum Development Council in 1988). To address the various problems that aroused in the universal education period, the Target Oriented Curriculum was advocated in the early 1990s under the recommendation of the 1990 *Education Commission Report No. 4*. The Target Oriented Curriculum brought about heated debates within the education circle in general and the mathematics education community in particular. The Ad hoc Committee on Holistic Review of the Mathematics Curriculum, directly under the Curriculum Development Council, was set up in 1997. The Committee released its final report toward the end of 1999. The new secondary and primary mathematics curricula were published in 1999 and 2000 respectively.

The Curriculum Development Council (2000) stated the aims of the primary mathematics curriculum as follows:

1. stimulate the interest of pupils in the learning of mathematics;
2. develop pupils' understanding and acquisition of basic mathematical concepts and computational skills;
3. develop pupils' creativity, and their ability to think, communicate and solve problems;
4. develop pupils' number sense and spatial sense, and their

ability to appreciate patterns and structures of number and shapes;

5. enhance pupils' lifelong learning abilities through basic mathematical knowledge.

(Curriculum Development Council, 2000, p. 4)

The objectives for the three domains of *Knowledge*, *Skills*, and *Attitudes* were further laid out. We see similar formats in secondary mathematics, on top of the general aim, objective for the three domains of "knowledge", "skill" and "attitude" were also given.

We see that not only the goals were widen to include various domains, vast difference of the entire approach can also be drawn from earlier curricula. For example, in the foreword of the 1985 secondary school mathematics syllabus, it was clearly stated that "These objectives reflect an emphasis which treats mathematics more as a tool than a way of thought" (Curriculum Development Committee, 1985, p. 5). It was said that this position was a result of a bounce-back from the Modern Mathematics reform.

Similar to many other regions, the two curricula were arranged in various dimensions (*Number*; *Algebra*; *Measures*; *Shape & Space*; and *Data Handling* for primary schools; and *Number & Algebra*; *Measures, Shape & Space*; and *Data Handling* for secondary schools). Another feature is the identification of the "foundation part" as a means to cater for individual difference and school-based curriculum tailoring. Less able students can focus their attention on the "formulation part". It was said that the "'foundation part' of the syllabus represents the topic that ALL students should strive to master" (Curriculum Development Council, 1999, p. 1; see also Curriculum Development Council, 2002, p. 29). At the moment, the Basic Competency Descriptors and the Basic Competency Assessment have been under development to assist students to proceed along the foundation part of the syllabus. Furthermore, the foundation part does not involve a rigid arrangement of tracking or streaming since the teacher and students can judge (without pre-registration or labeling) which portion one should focus one's learning. In other words, one can tailor a subset T with "Foundation Part $\subset$ T $\subset$ whole syllabus" for one's study scheme, as long as T constitutes a coherent part of the curriculum.

Enrichment topics were also suggested for abler students. Furthermore, "spare periods" were created. During the periods, teaches could teach freely. This measure is to counteract the rigid allocation of teaching time for each topic in previous curricula. This 10–15% of "buffer" allows teachers to conduct remedial teaching for the average students and/or further investigations (e.g., enrichment topics). It was further elaborated in the 2002 curriculum guide that "[t]he suggested time allocations are not mandatory" (Curriculum Development Council, 2002, p. 36). It is seen that more and more discretion are given to schools for curriculum tailoring.

With the launching of educational reform in 1999 — two years after the reunification of Hong Kong with China, the *Basic Education Curriculum Guideline* was published in 2002. Under the umbrella of the document *Learning to Learn* (Curriculum Development Council, 2001) The nine generic skills — collaboration skill, communication skill, creativity, critical thinking skill, information technology, numeration skill, problem solving skill, self management skill, and study skill — were advocated. Positive values and attitudes were also emphasized.

3.4 *Japan*

The Japanese mathematics curriculum is regularly revised every ten years. Modern mathematics was introduced in the 1970s, then we have "back to basics" in 1980s, individualization in 1990s and emphasis of mathematical activities in 2000s (see Japan Society of Mathematical Education [JSME], 2000).

In 1996, Japan Central Council for Education published its first report, *The Model for Japanese Education in the Perspective of the 21ˢᵗ Century.* It was stated that "helping children develop their zest for living is of the most importance and one should let them make use of most of their time in independent free trails and discoveries" (see N. Y. Wong & Tanaka, 2000). Accordingly, in 1998, the Ministry of Education started to revise the school curriculum. In the new curriculum, students of the 3ʳᵈ the 6ᵗʰ grade are required to take a new subject "Integrated Learning." To accommodate with this, the time allocated to arithmetic has to be reduced by 30%, which aroused some heated debates (Sawada, 2002; N. Y. Wong & Tanaka,

2000). In the new mathematics curriculum, Topics concerning basic knowledge and skills were carefully selected. The emphases were put on independent activities, enjoyment of doing mathematics, and connection between mathematics and daily life (Okubo, 2000).

Here, we list the overall objectives of mathematics for elementary school and lower secondary school for reference:

> Through mathematical activities concerning numbers, quantities and geometrical figures, children should get basic knowledge and skills, should get abilities to think logically and to think with good perspectives, should notice the pleasure of doing activities and appreciate the value of mathematical methods, and should get attitude to make use of mathematics in daily life situations.
>
> (Elementary school; see JSME, 2000, p. 7)

> For students to understand deeply the fundamental concepts, principles, and rules relating to numbers, quantities, figures and so forth. For students to acquire methods of mathematical expressions and strategies, and to improve their ability to relate phenomena mathematically. For students to enjoy mathematical activities, to appreciate the importance of mathematical approaches and ways of thinking, and to inculcate in them the right attitudes necessary to make use of mathematics.
>
> (Lower secondary school; see JSME, 2000, p. 21)

At upper secondary level, "at least one of 'Fundamentals of Mathematics' or 'Mathematics I' is required to be taken by all students. Mathematics I, II and III are regarded as core subjects and Mathematics A, B and C are regarded as optional subjects" (JSME, 2000, p. 5).

The contents of mathematics in elementary school were put into the categories of *Number & Calculations, Quantities & Measurements*, and *Geometrical Figures*. For Grades 4–6, an additional category *Mathematical Relations* was found.

In lower secondary level, the categories were *Numbers & Algebraic Expressions, Geometrical Figures*, and *Mathematical Relations*. In upper secondary level, one have *Fundamentals of Mathematics, Mathematics & Human Activities, Mathematical Considerations in Society*, and

Elementary Statistics.

The standards were basically descriptions of students' learning behavior such as "Compare the numbers of objects by manipulation such as correspondence" (under *Number & Calculations*, Grade 1, see N. Y. Wong & Tanaka, 2000, p. 50).

3.5 *Singapore*

Different mathematics syllabi were developed in Singapore. The "Syllabus B" was implemented before the Modern Mathematics reform in the 1960s. Afterwards, Singapore had its "Syllabus C" at the secondary level. "Syllabus D" was introduced in the early 1980s and since 1997 a series of new initiatives have been introduced, including the idea of national education. Information technology and the notion of "thinking schools and a learning nation" were also advocated. Twenty percent of the contents were also reduced to give way to information technology and higher-order thinking (Lee & Fan, 2002; see also http://www.moe.edu.sg, http://www.sgnews.gov.sg)

The aims of mathematics education were stated in the Singapore curriculum as follows:

Mathematics education aims to enable pupils to
- acquire and apply skills and knowledge relating to number, measure and space in mathematical situations that they will meet in life
- acquire mathematical concepts and skills necessary for a further study in Mathematics and other disciplines
- develop the ability to make logical deduction and induction as well as to explicate their mathematical thinking and reasoning skills through solving of mathematical problems
- use mathematical language to communicate mathematical ideas and arguments precisely, concisely and logically
- develop positive attitudes towards mathematics

including confidence, enjoyment and perseverance
- appreciate the power and structure of mathematics, including patterns and relationships, and to enhance their intellectual curiosity

(Curriculum Planning and Development Division, 2000a, 2000b, p. 9)

The framework of the curriculum comprised the five sections of concepts, skills, processes, attitudes, and metacognition.

It was also mentioned that "This framework encompasses the whole mathematics curriculum from primary to secondary school. At the primary level, concepts, skills and processes will be taught at a level appropriate to the cognitive development of the pupils. Attitudes and metacognition, though not given the same emphasis, should form part of the teaching methodology" (Curriculum Planning and Development Division, 2000a, p. 11). The Singapore mathematics curriculum is now under major revision and interested readers are referred to their official website for update developments.

4 Discussion and Conclusion

4.1 *"The world has changed": The rationale for change and the dilemmas of change*

With the above expositions of the mathematics curriculum documents in various regions, we get an overall picture of the mathematics curricula for the 21st century. Besides the "magic number" 2000 that governments all around the world see the need of changing the mathematics curriculum (in fact some regions revise their mathematics curricula regularly once every ten years), society is seen to have been changing rapidly and so there is pressing need for such changes (see e.g., N. Y. Wong, 1997). The change of job natures is one of them. As stated in Mathematical Sciences Education Board (1989), "The changing nature of work will make continuing education a lifelong reality for adults. Schools, therefore, will have to provide all students with a strong foundation for lifelong learning" (p.11). Thus, the notions of "lifelong learning" and "learning to learn" are once again advocated (see e.g., Curriculum Development Council, 2001).

One immediate cause for change is the lowering of academic standard, which is often seen as a consequence of universal education. The curriculum being too conventional, too packed, and still targeting at those who have potential to receive higher education in the field of science, are also some of the problems. Mathematics learning too boring, students' lack of confidence, assessment relying too much on paper and pencil, and curriculum too rigid to cater for individual differences are some more reasons for change (Gu, 2002; Okubo, 2000; N. Y. Wong, Lam, Leung, Mok, & K. M. Wong, 1999).

However, curriculum change is not an endeavor that follows a linear fashion. Obviously it faces confrontations and dilemmas. For instance, when one wants to upgrade the quality of education, there is a possibility of tightening educational control; and in many places in the world ("Eastern" regions in particular), when one tries to pay more emphasis on a certain facet of learning (e.g., higher-order thinking), the examination orientation would generate high stake in the related assessment exercises (Biggs, 1996; Pong & Chow, 2002; Zang & Ren, 1998).

In comparing the recent changes in mathematics curricula in Hong Kong and Shanghai, Gu (2002) identified the following key issues underlying the motive for changes: "academic and exam orientation, boring and difficult, not cater for individual differences and relying on conventional paper & pencil and high-stake assessments" (Gu, 2002, pp. 2–3). The dilemmas that the two places are facing include "internationalization/globalization vs. localization, discipline vs. student orientation, unification vs. school-based curriculum development, curriculum integration vs. differentiation, common core vs. individual differences, general vs. elite, cooperation vs. competition, transmission vs. creativity, assessment for selection vs. assessment for development, and anticipation for an idealistic curriculum vs. respect of current situation" (Gu, 2002, p. 3).

In the following sections, we will further analyze the challenges these curriculum changes have to meet.

4.2 *The components of change*

Let us look at some of the "magic words" we often found in the above-mentioned new curriculum documents:

- higher-order thinking
- generic skill
- value
- real life mathematics
- interest
- relevance
- confidence and attitude
- individual differences
- information technology
- holistic consideration/"through train"

As said in Mathematical Sciences Education Board (1990), the goal of mathematics education is expanding. We will start our discussion in the figure that was conceptualized by the authors (Figure 1).

Indeed, universal education (which originates from the notion of "mathematics for all") is an educational policy that has never been implemented in human history. The implication of such a move is far more than providing enough school places for all children. It has to meet a lot of challenges, individual differences being a prominent one among other things. The issues of individual differences include learners' differences in ability, learning styles, and motivations to learn. The education system also has to prepare students for different "walks of life," not just for the academic sector. On the one hand, there is pressing need for differentiation on the curriculum, including tracking, streaming, ability grouping, remedial teaching, enrichment topics, and possible acceleration. On the other hand, besides the possibility of reinforcing labeling effect and high-stake assessments, in anticipation of diversity, the call for the identification of a common core is equally loud. In order to help learners — "slow learners" in particular — to proceed along the curriculum, to maintain a minimum standard of the curriculum, and to "rescue" as many as possible those lagging behind, the idea of standardization of the curriculum is put forth. A basket of accompanying concepts like attainment targets, minimal competency, basic competency, progress map and hypothetical learning trajectory have sprung out (see, e.g., Masters & Forcester, 1996; Simon, 1995).

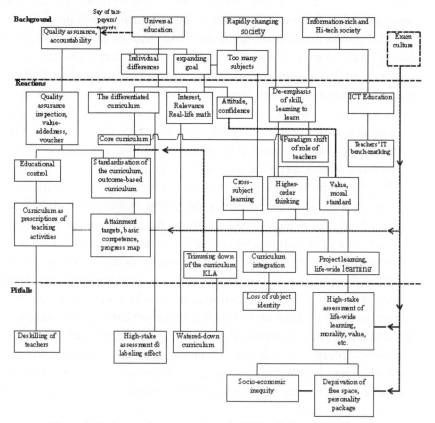

Figure 1. Background, components and pitfalls of educational change

Cultivation of learning interest among students is another key issue. This partially explains the emphasis on daily life or real life application of mathematics. However, many have alerted us the possible gap between "realistic mathematics" and "esoteric mathematics" (Cooper & Dunne, 1998). If the gap was not handled appropriately, it is likely that the mathematics content of learning will be watered down. Leung (2001) mentioned the dilemma between "working hard" and "pleasurable learning" as one of the characteristic features between "Western" and "Eastern" mathematics learning. Though in some regions like China, too much pressure is exerted on students, there have been criticism in some other regions like Hong Kong and Japan that caring too much about the pleasure of student learning could lead to the lowering of academic standard and shift students' motivation from intrinsic to extrinsic.

The standardization of curriculum can also be seen as a form of educational control. When the control is made too tight, there is a tendency of having an over-detailed prescription of student learning, student learning outcomes, teaching activities, and a broad scope of student activities. When the whole thing is distorted, there is a possibility of making teaching and learning too rigid, the curriculum too centralized, students receiving too much control, and deskilling of teachers. We will have more discussions on the issue in later sections.

In the rapidly changing society (including the workplace), governments in general and education policy makers in particular are aware of the need for making corresponding changes in curriculum structure, or even redefining what should be learned in school. One of the problems which was seen to be rather serious is having two many subjects in school. For instance, in Hong Kong, there are over one hundred subjects at secondary school level. Though students usually take eight to ten, there is a tendency of pushing new areas like moral education, civic education, sex education, environmental education, drug education, and life skills as mandatory courses in schools. To tackle this, the trimming down of curriculum was initiated in many regions. There are at least two facets of this policy. First, reducing the number of subjects or integrating some subjects — this brought about the notion of "key learning areas" though some criticized that sometimes irrelevant subjects were being "pooled together." (see Curriculum Development Council, 2001, pp. I1-I4). This may lead to the possibility of losing subject identities.

Second, the identification of core parts of the curriculum to leave room for cross-subject learning, higher-order thinking, generic skills, and developments for "leaning to learn." This is in accordance with the change to an "information-rich" society and the call for de-emphasis of skill with the advancement of ICT. Life-long and life-wide learning (including inquiry, projects and out of school experiences) are advocated. Low cost of ICT allows it to enter the classroom environment. The urge for "paradigm shift" of teachers from "transmitters" to "facilitators" — which is again in line with all of the above — has never been so strong (N. Y.

Wong, 2003).

Examination orientation in many regions (Confucian Heritage Culture [CHC] regions in particular) ruins most of the good wills. There is a strong tendency of turning everything into assessment items in the form of high-stake competitive tests. The expansion of the goal of education (which has the need in its own right), when blended with the "examination culture," is putting attitude, confidences, conduct, morality, and high-order thinking into different kinds of measurable scales. Performance in extra-curricular activities and participation in community service become criteria for university entrance, thus making students conforming to a "personality package" (Choi, 2001).

Socio-economic inequity due to the wide use of information technology and project learning could be another pitfall. The case is more serious when it is linked with high-stake tests leading to various kinds of selection.

4.3 *Implications on mathematics education: Pitfalls and bridges*

From the above discussion, we get a picture of the various components of the current educational reform, many of which were reflected in the mathematics curriculum.

4.3.1 *The "product-process" dichotomy*

Leung (2001) identified some characteristic distinctions between Western and Eastern mathematics curricula: product (content) versus process, rote learning versus meaningful learning, studying hard versus pleasurable learning, and extrinsic versus intrinsic motivation. Such dichotomies can be dated back earlier to the 1970s and they are still one of the central points of argument in "mathematics wars" in many regions. In the NACOME (National Advisory Committee on Mathematics Education, 1975) report, the dichotomies of "old or new, skills or concepts, concrete or abstract, intuitive or formal, inductive or deductive" (Hill, 1976, p. 442) were formally raised. Howson and Wilson (1986) queried the "process-based" curriculum (pp. 25–26) and concluded that one should strike a balance between content and process (pp. 35, 51). The issue was raised again in Senk and Thompson (2003):

> In particular, critics of the Standards worry about what they perceive to be an overemphasis on the process of obtaining an answer, rather than on the answer itself. They are encouraging students to invent solutions and algorithms, rather than emphasizing use of traditional algorithms, will lead to a decline in basic skills. ... The use of co-operative learning and discovery approaches instead of direct instruction has raised concerns that either teachers are not teaching or only some children are learning mathematics ... In contrast, people who generally support mathematics education reform often object to the drill and kill that characterizes many traditional programs. (p. 16)

However, we suppose that more discussions and investigations should be made on how mathematics should be learned (see e.g., Sfard, 1991, 1998). Putting it in simple terms, the questions are: how much true is knowledge acquired or self-constructed within individuals? Are these two paths of mathematization leading to different kinds mathematics "knowledge/understanding"? How is higher-order thinking and process abilities acquired/developed and could there be a path bridging basic skills and higher-order thinking? (N. Y. Wong, 2002)

The emphasis of (non-mathematical) generic skills (including creativity, values, and beliefs) added new elements to the "process-product" debate. Should general abilities like being carefulness, perseverance be regarded as "additional teaching duties" put on the teaching of mathematics (and other specific subjects)? Editorial Group from Thirteen Institutions (1980) listed five general abilities: being observant, memorization, imagination, thinking, and attentiveness. It was suggested that mathematics teachers should also take note of the developments of these abilities in their teaching. It is apparent in the above analyses of mathematics curricula in various regions of the world that process abilities are once again stressed. In some regions, we have specific standards on such abilities. Look at some of the points as advocated by the NCTM standard, Simon and Blume (1996) stated, "The standards documents promote a vision of classroom mathematics in which students engage in exploration of mathematical situations, ... Thus, students actively participate, taking on a role that is analogous to the role of mathematician, creating mathematics, evaluating mathematics that has been created by members of the classroom mathematics community, and negotiating shared approaches to and standards for these activities" (p. 3), we see a striking resemblance with the Modern Mathematics reform. It seems that history is repeating itself and swing between the two ends of "content" and "process" abilities like a pendulum (Sawada, 2002). "Nation at risk – sense of crisis among stakeholders – revolutionary reform – resistance from school – bounce-back – standard keeping declining – blaming the school/teacher – next round of 'Nation at risk'" seems to be the basic formula (N. Y. Wong, 2000).

The warning of dichotomisation (National Advisory Committee on Mathematics Education, 1975) is also overlooked. We think that the heart of the issue is not just the concern about striking a balance, but also about how to fully use "basic skills" as a foundation for the development of various process abilities, including construction which is a path of "mathematization" between realistic concrete objects to mathematics objects (N. Y. Wong, 2002).

In many regions, separating between "process-oriented dimension" and "product-oriented dimensions" appears in the curriculum whereas in others, requirements on process abilities were merged into the "product-oriented dimensions" (e.g., the U.K. National Mathematics Curriculum in 1995: Department for Education and the Welsh Office, 1995). The latter was the position of the Hong Kong curriculum, which was clearly stated in the final report of the Ad hoc Committee on Holistic Review of the Mathematics Curriculum (2000): "Since HOTs [Higher Order Thinking Skill] can only be developed through the learning of various mathematical knowledge in the content areas, they should be incorporated into the content-based learning dimensions to form a reference grid in designing the future mathematics curriculum". (p. 29) This could be one way out in handling the "product-process" dichotomy in the mathematics curriculum.

4.3.2 *Cross-subject learning: Lost of subject self-esteem?*

As pointed out in the Cockcroft Report that, "It is often suggested that mathematics should be studied in order to develop powers of logical thinking, accuracy and spatial awareness. The study of mathematics can certainly contribute to these ends but the extent to which it does so depends on the way in which mathematics is taught. Nor is its contribution unique; many other activities and the study of a number of other subjects can develop these powers as well. We therefore believe that the need to develop these powers does not in itself constitute a sufficient reason for studying mathematics rather than other things. (Cockcroft, 1982, p. 1)

We have a similar case in "ICT in education." Are we saying that the use of ICT would necessarily improve mathematics learning, or mathematics education should also shoulder the responsibility of bringing up our students in an "ICT environment"? (N. Y. Wong, 2003). There is a worry that the inclusion of more and more non-subject- specific educational goals in recent years could "dilute" the mathematical orientation of the curriculum. Such non-subject-specific goals include higher-order thinking skills, generic skills, development of personalities, and process abilities like "conceptualization, inquiry, reasoning, communication, application and problem solving" which were advocated in the Target Oriented Curriculum put forth in Hong Kong in the early 1990s (Curriculum Development Council, 1992, p. 12). There is a tendency to think that subject learning is "just" a means for developing these abilities.

When this is put to the extreme, mathematics learning can well be replaced by chess since both do equally well in the acquisition of problem-solving strategies (N. Y. Wong, 1992) (after all, D. Hilbert said that "Math is a game played according to certain simple rules with meaningless marks on paper"! – see, e.g. Rose, 1988). We think that it is time for us to reflect on the nature of mathematics, how mathematics took shape as a discipline in the long course of history, and the very aim of learning mathematics. For instance, seven areas of knowledge (logic and mathematics, physical science, mind, ethics and moral, esthetic experience, religion, and philosophy) were proposed by Hirst and Peters (1970, pp. 63–64) as starting points of designing the school curriculum.

Another similar issue is that of real-life application of mathematics or the notion of realistic mathematics. The notion of real-life mathematics was put forth to let students see how mathematics connects with other disciplines and different professions. It also lets them realize that "mathematics is everywhere" — we can find mathematics around us in daily life. As seen above, such an idea is found in the goals of mathematics curricula in many regions. However, on the one hand, there are criticisms that many so-called realistic situations (especially those provided in textbooks) are not realistic in students' experience. Most of these situations are designed by (middle-class) adults and generate another kind of social inequity. On the other hand, real-life situation may not be that mathematical. It is precisely the role of teachers to lead students to go through the path of mathematization, and of "turning" real-life objects into mathematical objects in order to bridge realistic mathematics with "esoteric mathematics." Some even considered it as an "ontological shift" (see e.g., Cooper & Dunne, 1998; K. M. Wong, 1997).

The Ad hoc Committee on Holistic Review of the Mathematics Curriculum (2000) gave a clear position of the issue: "The mathematics curriculum should be designed in such a way that mathematics learning progresses from concrete to abstract. The content in the mathematics curriculum should be arranged to let students get adequate prior experience with concrete objects before the formal treatment of mathematical concepts. Abstract concepts should also be backed up by an abundance of mathematical and non-mathematical (daily-life) examples" (p. 29).

In fact, before the holistic review, the Task Group on Review of Mathematics Syllabuses was already aware of the "dual nature of mathematics", that "mathematics [seen] as an exact science as well as an imaginative endeavor, as an abstract intellectual pursuit as well as a concrete subject with real-life applications; appreciate the beauty, the import, the power as well as the limitation of mathematics". (see N.Y. Wong, 1997; also, Sfard, 1991)

When mathematics is treated as a discipline that originates from various human activities, we can then see the real meaning of learning mathematics beyond just solving daily life "quasi-mathematical" problem. In such a way, students could begin to "develop an awareness of mathematics ... and they can gradually be able to conceptualize mathematically phenomena and problems met in daily life or in other disciplines. Furthermore, they can frame and formulate these problems in the mathematical language, to solve them with mathematical tools and then to make sense out of it in the mathematical way" (Ad hoc Committee on Holistic Review of the Mathematics Curriculum, 2000, p. 28).

4.3.3 *The expanding goal: An expanding control?*

Standardization is another curriculum trend in many regions, and is something more than just setting a minimum standard in some of the regions. As mentioned above, there is a tendency of prescribing all the details that are to be happening in the classroom. If we take the case in Hong Kong as an example, the primary mathematics curriculum has been evolving from a list of contents in the 1960s to the addition of teaching sequence in the 1970s. In the 1980s, teaching recommendations were inserted into the curriculum. Ironically, it is often the teachers who requested such a detailed disposition. In the standardization movement in Hong Kong in the early 1990s, at first, the TTRA ([Learning] **T**argets and **T**arget **R**elated **A**ssessments) was set up (Curriculum Development Council, 1992). Then, it was the teaching community who pressed the government to publish guidelines for teachers to teach in order to meet these standards. The TTRA was then turned into the Target Oriented Curriculum. In a sense, the teachers were surrendering their professional autonomy. Similar phenomenon was seen in the U.K. National Curriculum in which the programs of study downplayed attainment targets.

   With the goal being expanded, different aspects of learning became standardized. Affect, morality, and involvements in community activities were "checked." The description is extending from what is happening in the classroom to, to some extent, every corner of the children's life inside and outside school, making the "curriculum" all encompassing. We can get such an impression in the life-wide learning framework as proposed by the Hong Kong Curriculum Development Institute (Figure 2).

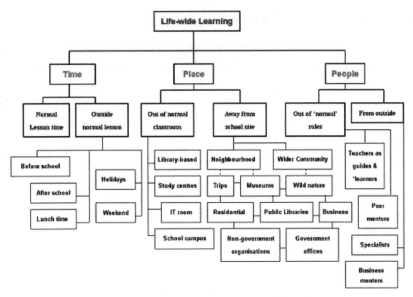

Figure 2. Life-wide learning contextual matrix.

Source. Life Wide Learning Section, Curriculum Development Institute, 2003

So, besides the criticism that standardization could fragment the curriculum (Kohn, 2000; Sacks, 1999), there is yet another issue of stripping away teachers' duty of teaching. Morrow and Torres (2000) pointed out that "… standardization of teaching and curriculum is closely linked to de-skilling of teachers and the logic of technical control on education" (p. 47). Blackmore (2000) also noted that "… increased standardization and universalization of curriculum and assessment as nation-states exert greater control through national curriculum frameworks" (p. 148) (see also Apple, 2000). This is, in fact, contrary to the call for "paradigm shift" of teachers in which teachers should make themselves thinkers, curriculum designers, researchers and educational decision makers (B. Clarke et al., 1996; Crawford & Adler, 1996).

Having everything centrally designed and prescribed should be the fatal cause of the phenomena of teacher de-skilling and anti-professionalism. Letting teachers thoroughly understand the principal rationale behind through professional discourse when there are new initiatives in learning could be a much better way than just asking them to implement the initiatives (Stigler & Hiebert, 1999; see also Ball, 1998).

4.4 *Globalization: Lost of local identity?*

Another phenomenon worth noticing is the cross-referencing of curriculum of other countries. Take the case of the holistic review of the mathematics curriculum in Hong Kong as an example, the ad hoc committee concerned paid great attention on whether the Hong Kong mathematics curriculum was in line with the world trend (Ad hoc Committee on Holistic Review of the Mathematics Curriculum, 2000, pp. 15 & 22). A comparative study was conducted to investigate the issue too (Leung et al., 1999). To some extent, this has its own need since we want our graduates to be recognized by other countries both for further studies and future employments. The Curriculum and Textbook Workgroup (2002) at the ICMI Comparative Study also observed that there is a diminishing difference between countries. In fact, when we compared the mathematics curricula in ten regions in 1997, a by-and-large distinction between "Western" and "Eastern" mathematics curricula was found. In brief, Eastern curricula were more centralized and focused more on "content". From the analyses in this chapter, such an "East–West" distinction has become blurred in this round of curriculum revision. In fact, key learning areas, standardization … seem to become common terminologies around the world (as we look at Tables 1 and 2, for instance). It simplistic terms, the Far eastern curricula started from highly centralized systems to the development of regional ones and go for curriculum differentiation. The Western ones seem to go in the reverse order. In addition, both content and process, both basic skills and higher order abilities are emphasized in both sides of the globe.

Though one can say that they are meeting in the "middle zone", cross-cultural comparisons repeatedly alerted us (see e.g. Watkins & Biggs, 2001) that good practices in the East may not necessarily work for the West. The Curriculum and Textbook Workgroup (2002) at the ICMI Comparative Study alerted us that "This is a danger of adopting a curriculum by shopping around.... The adoption of foreign ideas without critical evaluation can be detrimental to an education system" (p. 6). Hirabayashi also reminded us that "having a high achievement in international mathematics studies is not the only criterion" for a good curriculum (as quoted in Curriculum and Textbook Workgroup, 2002, p.6).

Ironically, some Eastern curricula are often being criticized of being too "Westernized" or even "Americanized" (Some even used the term "McDonalised", see Yang, 2002; see also Amos, Keiner, Proske, & Radtke, 2002; Burbules & Torres, 2000; Capella, 2000; Rizvi, 2000; Stromquist & Monkman, 2000). On the other hand, with the CHC learning phenomenon reinforced by the Third International Mathematics and Science Study (TIMSS) result that the four Little Dragons in Asia got superior scores; Western mathematics education began to "learn from the East". We also see mathematics textbooks in Eastern regions were also being transplanted to the West without careful consideration. What needs to be answered is: when we try to learn a lesson from others, did we consider their particular cultural context and values? More importantly, did we at the same time investigate the limitations and drawbacks of initiatives that were implemented elsewhere? How can we converge with a difference, taking into consideration curriculum initiatives in other places yet riding on the strengths of one's own cultural tradition could be one of the major challenges of curriculum development around the world.

4.5 *Concluding remark: Who is the "End User"?*

Curriculum reform could be an endeavor that is full of dilemmas. On the one hand, we need to meet the demands and expectation of stake-holders; on the other hand, we cannot simply make a compromise by "casting of votes." Dilemmas in curriculum reform in the age of "economic globalization" and "educational urbanization" is ever more intense. Mathematics for all carries the heavy duty of bringing up the whole younger generation who has diversified interest and who will enter different walks of life. When we over-emphasize the pragmatic value of education, aiming at producing a cohort of globally competitive human resource and a competitive workforce for the enterprise so as to make the society competitive, obviously the humanistic nature of education like caring, love, and individual growth could be overlooked. Along such a line of thought, we tend to worship testings, indicators, and international comparisons. Teaching (and the curriculum) is driven by testing objectives, testing items, and testing format. Backwash effect of assessment is intense (see e.g., Biggs, 1996). Value-addedness becomes just a tool of educational control and the "value" in the value-addedness formula is defined by those in power (potential employers, etc.). And fluctuation of results in international comparison brings about unnecessary accusation (see e.g., Hill, 1976). This blind belief on testing is the main cause of over-unification and conformity, squeezing the room of both student individualization and teachers' professional autonomy.

Though it seems that different parts of the world is settling down with the current wave of educational and curriculum reform, we believe that curriculum development is an ever on-going process. Appreciation and respect of students' individual differences, making it a divining force for learning, and the empowerment of the teacher could be the keys to reverse the above scenario. How curriculum change enhances but not manipulates teaching could be the major mission of educational policy makers and curriculum reformers (B. Clarke et al., 1996; Stigler & Heibert, 1999). Teachers' professional growth should proceed with curriculum development. Eventually, new notions like higher-order thinking, progress map, values ... are internalized among the teachers and exemplified naturally in day-to-day teaching. All these notions should not just be translated into steps in curriculum documents for teachers to follow. Curriculum should also be developed in full awareness of local context and local needs (N. Y. Wong et al., 1999). Let us conclude the chapter by a little Chan (Zen) story:

> Huang Bo was a great Chan master in the Tang dynasty (618-917) of China. One day when he was making a sermon in the assembly hall, he acclaimed, "Do you people know that there is no Chan master in the entire Tang Empire?" At that time a monk came out from the audience and said, "There are so many masters teaching in so many monasteries, why you said there is no Chan master?" Huang replied, "I did not say there is no Chan, I only said that there is no masters!" – Records of Green Cliff [碧岩录] (Chinese Buddhist Electronic Text Association, 2001, Vol. 48, p. 1051b)

References

Ad hoc Committee on Holistic Review of the Mathematics Curriculum. (2000). *Report on holistic review of the mathematics curriculum*. Hong Kong: Curriculum Development Council. Retrieved June 6, 2003 from http://cd.ed.gov.hk/maths/document/Adhoc. htm

Amos, K., Keiner, E., Proske, M., & Radtke, F.-O. (2002). Introduction. Globalisation autonomy of education under seiger? Shifting boundaries between politics, economy and education. *European Educational Research Journal, 1*(2), 193–213.

Apple, M. W. (2000). Between neoliberalism and neoconservatism: Education and conservatism in a global context. In N. C. Burbules & C. A. Torres (Eds.), *Globalization and education: Critical perspectives* (pp. 57–78). New York: Routledge.

Australian Education Council. (1990). *A national statement on mathematics for Australian schools*. Carlton, Victoria: Curriculum Corporation for the Australian Education Council.

Ball, S. J. (1998). *Global trends in educational reform and the struggle for the soul of the teacher!* Lecture by Wei Lun visiting professor. Hong Kong: The Chinese University of Hong Kong.

Basic Education Curriculum Material Development Centre, National Ministry of Education. (2001). *National mathematics curriculum standards at the compulsory education level (draft for consultation)* [In Chinese 义务教育阶段国家数学课程标准(征求意见稿)]. Beijing: Beijing Normal University.

Biggs, J. B. (Ed.). (1996). *Testing: To educate or to select? — Education in Hong Kong at the crossroads*. Hong Kong: Hong Kong Educational Publishing.

Blackmore, J. (2000). Globalization: A useful concept for feminists rethinking theory and strategies in education? In N. C. Burbules & C. A. Torres (Eds.), *Globalization and Education: Critical perspectives* (pp. 133–156). New York: Routledge.

Board of Studies. (2000). *Curriculum and standards framework II — mathematics* [CD-ROM]. Carlton, Victoria: Author.

Burbules, N. C., & Torres, C. A. (2000). Globalization and education: An introduction. In N. C. Burbules & C. A. Torres (Eds.), *Globalization and education: Critical perspectives* (pp. 1–26). New York: Routledge.

California State Board of Education. (1992). *Mathematics framework for California public schools: Kindergarten through grade twelve*. Sacramento: California Department of Education.

California State Board of Education. (1999). *Mathematics framework for California public schools: Kindergarten through grade twelve.* Retrieved June 6, 2003 from http://www.cde.ca.gov/cdepress/ math.pdf

Capella, J.-R. (2000). Globalization, a fading citizenship. In N. C. Burbules & C. A. Torres (Eds.), *Globalization and education: Critical perspectives* (pp. 227–252). New York: Routledge.

Chinese Buddhist Electronic Text Association. (2001). *Chinese electronic tripitaka series* (Vol. 48) [In Chinese 电子佛典系列] [CD ROM]. Taipei: Author.

Choi, P. K. (2001, November). *Counting our losses: The sacrifice of education to economic globalization.* Paper presented at the public conference in re-inventing Hong Kong in the age of globalization, Chung Chi College and Faculty of Social Science, The Chinese University of Hong Kong, Hong Kong.

Clarke, B., Clarke, D., & Sullivan, P. (1996). The mathematics teacher and curriculum development. In A. J. Bishop, K. Clements, C. Keitel, J. Kilpatrick, & C. Laborde (Eds.), *International handbook of mathematics education* (pp. 1207–1233). Dordrecht, The Netherlands: Kluwer Academic Publishers.

Cockcroft, W. H. (Chairperson). (1982). *Mathematics counts (Report of the Committee of Inquiry into the Teaching of Mathematics in Schools).* London: H. M. S. O.

Cooper, B., & Dunne, M. (1998). Anyone for tennis? Social class differences in children's responses to National Curriculum Mathematics Testing. *The Sociological Review, 46*(1), 115–148.

Crawford, K., & Adler, S. (1996). Teachers as researchers in mathematics education. The mathematics teacher and curriculum development. In A. J. Bishop, K. Clements, C. Keitel, J. Kilpatrick, & C. Laborde (Eds.), *International handbook of mathematics education* (pp. 1187–1205). Dordrecht, The Netherlands: Kluwer Academic Publishers.

Curriculum and Textbook Workgroup. (2002). *Draft report. ICMI Comparative Study.* Hong Kong: The University of Hong Kong.

Curriculum Development Committee. (1985). *Syllabuses for secondary schools: Mathematics (Form I-V).* Hong Kong: Government.

Curriculum Development Council. (1992). *Learning targets for mathematics (Primary 1 to Secondary 5).* Hong Kong: Government Printer.

Curriculum Development Council. (1999). *Syllabuses for secondary schools — mathematics (Secondary 1-5).* Hong Kong: Education Department.

Curriculum Development Council. (2000). *Mathematics education key learning area: Mathematics curriculum guide (Primary 1-6).* Hong Kong: Education Department.

Curriculum Development Council. (2001). *Learning to learn: The way forward to curriculum development.* Hong Kong: Education Department.

Curriculum Development Council. (2002). *Basic education curriculum guide: Building on strengths (Primary 1–Secondary 3).* Hong Kong: Education Department.

Curriculum Planning and Development Division. (2000a). *Mathematics syllabus: Primary.* Singapore: Ministry of Education.

Curriculum Planning and Development Division. (2000b). *Mathematics syllabus: Lower secondary.* Singapore: Ministry of Education.

Curriculum Reform Committee. (2001). *Curriculum standard for nine year compulsory education (for consultation)* [In Chinese 九年制义务教育数学科课程标准(征求意见稿)]. Shanghai: Shanghai Educational Press.

Department for Education and Employment and Qualifications and Curriculum Authority. (2000). *National curriculum (Mathematics).* Retrieved June 6, 2003 from http://www.nc.uk.net

Department for Education and the Welsh Office. (1995). *Mathematics in the national curriculum.* London: H. S. M. O. Retrieved June 6, 2003 from http://www.dfee.gov.uk/nc/index.html

Department of Education and Sciences and the Welsh Office. (1989). *Mathematics in the national curriculum.* London: H.S.M.O.

Department of Education and Sciences and the Welsh Office. (1991). *Mathematics for ages 5 to 16.* London: H. S. M. O.

Editorial Group from Thirteen Institutions. (1980). *The teaching of secondary school mathematics* [In Chinese 中学数学教材教法总论]. Beijing: People's Educational Press.

Goodlad, J. I. (1979). *Curriculum inquiry: The study of curriculum practice.* New York: McGraw-Hill.

Gu, L. (2002). An initial comparison of the development approaches of the Shanghai and Hong Kong school mathematics curricula [In Chinese 沪港两地学校数学课程发展思路的初步研究]. In Secondary Mathematics Subject Committee, Chinese Education Association (Ed.), *Mathematics classroom teaching reform for the full implementation of quality education* [In Chinese 全面推进素质教育, 改革数学课堂教学] (pp. 1–19). Beijing: People's Educational Press.

Hill, S. (1976). Issues from the NACOME report. *Mathematics Teacher,* 69(6), 440–446.

Hirst, P. H., & Peters, R. S. (1970). *The logic of education.* London: Routledge & Kegan Paul.

Howson, G., & Wilson, B. (Eds.). (1986). *School mathematics in the 1990s.* Cambridge: Cambridge University Press.

Jackson, A. (1997a). The Math Wars: California battles it out over mathematics reform (Part I). *Notices of the American Mathematical Society, 44*(6), 695–702.

Jackson, A. (1997b). The Math Wars: California battles it out over mathematics reform (Part II). *Notices of the American Mathematical Society, 44*(7), 817–823.

Japan Society of Mathematical Education. (2000). *Mathematics program in Japan.* Tokyo: Author.

Kohn, A. (2000). *The case against standardized testing: Raisin the scores, ruining the schools.* Portsmonth, NH: Heinemann.

Laborde, C. (2002, August). The mathematics curriculum in France at the beginning of the new century. Paper presented at the ICM (International Congress of Mathematician) 2002 Satellite Conference "International Conference on the Reform of Curriculum and Education in the 21st Century," Southwest China Normal University, Chongqing, China.

Lee, P. Y, & Fan, L. (2002, August). *The development of Singapore mathematics curriculum: Understanding the changes in syllabus, textbooks and approaches.* Paper presented at the ICM (International Congress of Mathematician) 2002 Satellite Conference "International Conference on the Reform of Curriculum and Education in the 21st Century," Southwest China Normal University, Chongqing, China.

Leung, F. K. S. (2001). In search of an East Asian identity in mathematics education. *Educational Studies in Mathematics, 47,* 35–51.

Leung, F. K. S., Lam, C. C., Mok, I. A. C., Wong, K. M., & Wong, N. Y. (1999). Comparative study on the mathematics curricula of major Asian and Western countries. Final report of a research commissioned by the Education Department, Hong Kong. Retrieved June 6, 2003 from http://cd.ed.gov.hk/maths/document/

Research1.htm

Life-wide Learning Section, Curriculum Development Institute. (2003). Life-wide learning contextual matrix. Retrieved June 6, 2003 from http://cd.emb.gov.hk/lwl/eng /what_lwl/matrix/matrix.htm

Masters, G., & Forcester, M. (1996). *Assessment resource kit: Progress maps*. Melbourne, Australia: Australian Council for Educational Research.

Mathematical Sciences Education Board, National Research Council. (1989). *Everybody counts* (Report to the Nation on the future of mathematics education). Washington, DC: National Academy Press.

Mathematical Sciences Education Board, National Research Council. (1990). *Reshaping school mathematics: A philosophy and framework for curriculum*. Washington, DC: National Academy Press.

Ministère de l'éducation nationale, de la Recherche et de la Technologie. (1999). *Accompagnement des programme* [Document accompanying the curricula]. Paris: Gouvernment de France. Retrieved September 9, 2000 from http://www.cndp.fr/college/frameset.asp?rub=col_txtoff.

Ministère de l'éducation nationale, de la Recherche et de la Technologie. (2000). *Lycée: Mathématique* [Senior secondary: Mathematics]. Paris: Gouvernment de France. Retrieved September 9, 2000 from http://www.cndp.fr/lycee/math.

Ministère de l'éducation nationale, de la Recherche et de la Technologie. (2002). *Les programmes pour l'ecole primaire* [Curricula for primary schools]. Paris: Gouvernment de France. Retrieved January 1, 2003 from http://www.cndp.fr/ecole.

Ministry of Education, Taiwan. (2001). *National 1st – 9th Grades curriculum alignment provisional syllabus: Mathematics learning dimension* [In Chinese 国民中小学九年一贯课程暂定纲要(数学学习领域)]. Taipei: Author.

Morrow, R. A., & Torres, C. A. (2000). The state, globalization, and educational policy. In N. C. Burbules & C. A. Torres (Eds.), *Globalization and education: Critical perspectives* (pp. 27–56). New York: Routledge.

National Advisory Committee on Mathematics Education. (1975). *Overview and analysis of school mathematics, Grades K12*. Washington, DC: Conference Board of the Mathematical Sciences.

National Commission on Excellence in Education. (1983). *A nation at risk: The imperative for educational reform*. Washington, DC: US Government Printing Office.

National Council of Supervisors of Mathematics. (1977). *Position paper on basic mathematical skills*. Washington, DC: National Institute of Education.

National Council of Teachers of Mathematics. (1980). *An agenda for action: Recommendations for school Mathematics of the 1980's*. Renton, VA: Author:

National Council of Teachers of Mathematics. (1989). *Curriculum and evaluation standards for school mathematics*. Reston, VA: Author.

National Council of Teachers of Mathematics. (2000). *Principles and standards for school mathematics*. Reston, VA: Author. Retrieved June 6, 2003 from http://standards.nctm.org

Okubo, K. (2000, August). *New directions in mathematics education in Japan*. Paper presented at the 9th International Congress of Mathematics Education (Topic Study Group 22), Tokyo/Makuhari, Japan.

Pong, W. Y., & Chow, J. C. S. (2002). On the pedagogy of examinations in Hong Kong. *Teaching and Teacher Education, 18*, 139-149.

Raizen, S. A., McLeod, D. B., & Rowe, M. B. (1997). The changing conceptions of reform.

In S. A. Raizen & E. D.Britton. (Eds.). *Bold ventures, Vol. 1: Patterns among U.S. innovations in science and mathematics education* (pp. 97–130). Dordrecht, The Netherlands: Kluwer Academic Publishers.

Rizvi, F. (2000). International education and the production of global imagination. In N. C. Burbules & C. A. Torres (Eds.), *Globalization and education: Critical perspectives* (pp. 205–226). New York: Routledge.

Robitaille, D. F., & Garden, R. A. (1989). *The IEA Study of Mathematics II: Contexts and outcomes of school mathematics*. Oxford: Pergamon Press.

Robson, R., & Latiolais, M. P. (1999). Standards-based education and its implications for mathematics faculty. *MAA (Mathematical Association of America) Online*. Retrieved June 6, 2003 from http://www.maa.org/features/robson.html

Robson, R., & Latiolais, M. P. (2000). Standards-based education. *Focus, May/June*, 12–13.

Rose, N. (1988). *Mathematical Maxims and Minims*. Raleigh NC: Rome Press Inc.

Sacks, P. (1999). *The standardized minds: The high price of America's testing culture and what we can do to change it*. Cambridge, MA: Perseus Publishing.

Sawada, T. (2002, August). *The reform of mathematics curriculum and its issue in Japan. Standards 2002*. Paper presented at the ICM (International Congress of Mathematician) 2002 Satellite Conference "International Conference on the Reform of Curriculum and Education in the 21st Century", Southwest China Normal University, Chongqing, China.

Schumann. H. (2002, June). *The German educational system and math curriculum*. Paper presented at the Hong Kong Mathematics Education Conference-02. Retrieved June 6, 2003 from http://www.ph-weingarten.de/homepage/lehrende/schumann/hong-kong/german.pps

Senk, S. L., & Thompson, D. R. (2003). School mathematics curricula: Recommendations and issues. In S. L. Senk & D. R. Thompson (Eds.), *Standards-based school mathematics curricula: what are they? What do students learn?* (pp. 3–27). Mahwah, NJ: Lawrence Erlbaum Associate.

Sfard, A. (1991). On the dual nature of mathematical conceptions: Reflections on processes and objects as different sides of the same coin. *Educational Studies in Mathematics, 22*(1), 1–36.

Sfard, A. (1998). On two metaphors for learning and the danger of choosing just one. *Educational Researcher, 27*(2), 4–13.

Simon, M. A. (1995). Reconstructing mathematics pedagogy from a constructivist perspective. *Journal for Research in Mathematics Education, 26*, 114–145.

Simon, M. A., & Blume, G. W. (1996). Justification in the mathematics classroom: A study of prospective elementary teachers. *Journal of Mathematical Behavior, 15*, 3–31.

Standards 2002 Writing Group. (2002, August). *Conception of the framework in Chinese standards of Senior High School Mathematics* (S. Wang, L. Wang, J. Li, & D. Zhang, Trans.). Paper presented at the ICM (International Congress of Mathematician) 2002 Satellite Conference "International Conference on the Reform of Curriculum and Education in the 21st Century", Southwest China Normal University, Chongqing, China.

Stigler, J. W., & Hiebert, J. (1999). *The teaching gap: Best ideas from the world's teachers for improving education in the classroom*. New York: Free Press.

Stromquist, N. P., & Monkman, K. (Eds.). (2000). *Globalization and education: Integration and contestation across cultures* (2nd edition). Lanham, MD: Rowman &

Littlefield.

Tanner, D., & Tanner, L. N. (1980). *Curriculum development: Theory into practice* (2nd ed.). New York: Macmillan.

Thwaites, B. (1972). *The school mathematics project: The first ten years.* Cambridge: Cambridge University Press.

Universität Würzburg. (2001) *Mathematics Education in Germany.* Retrieved June 6, 2003 from http://www.mathematik.uni-wuerzburg.de/History/meg

Watkins, D. A., & Biggs, J. B. (Eds.). (2001). *Teaching the Chinese learner: Psychological and pedagogical perspectives.* Hong Kong: Comparative Education Research Centre, The University of Hong Kong.

Wong, K. M. (1997). Do real-world situations necessarily constitute "authentic" mathematical tasks in the mathematics classroom? *Curriculum Form, 6*(2), 1–15.

Wong, N. Y. (1992). Mathematics in the 1990s [In Chinese 九十年代的数学教育]. *Mathmedia* [In Chinese 数学传播], *64,* 79–87.

Wong, N. Y. (1997). The Hong Kong mathematics curriculum: Anticipating a change. *Curriculum Forum, 6*(2), 56–65.

Wong, N. Y. (2000, October). *Education: A hundred year endeavor or a matter of days?* [In Chinese 百年树人, 还是只争朝夕?]. *MingPao Monthly* [In Chinese 明报月刊], 35–37.

Wong, N. Y. (2002). *Form "entering the way" to "exiting the way": In search of a bridge to span "basic skills" and "process ability".* In F. Lopez-Real (Ed.), Pre-conference proceedings of the ICMI Comparative Study (pp. 167–174). Hong Kong: The University of Hong Kong.

Wong, N. Y. (2003). Influence of technology on the mathematics curriculum. In A. J. Bishop, M. A., Clements, C. Keitel, J. Kilpatrick, & F. K. S. Leung (Eds.), *Second international handbook of mathematics education* (Vol. 1, pp. 271-321). The Netherlands: Kluwer Academic Publishers.

Wong, N. Y., Lam, C. C., Leung, F. K. S., Mok, I. A. C., & Wong, K. M. (1999). *An analysis of the views of various sectors on the mathematics curriculum.* Final report of a research commissioned by the Education Department, Hong Kong. Retrieved June 6, 2003 from http://cd.ed.gov.hk/maths/document/Research2.htm

Wong, N. Y., & Tanaka, S. (2000). Primary Japanese mathematics in the first decade of the 21st century — The course of study. *EduMath, 10,* 48–60.

Wong, N. Y., & Wong, K. M. (1997). The mathematics curriculum standards in ten regions [In Chinese 十地区数学教育课程标准]. *Mathmedia* [In Chinese 数学传播], *82,* 28–44.

Yang, S. K. (2002, December). *Educational research under the impact of globalization* [In Chinese 全球化冲击下的教育研究]. Keynote speech presented at the Hong Kong Educational Research Association 2002 International Conference "Globalization: New Horizons for Educational Change," Hong Kong.

Zang, X., & Ren, Z. (1998). High-stake testing from the Chinese perspective. *Mathematics Education Dialogues*, May/June, 468.

Chapter 3

Thinking Mathematically by Chinese Learners: A Cross-National Comparative Perspective[1]

CAI Jinfa   CIFARELLI Victor

Based on the findings from a number of cross-national comparative studies of US and Chinese students, we provided a retrospective review of these studies and presented a profile of Chinese learners' mathematical thinking in problem solving and problem posing. In particular, we identified several characteristics of Chinese learners' mathematical thinking in problem solving as well as pointed out some future directions to refine and extend this list of characteristics of Chinese learners. This chapter not only helps us understand the nature of Chinese students' mathematical thinking from a cross-national comparative perspective, but also provides information to refine instructional programs so that Chinese students' mathematical thinking can be better nurtured and developed.

Key words: mathematical thinking, characteristics of Chinese learners, cross-national comparisons, problem solving, problem posing

1 Introduction

Comparing is one of the most basic intellectual activities. We consciously make comparisons in order to understand where we stand, both in relation to others as well as to our own past experiences. There has been a long history of international comparative studies in education

[1] The research discussed in this paper was supported by grants from the Spencer Foundation and the University of Delaware Research Foundation to Cai Jinfa. The preparation of this paper was supported, in part, by a grant from the National Science Foundation (ESI-0114768) to Cai Jinfa. Any opinions expressed do not represent the views of either foundation.

(Alexander, 2000). Cross-national comparative studies in education not only provide information on students' achievement examined in the context of the world's varied educational institutions, but also help identify effective aspects of education practice. In the past decade, we have ccnducted a series of cross-national studies to assess and understand US and Chinese students' thinking in mathematical problem solving and problem posing (Cai, 1995, 1998, 2000a, 2000b; Cai & Hwang, 2002). The purposes of these studies are to reveal the similarities and differences between US and Chinese students' mathematical thinking, and then to provide information about how we can improve students' learning in mathematics.

In this chapter, we provide a retrospective review of these studies and present a profile of Chinese learners' mathematical thinking in problem solving and problem posing. In particular, we try to characterize the nature of Chinese learners' mathematical thinking from a cross-national comparative perspective. We draw on findings from a series of cross-national studies of US and Chinese students to describe and understand Chinese learners' mathematical thinking. While these studies are interrelated and sequential, they also serve as an assessment of US and Chinese students' mathematical thinking within a multi-dimensional framework (Cai, 1995, 2000a; Cai & Silver, 1995) that addresses cognitive processes of solving problems (Cai, 1995, 1998, 2000a, 2000b) as well as processes that underlie problem posing (Cai, 1998; Cai & Hwang, 2002). The first part of the chapter provides a brief overview about aspects of mathematical thinking and thus serves as a rationale for the various analyses that were undertaken in studies reviewed. We then suggest a profile of Chinese learners' mathematical thinking in problem solving and problem posing.

2 A Retrospective Review

While there is no consensus on what mathematical thinking is, it is widely accepted that there are many aspects of mathematical thinking that warrant examination (Ginsburg, 1983; Schoenfeld, 1997; Sternberg & Ben-Zeev, 1996). Studies of mathematics learning over the years have included a focus on identifying those ways that students demonstrate a propensity to "think mathematically" in their actions. For example, Pólya found that capable problem solvers employ heuristic reasoning strategies to solve problems (Pólya, 1945). Being able to self-generate useful analogies while solving a problem is an example of a heuristic that capable solvers demonstrate as they solve problems. In addition, Krutetskii (1976) found that able students are more likely than less able students to use generalizations in their mathematical problem solving. Other researchers have described and explained what it means to "think mathematically" (Burton, 1984). More recently, mathematical thinking has been characterized in terms of the learner being able to develop strong understandings in mathematical situations (Kieran & Pirie, 1991).

All of these studies suggest that we need to be very broad in assessing the mathematical thinking of students. For example, while we know that it is important for students to have algorithmic knowledge to solve many kinds of problems, this does not ensure that they have the conceptual knowledge to solve non-routine or novel problems (Hatano, 1988; Steen, 1999; Sternberg, 1999). In order to understand the differences in students' learning and mathematical thinking, we must use a variety of assessment tasks, thereby addressing the different facets of mathematical thinking. Hence, it is crucial that studies of mathematical thinking include tasks that measure both students' high-level thinking skills as well as their routine problem-solving skills that involve procedural knowledge.

In addition, studies of mathematical thinking need to focus more on the ways that students conceptualize a problem and develop appropriate solution strategies rather than whether or not they can carry out a formal algorithm to reach a solution. Furthermore, it is important to examine cognitive aspects of problem solving, such as the students' solution strategies, their mathematical misconceptions/errors, mathematical justifications, and representations. In fact, the examination of solution strategies can reveal qualitative aspects of students' mathematical thinking and reasoning such as how they go about formulating goals and purposes in their problem solving (Sternberg, 1991). Similarly, the examination of solution justifications and representations reveals the ways that students process a problem and express their mathematical ideas and thinking processes.

Therefore, in order to understand the international differences in students' mathematical thinking, it is desirable to use various types of assessment tasks to measure different facets of mathematical thinking. The use of both quantitative and qualitative assessment methods enables the researcher to broaden somewhat the scope of the analysis. Our studies incorporate such a comprehensive focus on the mathematical thinking of students.

2.1 *Examining students' multi-facets of mathematical thinking*

As an example of multi-dimensional assessment, Cai (1995) used three types of problem tasks to examine US and Chinese students' mathematical performance. These consisted of: (1) 20 multiple-choice tasks measuring computation skills; (2) 18 multiple-choice tasks measuring simple problem-solving skills; and (3) seven open-ended tasks measuring complex problem-solving skills. It was found that Chinese students outperformed US students on computation and simple problem-solving tasks but not on open-ended tasks that assessed complex problem solving. When differences for each of the open-ended tasks were examined, the performance patterns were not consistent across these tasks. For some of the open-ended assessment tasks, US students had higher mean scores than Chinese students. For other tasks, Chinese students had higher mean scores than US students.

In a later study, Cai (2000a) elaborated his ideas about the processes involved in complex problem solving. Specifically, in addition to assessing the computational and simple problem solving skills of students, Cai incorporated some new tasks to assess complex problem solving skills, tasks focused on the degree of novelty that must be used in order to find solutions. *Process-constrained* tasks refer to problems that can be solved by executing a "standard algorithm". In contrast, *process-open* tasks are problems that usually cannot be solved by an algorithm, and more typically require novel exploration of the problem situation. Furthermore, a process-open task usually lends itself to a variety of acceptable solutions. The study used six process-constrained and six process-open tasks to measure the students' complex problem-solving skills.

Table 1 shows the mean percent scores of the US and Chinese students on the computation tasks, simple problem solving tasks, the process-constrained and the process-open performance assessment tasks. The Chinese sample had significantly higher mean scores than the US sample on the computation tasks, simple problem solving tasks, and the process-constrained tasks. However, the US sample had significantly higher mean scores than the Chinese students on the process-open tasks. For the US sample, the mean score on the process-open tasks is the highest score that they achieved, while the mean score on the computation tasks is the lowest. For the Chinese sample, however, the mean score on the process-open tasks is the lowest score that they achieved, while the mean score on the computation tasks is the highest.

Table 1
Mean Percentage Scores of US and Chinese Students on Four Types of Tasks

Nations	Computation	Simple Problem Solving	Process-Constrained Complex Problem Solving	Process-Open Complex Problem Solving
US ($n = 232$)	48%	57%	54%	61%
China ($n = 310$)	88%	77%	75%	57%

From these findings, we see some of the challenges involved in cross-cultural assessments of mathematical thinking. The Chinese students did significantly better than the US students in 3 of the 4 types tasks; however, we found it surprising that the US students performed better in the process-open task, which we assumed to be the most novel task. Hence, even these multi-dimensional analyses sometimes can yield puzzling information and may require more probing to explain the differences. In addition to the quantitative analysis of performance, the study included a qualitative phase, whereupon the student responses for each assessment task were examined for cognitive aspects of performance such as students' preferred solution strategies, mathematical errors, and mathematical representations. This analysis identified several aspects of solution performance that helped to clarify and explain the quantitative performance measures and also suggested some hypotheses, which served to motivate the later studies. The next section discusses the qualitative aspects of the analysis to examine cognitive processes of solving problems.

2.2 *Examining cognitive processes of solving problems*

Given the fact that simple comparisons of status using international ranking provide little guidance for understanding and improving students' mathematics learning, it would be important to understand the international performance differences in other terms. Certainly, information about how students approach the solution of a given problem is more important than whether or not they are able to recognize the correct solution from among several candidates. While it is useful to know the performance differences in terms of mean scores or average correctness, we also need to describe student performance in qualitative terms to understand the nature of the international differences in students' mathematical thinking and reasoning. In a number of studies, we have used both quantitative and qualitative analysis methods to describe US and Chinese students' mathematical thinking and reasoning. For example, in the quantitative analysis of the earlier study (Cai, 1995), each student response was assigned a numerical score from 0 to 4. In contrast, the qualitative analysis focused on four critical cognitive aspects: solution strategies, mathematical misconceptions/errors, mathematical justifications, and representations (Cai, 1995).

The examination of solution strategies can provide qualitative aspects of information regarding students' mathematical thinking and reasoning (Sternberg, 1991). Learning can be viewed as a qualitative change in a student's way of experiencing and understanding of mathematics (Marton & Ramsden, 1988). The study of misconceptions provides information with respect to the characteristics and treatment of misconceptions and the extent to which students modify their misconceptions. The examination of solution justifications and representations reveals the ways that students process problems and also sheds light on the ways that students communicate their mathematical ideas and thinking processes.

Quantitative and qualitative analysis methods are not only interrelated but also complementary. In the quantitative analysis, each student response to a task is assigned a score based on a set of well-specified criteria of mathematical problem solving and reasoning. However, this procedure may conceal some aspects of students' performance. For example, different students can use different strategies to obtain a particular score level, and thus, individual student differences in solution strategies will not be evident using the quantitative analysis. Similarly, students may exhibit different mathematical misconceptions at a particular score level.

To complement the quantitative analysis, the qualitative analysis provided a more detailed description of the kinds of strategies associated with high-level scores and the kinds of errors associated with lower-level responses. For example, while the quantitative analysis found that the US and Chinese students had similar overall performance on novel tasks of complex problem solving (Cai, 1995), a detailed cognitive analysis of students' written responses revealed both similarities as well as subtle differences among the students' solutions. The Number Theory Problem, shown in Appendix, is one of the open-ended problems used in Cai (1995).

In this problem, students must solve for an unknown number that satisfies several problem conditions set in a story context. Specifically, the student must find the total number of blocks in a set given that 1 block is remaining when the whole set is partitioned into either groups of size 2, 3, or 4. Thus, a correct numerical answer should have a remainder of 1 when divided by 2, 3, or 4. An implicit condition of the problem is that the same set of blocks is partitioned each time. The Number Theory Problem has more than one correct answer. In fact, if we add 1 to any multiple of 12, we get a correct answers for the problem (i.e., $1 + 12n$, $n = 0, 1, 2, \ldots$, are all correct answers for the Number Theory Problem).

2.2.1 *Correctness of answers*

The results from this study showed that over one half of the US and Chinese students got correct answers. In particular, 56% of the US sample had correct answers to the Number Theory Problem; this success rate is almost the same as that of the Chinese sample (54%). However, the frequency distributions were significantly different for US and Chinese students who provided the correct answer of 13 and those who gave correct answers other than 13. A larger percentage of Chinese than US students tended to provide correct answers other than 13. Correct answers other than 13 included 1, 25, 49, etc. For those US and Chinese students who provided correct answers other than 13, the majority of them had 25 as the correct answer. It is interesting to note that only two US students and seven Chinese students provided more than one correct answer in their response.

2.2.2 *Representations*

Students used various representations in their solutions of solving the Number Theory Problem. The frequencies in which US and Chinese students used various representations were also significantly different. Three categories were used to classify the representations: verbal, symbolic, and visual. The student response was coded as a verbal representation if he/she used mainly written words to explain how they found the answer. The response was coded as a visual representation if the student used mainly a picture or drawing to explain how he/she found the answer. The response was coded as a symbolic representation if the student used mainly mathematical expressions to explain how he/she found the answer. Figure 1 shows the percentage distributions of US and Chinese students' representations for solving the Number Theory Problem. A larger percentage of Chinese than US students used symbolic representations; while a larger percentage of US than Chinese students used verbal representations and visual representations.

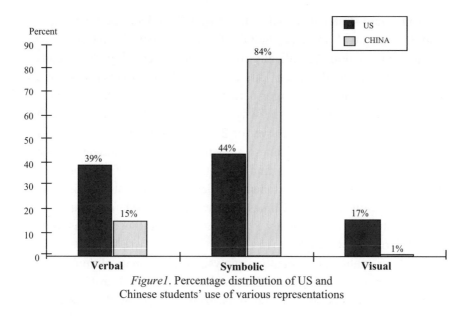

Figure1. Percentage distribution of US and
Chinese students' use of various representations

2.2.3 *Solution strategies*

The Number Theory Problem evoked a variety of solution strategies.
Table 2 describes each of the solution strategies and shows the
percentages of US and Chinese students using each strategy. Only a
slightly larger percentage of US students (52%) than Chinese students
(45%) had used apparent strategies, with the difference not statistically
significant. However, for those US and Chinese students with apparent
strategies, the frequency distributions of strategies used were
significantly different. Strategy 1 through strategy 6 involved common-
multiple approaches and strategies 7 and 8 used variations of a "trial and
error" approach. For those US and Chinese students with apparent
strategies, a larger percentage of Chinese than US students used common
multiple approaches (strategy 1 through 6) to obtain solutions. A larger
proportion of US students than Chinese students used "trial and error"
approaches (strategies 7 and 8).

Moreover, US and Chinese students tended to use different
variations of the common multiple approaches. For example, two
common multiple approaches that were most frequently used by Chinese

students were strategies 2 and 5; those by US students were strategies 1 and 3. Strategies 1 and 2 are literally the same except for the final result of the computation. Specifically, the use of strategy 1 yields a correct answer of 13, and the use of strategy 2 yields a correct answer of 25. This may explain why a larger percentage of US than Chinese students provided the answer of 13 and why a larger percentage of Chinese than US students provided the answer of 25. Twenty-eight US students used strategy 3, but only two Chinese students used it. In strategy 3, visual representations were used to find a common multiple of 2, 3, and 4. As we see above, overall, US students tended to use visual representations more frequently than did Chinese students. A considerable number of Chinese students used strategy 5 in which a "short division" was used to find the common multiple.

In later studies, this cognitive analysis of mathematical thinking was extended by considering both the problem solving and problem posing actions of students. By including problem posing in the analysis of mathematical thinking, we were able to get a more extensive picture of the mathematical thinking processes of Chinese and US students. The following section includes discussion of the critical role that problem posing plays in mathematical thinking as well as findings from recent studies that examined the problem solving and problem posing processes of US and Chinese students.

Table 2
Description of Solution Strategies and Percentages of US and Chinese Students

Description	Percentage of Students	
	US ($n = 129$)	China ($n = 193$)
Strategy 1: The student found 12 as a common multiple of 2, 3, and 4 by direct computation ($2 \times 6 = 12$, $3 \times 4 = 12$, $4 \times 3 = 12$), and then added one to the common multiple.	19	2
Strategy 2: The student found 24 as a common multiple of 2, 3, and 4 by direct computation ($2 \times 3 \times 4 = 24$), and then added one to the common multiple.	1	42
Strategy 3: The student constructed three separate diagrams showing sets of blocks, each divisible into groups of 2, 3, or 4; attempted to make the sets all the same size, and then added 1 block to each of the sets. For example, the first set of blocks had 12 blocks which were grouped in groups of 2; the second set of blocks had 12 blocks which were grouped in groups of 3; and the third set of blocks had 12 blocks which were grouped in groups of 4. Then, 1 block was added to each set to obtain a total of 13.	22	1
Strategy 4: The student listed the multiples of 2, of 3, and of 4; identified the common multiple; and then added one. For example, the student did as follows: 2, 4, 6, 8, 10, 12, 14, 16, ... 3, 6, 9, 12, 15, 18, ... 4, 8, 12, 16, 20, 24, ... $12 + 1 = 13$, so the answer was 13.	2	1
Strategy 5: The student used "short division" to find the common multiple of 2, 3, and 4, then added 1 to the common multiple to obtain a solution.	2	32
Strategy 6: Other common multiple approaches.	12	5
Strategy 7: The student showed a number (e.g., 13) divided by 2, by 3, and by 4 in three separate long divisions, indicating that all the divisions had a remainder of 1. In this way, the student verified a correct answer by the divisions without showing how he or she obtained the dividend.	29	13
Strategy 8: The student systematically or randomly guessed numbers of blocks and checked if the guesses satisfied the conditions of the problem.	13	4

2.3   *Examining both mathematical problem solving and problem posing*

Mathematical problem posing is one of the key components of mathematical exploration. In scientific inquiry, formulating a well-defined problem is often the key to finding solutions to the problem. It is important to include a focus on both problem solving and problem posing in examinations of students' mathematical thinking because such analyses inform us when the students shift their thinking among different perspectives. For example, examining US and Chinese students' problem solving can help us understand the solution strategies and representations students used to solve problems. In contrast, the examination of US and Chinese students' mathematical problem posing can help us understand how US and Chinese students self-generate the problems they see fit to solve. Since US students are much more likely than Chinese students to use visual-based strategies and representations in problem solving, is it possible that US students would be more likely than Chinese students to use visual representations to generate problems to solve? Assessments beyond problem solving allow us to determine those similarities and differences that exist between students in the two nations in the areas of problem posing. In addition, such assessments also allow us to examine the generality of the relatedness of students' performance in problem solving and problem posing from a cross-national perspective.

In a recent study, we examined the nature of US and Chinese students' generalized and generative thinking in mathematical problem solving and problem posing (Cai & Hwang, 2002). This study addressed three key sets of questions. First, given the existing evidence that Chinese students use more abstract strategies in problem solving than do their US counterparts, is it reasonable to expect that they would also be more successful solving problems that are most efficiently and accurately solved using abstract strategies? Second, might US students outperform Chinese students on problem posing tasks by producing a larger variety of problems? Related to this, should US students be expected to produce more problems involving pictures? Finally, from a cross-national perspective, can any general statements be made regarding the link between students' problem posing and problem solving?

Using three pairs of problem solving and problem posing tasks, the study focused on the students' mathematical performance on tasks of varying levels of difficulty. For each of the problem-posing tasks, students were asked to pose one easy problem, one moderately difficult problem, and one difficult problem. For each of the problem-solving tasks, students were asked to answer several questions based on the given pattern. In particular, students needed to employ their generalization skills in order to answer the last question in each problem-solving task efficiently. Appendix shows one-pair of the Door Bell problem-solving and Door Bell problem-posing tasks.

By designing the problem-posing task to have a mathematical structure similar to that of the problem-solving task, the data was then made possible to examine the relatedness of student solution processes in solving the pattern problem and the problems the students posed in the problem-posing task. The following sections summarize the results from the pair of the Doorbell situation.

2.3.1 *Door bell posing task*

Given the existing evidence from prior studies that US students use more concrete and pictorial strategies in problem solving than do their Chinese counterparts, is it reasonable to expect that they would also be likely to pose more problems involving pictures? This study provided no evidence showing that US students were more likely than Chinese students to pose picture related problems. The US students did pose more drawing problems than did their Chinese counterparts (9% of all US problems vs. 7% of all Chinese problems). However, the magnitude of the difference did not reflect the much wider gap in US students' preferred visual solution strategies. In fact, the US students were much more likely than their Chinese counterparts to generate extension problems across the posing tasks. Moreover, the percentage distributions of the various posed problem types were quite different between the two samples. Table 3 shows the percentages of US and Chinese students' various posed problem types.

Regarding the kinds of Doorbell problems generated, students in both samples tended to move away from generating problems solely based on the given information, instead they generated problems of greater difficulty. The most frequently generated problems for US students involved finding the number of guests at a particular ring for the easy and moderate problems, and computing the total number of guests after a specific ring for the difficult problem. In contrast, the most frequently generated problems among Chinese students were non-extension problems for the easy problem (e.g., How many guests entered on the fourth ring?), and problems asking for the number of guests entering on a non-given ring (e.g., 10th ring or 100th ring) for moderate and difficult problems.

Table 3
Types of Problems Posed for the Doorbell Situation

	98 US Students			155 CH Students		
	P1	P2	P3	P1	P2	P3
Extension Problems						
# of Guests on a Ring	33	27	17	21	30	27
Ring # for Some Guests	0	2	1	1	3	1
Total # of Guests for Several Rings	7	19	26	4	7	11
Total # of Rings for Some Guests	0	0	6	0	3	6
Rule-Based Problems	13	7	0	6	3	3
Total % of Extension Problems	*53*	*55*	*50*	*32*	*46*	*48*
Non-Extension Problems	*20*	*5*	*2*	*41*	*20*	*9*
No/Irrelevant Problems	*27*	*40*	*48*	*27*	*34*	*43*

Looking at the variety of problems posed by individual students, we see some similarity between the US and Chinese samples for each of the problem situations. The percentages of US and Chinese students who generated at least two distinctive problems for the Doorbell task were almost identical (51% for US and 50% for China). A slightly larger percentage of US students (16%) than Chinese students (9%) generated three distinctive problems, though the difference is not statistically significant. Hence, in answer to question two, there is no evidence that the US students tended to generate a larger variety of problems than the Chinese sample. In fact, the percentages of US and Chinese students who generated multiple distinctive problems are almost identical.

2.3.2 *Door bell solving task*

Given the existing evidence from prior studies that Chinese students use more abstract strategies in problem solving than do their US counterparts, is it reasonable to expect that they would also be more successful solving problems that are most efficiently and accurately solved using abstract strategies? In solving the Doorbell Problem, the US and Chinese students had almost identical success rates (70%) when they were asked to find the number of guests who entered on the 10th ring. However, the success rate for Chinese students (43%) was significantly higher than that of the US students (24%) when they were asked to find the ring number at which 99 guests would enter the room.

The strategies that students used to solve the Doorbell problem were classified into three categories: concrete, semi-abstract and abstract. Students who chose an abstract strategy to solve the Doorbell Problem generally followed one of two paths. Some noticed that the number of guests who entered on a particular ring of the doorbell was equal to twice the ring number minus one (i.e., $y = 2n - 1$, where y represents the number of guests and n represents the ring number). Others recognized that the number of guests who entered on a particular ring equaled the ring number plus the ring number minus one (i.e., $y = n + (n - 1)$). Those students who used a semi-abstract strategy showed a number of steps of computation to yield a correct answer. Below are two examples of semi-abstract strategies for finding the ring number at which 99 guests entered:

Example 1: $99 - 9 = 90$. $90 \div 2 = 45$. $45 + 5 = 50$.
Example 2: $99 - 7 = 92$. $92 \div 2 = 46$. $46 + 4 = 50$.

Finally, those who used a concrete strategy made a table or a list or noticed that each time the doorbell rang, two more guests entered than on the previous ring and so added 2's sequentially to find an answer.

In general, the findings confirmed the previously reported tendency for Chinese students to use abstract strategies and symbolic representations and for US students to use concrete strategies and drawing-based representations. Figure 2 shows the percentages of US and Chinese students' choosing appropriate concrete, semi-abstract and abstract solution strategies to answer Questions 1 and 3. Forty-four percent of the Chinese students with appropriate strategies used abstract strategies to find the number of guests who entered on the 10th ring (Question 1), while only 1% of the US students with appropriate strategies used abstract strategies. In the US sample, the vast majority used concrete strategies to answer Question 1. Although a larger percentage of US than Chinese students (48% vs. 42%) used appropriate strategies to find the ring number at which 99 guests entered, the Chinese students were much more likely to use abstract strategies. Indeed, 65% of Chinese students choosing an appropriate strategy for Question 3 used an abstract strategy as compared to only 11% of the US sample. Instead, the majority (75%) of US students chose concrete strategies, compared to 29% of the Chinese students.

Table 4 shows the success rates of US and Chinese students who used various solution strategies to answer Question 3. The Chinese students' use of an abstract strategy in the last question is clearly associated with their higher success rates for answering Questions 1 and 3. In fact, with one exception, every Chinese student who used an abstract strategy for Question 3 answered both Question 1 and 3 correctly. In contrast, the US sample does not display such a strong relationship between students' problem-solving strategies and their problem-solving performance. This finding may well be related to the fact that only a few of the US students used abstract strategies to answer Question 3. However, one thing that was clear across both samples, and which might be expected by intuition, was that students who used strategies that were inappropriate or gave no explanation were least likely to answer Question 3 correctly.

The disparities in the US and Chinese students' problem-solving success rates may be related to their use of different strategies. Within the Chinese sample, those who used abstract strategies had much higher success rates for all questions than those who used concrete strategies. If we limit our analysis to those US and Chinese students who used concrete strategies, the success rates between the two samples become very similar. Therefore, the results from both problem-solving tasks provide evidence that the Chinese students' preference for abstract strategies seems to help them outperform the US students on problems amenable to abstract strategies.

Strategies for Finding the Number of Guests that Entered on the 10th Ring (Question 1)

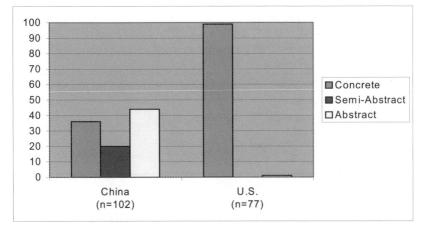

Strategies for Finding the Ring Number When 99 Guests Entered (Question 3)

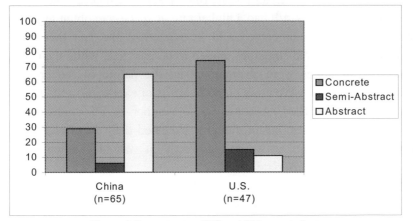

Figure 2. Percentages of US and Chinese students
using concrete, semi-abstract, and abstract strategies

Table 4

Association of US and Chinese Students' Success Rates for Questions 1 and 3 and Their Use of Strategies for the Doorbell Problem

	% of Students	
	Question 1 (Guests on the 10th ring)	Question 3 (Ring # for 99 guests)
CHINESE SAMPLE		
Concrete Strategies (n=19)	74	37
Semi-Abstract Strategies (n=4)	50	75
Abstract Strategies (n=42)	98	98
Inappropriate or No Strategies (n=90)	57	18
US SAMPLE		
Concrete Strategies (n=35)	83	46
Semi-Abstract Strategies (n=7)	71	43
Abstract Strategies (n=5)	60	60
Inappropriate or No Strategies (n=51)	63	2

The curious results regarding appropriate strategy choice in both problems point to one possible reason for this advantage. In answering the last question of the Door Bell problem, the US students actually chose an appropriate strategy more often than the Chinese students. Yet, the Chinese students still had a higher rate of success in obtaining correct answers. This phenomenon could be related to the fact that the US students' appropriate strategies tended to be concrete, while the Chinese students' strategies were abstract. Given the nature of the problems, concrete strategies were more prone to errors of execution, and thus were less likely to succeed. A considerable number of US students chose appropriate strategies, but presumably executed them incorrectly. When the Chinese students answered incorrectly, it was most often because they chose an inappropriate strategy.

2.3.3 *Relatedness between problem posing and problem solving*

The study (Cai & Hwang, 2002) showed a stronger link between problem solving and problem posing for the Chinese sample, while the link is weaker for the US sample. We compared the performance of students who posed at least two extension problems and students who posed fewer than two. For both samples, students with at least two extension problems consistently outperformed those with fewer than two extension problems across the four questions of the problem. In the Chinese sample, 81% and 56% of those who posed at least two extension problems gave correct responses to Questions 1 and 3, respectively, while only 60% and 33% of the others did so. The US sample exhibited the same pattern.

There was also a link between the variety of problems students posed and their success with problem solving, though the relationship was more apparent in the Chinese sample. In both samples, students who had posed type-0 problems (meaning that the problems they posed were either nonsense, irrelevant, or non-responses), on average, had the lowest percentage of correct answers in problem solving, particularly when compared to their peers with at least 2 types of problems posed. The difference was much larger in the Chinese sample than in the US sample. For example, nearly 75% of the Chinese students who posed at least two types of problems correctly found the number of guests on the 10th ring or the ring number when 99 guests entered. Only 40% of the students who posed type-0 problems had a correct answer for either of these questions. For the US sample, over 50% of the students who posed at least two types of problems correctly found the number of guests on the 10th ring or the ring number when 99 guests entered. Only 40% of the students who posed type-0 problems had a correct answer for either question.

For the Chinese students, 42% of those posing fewer than two extension problems used abstract strategies to answer the last Doorbell question. However, 79% who posed at least two extension problems chose abstract strategies for that question. A relationship between the variety of problems posed and the kind of strategy used in problem solving was also evident in the Chinese sample, but not in the US sample. Chinese students who had generated at least two distinct types of problems tended to use abstract strategies to solve problems, whereas their peers who posed fewer than two types of problems tended to use wrong or unidentified strategies, or gave no explanation in problem solving. In particular, nearly 55% of the Chinese students who had generated at least two distinct types of problems used abstract strategies in their problem solving; only about 10% of those who had generated fewer than two distinct types of problems used abstract strategies.

In summary, there was a stronger link between problem solving and problem posing for the Chinese sample, while the link is much weaker for the US sample. However, the differential nature of the relationships for US and Chinese students does not imply a lack of generality in the links between problem solving and problem posing. Instead, the stronger link between variety of posed problems and problem-solving success for the Chinese sample might be attributable to the fact that the US students almost never used abstract strategies. Posing a variety of problem types seems to be strongly associated with abstract strategy use in the Chinese sample. In the US sample, only a few students used abstract strategies for Question 3 of the Doorbell Problem. At most, the data from that question suggest that the variety of problem types posed is weakly associated with abstract strategy use. The findings of this study are limited due to the fact that only a few US sixth grade students used abstract strategies. Since older students (e.g., seventh, eighth or ninth graders) are more likely than sixth graders to use abstract strategies, future studies are needed to use older students as subjects. Their responses could be useful in clarifying the relationships between the use of strategies and problem-solving success, as well as further exploring and illuminating the links between problem solving and problem posing.

3 An Initial Profile

In the previous section of this chapter, we reviewed the results from several studies of the mathematical thinking processes of Chinese and US students. The focus was on the ways that these studies enabled us to capture the quantitative and qualitative aspects of mathematical performance. It is clear that there are remarkable differences between US and Chinese students' mathematical thinking involved in problem solving and problem posing. In this section, we will attempt to identify several characteristics of Chinese learners' mathematical thinking based on the available evidence. In the process of discussing these characteristics, we will speculate possible contextual reasons that nurtured Chinese learners.

3.1 *Performing unevenly on various tasks*

As was shown above, Chinese students performed unevenly on various tasks. The success rates for Chinese students on the computation tasks and simple problem-solving tasks are much higher than those on the complex problem solving tasks. For example, the mean percentage for computation tasks is 88% to 77% for simple problem solving, 75% for the process-constraint complex problem solving, and 57% for the process-open complex problem solving (see Table 1). Such a performance pattern of the Chinese students was also shown in the following Division Problem: *Students and teachers at Gunming elementary school will go by bus for Spring sightseeing. There is a total of 1128 students and teachers. Each bus holds 36 people. How many buses are needed?* In solving the Division Problem, one not only needs to correctly apply and execute division computation (computation phase), but also to interpret correctly the computational results with respect to the given situation (sense-making phase). Chinese students outperformed US students on the computation phase, but not on the sense-making phase. Moreover, Chinese students' success rate in the computation phase was much higher than that in the sense-making phase.

A number of researchers have found that having expertise in routine application does not imply expertise in complex and novel problem solving. Routine applications can often be solved using procedural knowledge; in contrast, complex and novel problem solving usually requires that the solver use conceptual knowledge in order to find a solution. Chinese students' varied performance on different tasks provides further evidence to support the assertion. In addition, Chinese students' differential performance on various tasks may reflect the different emphasis in curriculum and instruction. As was indicated in Zhang, Li, and Tang (this volume), basic knowledge and skills are two of the important emphases in Chinese curriculum and instruction.

Do Chinese students really outperform US students in mathematics? Since a number of cross-national studies consistently showed that Chinese students outperformed US students on tasks requiring the applications of mathematical knowledge and skills routinely learned in school, many people might answer "yes" to the question. However, the Chinese students' differential performance patterns on various tasks show the complexity of the issues that must be addressed in order to answer this question. In fact, the performance differences between US and Chinese students appear to be related to the nature of the assessment tasks. For example, on mathematical problem-posing tasks, there were essentially no differences between US and Chinese students.

3.2 *Using generalized strategies and symbolic representations*

Across the studies and tasks, we consistently found that Chinese students demonstrated a strong preference for using abstract strategies in their problem-solving actions, while the US students were more likely to employ the use of concrete drawing strategies while they solved problems. Even US eighth graders are more likely than Chinese fourth graders to use concrete drawing strategies (Cai, 2004). In one of our studies (Cai, 2000b), we examined the solution strategies and representations used by US and Chinese students' to solve two problems related to arithmetic average. We also examined the relationship between the students' solution representations and their problem-solving performance. Among the findings was that the students' use of abstract strategies and symbolic representations greatly aided their mathematical performance. In particular, for the US sample, students who used arithmetic representations performed significantly better than those who used verbal and pictorial representations on a problem-solving measure. For the Chinese sample, students using algebraic representations performed slightly better than those using arithmetic, verbal, and pictorial representations. Overall, Chinese students performed better than US students on each of the averaging problems and on the problem-solving measure. However, if the analysis is limited to US students using symbolic (algebraic or arithmetic) representations, there is no mean difference between US and Chinese students' performance. These findings not only support the argument that the representations students use can serve as an index of how well they might solve particular problems (Dreyfus, & Eisenberg, 1996; Janvier, 1987), they also suggest that Chinese students' superior performance on the averaging problems may be due, in part, to their use of more sophisticated representations (e.g., algebraic).

In another study (Cai & Hwang, 2002), we identified the advantages of students' using abstract strategies. Within the Chinese sample, those who used abstract strategies had much higher success rates for all problems than those who used concrete strategies. Since we did not found the US students used abstract strategies, it is impossible in the study to provide a reliable picture of how US students choosing abstract strategies compare to those choosing concrete strategies. However, if we limit our analysis to those US and Chinese students who used concrete strategies, the success rates between the two samples become very similar for each of the problems. Therefore, the Chinese students' preference for abstract strategies seems to help them outperform the US students on problems amenable to abstract strategies. Indeed, across problem-solving tasks, the performance gap between US and Chinese students widens as the questions become more abstract. For example, in solving the Door Bell Problem (see Appendix), the US and Chinese students had almost identical success rates when they were asked to find the number of guests who entered on the 10th ring. However, the success rate for Chinese students (43%) was significantly higher than that of the US students (24%) when they were asked to find the ring number at which 99 guests would enter the room.

We are still in the beginning stage of understanding the possible reasons why US and Chinese students have different preferences for using strategies and representations. However, it seems apparent that teachers' mathematical beliefs greatly influence their teaching practice and thus influence the US and Chinese students' choices of strategy use and representations. We recently interviewed a group of experienced teachers including 11 US teachers and a group of 9 Chinese teachers (Cai, in press-a). In the interview, we asked each teacher to score a set of 28 student responses using a five-point scale from 0-4, with a rating of 0 to describe a low level of mathematical sophistication demonstrated by the student's reasoning and a rating of 4 to indicate highly sophisticated reasoning on the part of the student. Each student response had a correct answer (or a reasonable estimate for the answer) and an appropriate strategy that yielded the correct answer (or estimate); however, the representations and solution strategies used by students in these responses indicated the different strategies and approaches taken by students in their reasoning. Each teacher was asked to explain the reasons for their scoring. Both US and Chinese teachers scored extremely high for the student responses involving abstract strategies; for those responses involving concrete drawing strategies, Chinese teachers scored them significantly lower than the US teachers. According to the Chinese teachers, being able to solve a problem is good, but it is just the first step of the learning. Chinese teachers want students to learn generalized problem-solving methods that transfer to other problem situations. However, there is no evidence from the interviews that US teachers have such a goal. Instead, US teachers' goal is to have students solve a problem no matter what strategies they use.

3.3 *Using more conventional strategies*

While students' solution strategies can be examined in terms of abstractness vs. concreteness, they can also be examined in terms of mathematical conventionality. A conventional strategy is one that is usually taught in the classroom; in contrast, a non-conventional strategy may not necessarily be taught in the classroom and may evolve from the students' novel explorations. For some tasks, students' solution strategies are better examined in terms of their abstractness while for others, the degree of conventionality exhibited by a student's strategies better captures their underlying reasoning. The results from a number of studies showed that Chinese students are more likely than US students to use conventional strategies. For example, when US and Chinese sixth-grade students were asked to solve a Pizza Ratio Problem (see Appendix), in which they needed to determine if each girl or each boy gets more pizza when seven girls share two pizzas and three boys share one pizza equally, they used eight different ways to justify that each boy gets more than each girl (Cai, 2000a). For those who used appropriate strategies, over 90% of the Chinese students used the following conventional strategy: *Each boy will get 1/3 of a pizza and each girl will get 2/7 of a pizza. If you compared 1/3 with 2/7, you would know that 1/3 is bigger than 2/7 by transforming them into common fractions (1/3 = 7/21 and 2/7 = 6/21. 7/21 — 6/21 = 1/21) or decimals (1/3 = .33 and 2/7 = .29. .33 — .29 = .04)*. However, only about 20% of the US students used such a conventional strategy. In contrast, the vast majority of the US students used one of the following non-conventional strategies.

Solution 1: Three girls share one pizza, and another three girls share another pizza. Each of these six girls will get the same amount of the pizza as each of the three boys. But one of the girls has no pizza. So, each boy will get more.

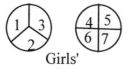 G

Solution 2: Three girls share one pizza and the remaining four share one pizza. Each piece that each of the remaining four girls get is smaller than the boys get. So the boys get more.

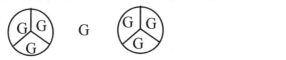

Girls'   Boys'

Solution 3: 7 Girls get two pizzas, and 3 boys get one pizza. The girls have twice as many pizza as boys. But the number of girls is more than twice as many than boys. So the boys get more.

Solution 4: Each pizza was cut into 4 pieces. Each girl gets 1 piece with 1 piece left over. Each boy gets 1 piece with 1 piece left over. The one piece left over must be shared by the 7 girls, but the 1 piece left over will be shared by three boys. So the boys get more.

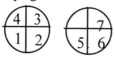

Girls'   Boys'

This example shows a dilemma we face. While the conventional strategy is apparently quite efficient and can be easily applied to solve other similar problems, this conventional strategy shows little originality. In contrast, while non-conventional strategies show the originality of students' thinking, they also are task specific and less applicable for solving other similar problems, especially those that involve bigger numbers. The results from this particular example may suggest the effectiveness of Chinese classroom instruction on developing students' efficient strategies and the effectiveness of US classroom instruction on developing original mathematical thinking. Ideally, we would hope that instruction can foster students' learning of efficient problem solving-strategies and develop their mathematical thinking with originality. If that is one of the goals for school mathematics, we have to seriously investigate the classroom instruction in both nations so that one can benefit from the other.

3.4 *Generating more solutions if they are asked to*

Collectively, US student are likely to give more variety of solutions than Chinese students. However, when each student is asked to provide multiple solutions, Chinese students tended to generate more solutions than US students. For example, when US 7th and 8th graders and Chinese 6th graders were asked to generate three different solutions to the Pizza Ratio Problem mentioned before, about 40% of Chinese students generated two or three different solutions, but only about 20% of the US students generated two or three different solutions. Interestingly, in Chinese students' second or third solutions, they rarely used one of the four solutions mentioned above. Instead, the second or third solution provided by Chinese students is one of the following two: (1) 7/2 = 3.5 and 3/1 = 3. Therefore 3.5 girls will share one pizza and 3 boys will share one pizza. Thus, each boy gets more; or (2) If there were six girls, each girl and each boy would have the same. But you have 7 girls, so each girl gets less than each boy.

In another task, US and Chinese sixth graders were asked to come up with two solutions to the following problem: *Margarita and Sam worked at the local park. Margarita earned $15 a day selling food. Sam earned*

$10 a day cleaning tables. Margarita worked a <u>different</u> number of days than Sam. Margarita and Sam earned the <u>same</u> total amount of money. How many days could each person have worked? Nearly 70% of the Chinese students came up with two different solutions, as compared to about 50% of the US students. While none of the US students came up with more than two solutions, some of the Chinese students came up with more than two different solutions. On the other hand, while only 5% of the Chinese students provided two repeated solutions, about 20% of the US students did so.

Even though Chinese students are more likely to generate multiple solutions to the Pizza Ratio Problem if they are asked to, their solutions are still quite conventional. The finding that Chinese students generate more solutions may be explained by the Chinese curriculum emphasis. The Chinese mathematics curriculum emphasizes a diversity of approaches to solve mathematics problems. Textbooks serve to support this approach by demonstrating both arithmetic and algebraic solutions to problems. In contrast, the US mathematics curriculum places greater emphasis on teaching particular methods and heuristics to solve mathematics problems.

3.5 *Committing errors involving unjustified symbol manipulations*

While there are remarkable differences between US and Chinese students' solution strategies and representations in problem solving, the types of errors both US and Chinese students committed are very similar. One of the errors committed is related to the unjustified symbol manipulation. Students just picked some numbers from a problem and worked with them in ways irrelevant to the problem context. An example of the unjustified symbol manipulation error for the Number Theory Problem is to add all numerals in the problem unreasonably in trying to solve the problem $(2 + 3 + 4 + 1 + 1 + 1 = 12)$. For both US and Chinese students, this unjustified symbol manipulation is the most frequently committed errors in solving this particular problem.

Similarly, a considerable number of US and Chinese students committed the unjustified symbol manipulation errors to solve the Hats Average Problem (see Appendix). For example, a student simply added up all numerals given in the Hats Average Problem and recorded the sum in the answer space. The student counted the number of hats sold in week 1 (9), week 2 (3), and week 3 (6). Then the student wrote down all numerals in the problem, such as 1 in "Week 1", 2 in "Week 2", 3 in "Week 3", 4 in "Week 4", and 4 and 7 in "How many hats must Angela sell in Week 4 so that the <u>average</u> number of hats sold is 7?" Finally, the student added <u>all</u> the numbers that appeared in the problem ($9 + 3 + 6 + 1 + 2 + 3 + 4 + 4 + 7 = 39$) and put 39 as the answer.

Another common error for both US and Chinese students was their "incorrect use of the computational algorithm". For example, there are six incorrect ways US and Chinese students applied the averaging algorithm in an attempt to solve the Hats Average Problem.

1. The student added the number of hats sold in week 1 (9), week 2 (3), and week 3 (6), then divided the sum by 3, to get an answer of 6. However, the average was 7. Therefore, the student added 3 to the sum of the numbers of hats sold in the first three weeks, then divided it by 3, to get 7, and then gave the answer 3.
2. The student added the number of hats sold in week 1 (9), week 2 (3), and week 3 (6), then divided the sum by 3, and got 6, $6 + 1 = 7$. So the student gave the answer 1.
3. The student added the number of hats sold in week 1 (9), week 2 (3), and week 3 (6), then divided the sum by 3. The student then gave the quotient (6) as the answer.
4. The student added the number of hats sold in week 1 (9), week 2 (3), week 3 (6), and the average (7), then divided the sum by 4. The student then gave the whole number quotient (6) as the answer.
5. The student added the number of hats sold in week 1 (9), week 2 (3), and week 3 (6), then divided the sum by 4. The student then gave the quotient (4.5) as the answer.
6. The student added the number of hats sold in week 1 (9), week 2 (3), and week 3 (6), then divided the sum by 7. The student then gave the whole number quotient (2) as the answer.

In the last four incorrect applications, students attempted to directly apply the averaging algorithm to find the answer (add-then-divide).

These students seemed to have neglected either problem condition that the average of the hats sold in four weeks should be 7 or the question that they were asked to answer (i.e., How many hats must Angela sell in Week 4 so that the average number of hats sold is 7?). In the first two incorrect applications, however, students did more than directly applying the averaging algorithm. These students manipulated the numbers to produce an answer of seven. It appears that they realized that the average of the hats sold in four weeks should be 7 and so they tried to do something more than directly applying the averaging algorithm. Regardless of whether or not these students tried to make the average seven, all seem to have lacked the necessary conceptual understanding of the averaging algorithm. It appears, though, that they knew the computational procedure for calculating an average if they are given the information in a standard "add-then-divide" algorithm. Thus, it is likely that the difficulties for US and Chinese students are not due to their lacking of procedural knowledge but rather that they possessed an incomplete conceptual understanding of the averaging algorithm.

Similar errors were documented by Lee, Zhang, and Zheng (1997) when a group of Chinese fourth graders, seventh graders, eighth graders, and twelfth graders were asked to solve an absurd problem: *There are 26 sheep and 10 goats in a ship. How old is the captain?* About 90% of the Chinese fourth graders, 82% of the seventh and eighth graders, and 34% of the twelfth graders "solved" this problem by combining numbers in it without realizing the absurd nature of the problem (Lee et al., 1997). When these Chinese students were asked why they did not recognize that the problem was meaningless, many students responded that "any problem assigned by a teacher always has a solution."

More research is needed to help students overcome difficulties described above, but one thing might be clear, though, that mathematical instruction cannot simply focus on teaching students to manipulate numbers or symbols without meaningful connections. Instead, we have to strive for developing both students' procedural knowledge and conceptual understanding behinds the procedures.

3.6 *Less willing to take risks in problem solving*

Analyses of students' responses gave a strong impression that US students are much more willing to take risks than Chinese students in problem solving. For those who did not have a clue to solve a problem, Chinese students were likely to skip the problem and leave it a blank, but US students usually put something down even though the things they wrote might be meaningless. For example, although a larger percentage of the Chinese students (43%) than US students (24%) correctly found the ring number when 99 guests entered for the Door Bell Solving Problem (Cai, 2000a), a considerable number of US and Chinese students did not answer the question correctly. For those Chinese students who did not answer the question correctly, nearly half of them left it blank. However, for those US students who did not answer the question correctly, only about 10% of them left it blank. That means that about 90% of the US students who did not answer the question correctly included written work on their papers. Although we did not have first hand knowledge why so many Chinese students left the problem blank, our conversation with some Chinese teachers suggest that if students are unable to solve a problem, they rather leave it in blank than take a risk to guess a solution.

The response to the following problem provided further evidence that Chinese students are less willing to take risks in problem solving: $5 + (-4) = ?$ Four possible answers were provided. This is one of the 20 computation tasks in an earlier study (Cai, 1995). This is the only task in which US sixth-grade students performed better than Chinese sixth-grade students. For both nations, addition involving negative numbers was not covered in the regular curriculum. Teachers' questionnaires indicated that the tested sixth grades in both nations have not learned the operation of addition when negative numbers are involved. Therefore, both US and Chinese sixth graders did not know how to solve this problem. What really interesting is that about 15% of the Chinese students did not guess possible answers by simply choosing one of the four provided answers.

4 Conclusions

Based on a number of cross-national comparative studies of US and Chinese students, we tried to characterize Chinese learners' mathematical thinking. In particular, we identified six characteristics of Chinese learners' mathematical thinking. Chinese students performed unevenly on various tasks — better on tasks assessing computation skills and basic knowledge than on tasks assessing open-ended complex problem solving. Chinese students are more likely to use generalized strategies and symbolic representations. Chinese students usually provide more conventional solutions. Chinese students can generate more solutions if they are asked for. Like US students, a considerable number of Chinese students committed errors involving unjustified symbol manipulations. Chinese students are less willing to take risks in problem solving.

The "golden ring" of educational research is to improve the learning opportunities for all students. The purpose, then, of international studies is to provide information about how we can improve students' learning in mathematics (Cai, 2001). There is no doubt that the more information that we obtain about what students know and think, the more opportunities we are able to provide meaningful learning opportunities for students. It is an initial attempt to characterize Chinese learners' mathematical thinking. Future studies are needed to refine and extend this list of characteristics of Chinese learners. And also, it should be indicated that in this chapter our focus is not to examine possible reasons why US and Chinese students think differently. Although some studies have been conducted to understand why US and Chinese students think differently (e.g., Cai, 2004, in press-a, in press-b), continuous effort is needed to systematically examine the impact of teaching and curriculum variables on students' thinking. Nevertheless, this chapter not only helps us understand the nature of Chinese students' mathematical thinking from a cross-national comparative perspective, but also provides information to refine instructional program so that Chinese students' mathematical thinking can be better nurtured and developed.

References

Alexander, R. (2000). *Culture and pedagogy.* Blackwell Publishing.

Burton, L. (1984). Mathematical thinking: The struggle for meaning. *Journal for Research in Mathematics Education, 15*(1), 35-49.

Cai, J. (1995). *A cognitive analysis of U.S. and Chinese students' mathematical performance on tasks involving computation, simple problem solving, and complex problem solving.* (Journal for Research in Mathematics Education monograph series 7), Reston, VA: National Council of Teachers of Mathematics.

Cai, J. (1998). An investigation of U.S. and Chinese students' mathematical problem posing and problem solving. *Mathematics Education Research Journal, 10*(1), 37-50.

Cai, J. (2000a). Mathematical thinking involved in U.S. and Chinese students' solving process-constrained and process-open problems. *Mathematical Thinking and Learning: An International Journal, 2,* 309-340.

Cai, J. (2000b). Understanding and representing the arithmetic averaging algorithm: An analysis and comparison of U.S. and Chinese students' responses. *International Journal of Mathematical Education in Science and Technology, 31*(6), 839-855.

Cai, J. (2001). Improving mathematics learning: Lessons from cross-national studies of U.S. and Chinese students. *Phi Delta Kappan, 82*(5), 400-405.

Cai, J. (2004). Why do U.S. and Chinese students think differently in mathematical problem solving? Exploring the impact of early algebra learning and teachers' beliefs. *Journal of Mathematical Behavior, 23*(2), 133-165.

Cai, J. (in press-a). U.S. and Chinese teachers' cultural values of representations in mathematics education. In K. D. Graf, F. K. S. Leung, & F. Lopez-Real (Eds.), *Mathematics education in different cultural traditions: A comparative study of East Asian and the West.* Dordrecht, The Netherlands: Kluwer Academic Publishers.

Cai, J. (in press-b). U.S. and Chinese teachers' knowing, evaluating, and constructing representations in mathematics instruction. *Mathematical thinking and Learning: An International Journal.*

Cai, J., & Hwang, S. (2002). Generalized and generative thinking in U.S. and Chinese students' mathematical problem solving and problem posing. *Journal of Mathematical Behavior. 21*(4), 401-421.

Cai, J., & Silver, E. A. (1995). Solution processes and interpretations of solutions in solving a division-with-remainder story problem: Do Chinese and U.S. students have similar difficulties? *Journal for Research in Mathematics Education, 26*(5), 491-497.

Dreyfus, T., & Eisenberg, T. (1996). On different facets of mathematical thinking. In R. J. Sternberg, & T. Ben-Zeev (Eds.), *The nature of mathematical thinking* (pp. 253-284). Hillsdale, NJ: Erlbaum.

Ginsburg, H. P. (Ed.) (1983). *The development of mathematical thinking*. New York: Academic Press.

Hatano, G. (1988). Social and motivational bases for mathematical understanding. In G. B. Saxe & M. Gearhart (Eds.), *Children's mathematics* (pp. 55-70). San Francisco, CA: Jossey Bass.

Janvier, C. (1987). *Problems of representation in the teaching and learning of mathematical problem solving*. Hillsdale, NJ: Erlbaum.

Kieran, T., & Pirie, S. B. (1991). Recursion and the mathematical experience. In L. P. Steffe (Ed.), *Epistemological foundations of mathematical experience* (pp. 78-101) New York: Springer-Verlag.

Krutetskii, V. A. (1976). *The psychology of mathematical abilities in schoolchildren*. Chicago, IL: University of Chicago Press.

Lee, P. Y., Zhang, D., & Zheng, Z. (1997). Examination culture and mathematics education. *EduMath, 4*, 96-103.

Marton, F., & Ramsden, P. (1988). What does it take to improve learning? In P. Ramsden (Ed.), *Improving learning: New perspectives* (pp. 268-286). London: Kogan Page.

Pólya, G. (1945). *How to solve it*. Princeton, NJ: Princeton University Press.

Schoenfeld, A. H. (Ed.) (1997). *Mathematical thinking and problem solving*. Mahwah, NJ: Erlbaum.

Steen, L. A. (1999). Twenty questions about mathematical reasoning. In: L. V. Stiff & F. R. Curcio, (Eds.), *Developing mathematical reasoning in grades K – 12* (pp. 270-285). Reston, VA: National Council of Teachers of Mathematics.

Sternberg, R. J. (1991). Cognitive theory and psychometrics. In R. K. Hambleton & J. N. Zaal (Eds.), *Advances in educational and psychological testing: Theory and applications* (pp. 367-393). Boston: Kluwer Academic Publishers.

Sternberg, R. J. (1999). The nature of mathematical reasoning. In L. V. Stiff & F. R. Curcio (Eds.), *Developing mathematical reasoning in grades K – 12* (pp. 37-44). Reston, VA: National Council of Teachers of Mathematics.

Sternberg, R. J., & Ben-Zeev, T. (Eds.) (1996). *The nature of mathematical thinking*. Hillsdale, NJ: Erlbaum.

Appendix

Tasks

The Number Theory Task

Yolanda was telling her brother Damian about what she did in math class.

Yolanda said, "Damian, I used blocks in my math class today. When I grouped the blocks in groups of 2, I had 1 block left over. When I grouped the blocks in groups of 3, I had 1 block left over. And when I grouped the blocks in groups of 4, I had 1 block left over.

Damian asked, "How many blocks did you have?"
What was Yolanda's answer to her brother's question?
Show how you found your answer.

Doorbell Problem-Solving Task

Sally is having a party, the first time the doorbell rings, 1 guest enters.
The second time the doorbell rings, 3 guests enter.
The third time the doorbell rings, 5 guests enter.
The fourth time the doorbell rings, 7 guests enter.
Keep on going in the same way. On the next ring a group enters that has 2 more persons than the group that entered on the previous ring.

1. How many guests will enter on the 10th ring? Explain how you found your answer.
2. In the space below, write a rule or describe in words how to find the number of guests that entered on each ring.
3. 99 guests entered on one of the rings. What ring was it? Explain or show how you found your answer.

Doorbell Problem-Posing Task

Sally is having a party, the first time the doorbell rings, 1 guest enters.
The second time the doorbell rings, 3 guests enter.
The third time the doorbell rings, 5 guests enter.
The fourth time the doorbell rings, 7 guests enter.

Keep on going in the same way. On the next ring a group enters that has 2 more persons than the group that entered on the previous ring.
For his student's homework, Mr. Johnson wanted to make up three problems BASED ON THE ABOVE SITUATION: an easy problem, a moderate problem, and a difficult problem. These problems can be solved using the information in the situation.

Help Mr. Miller make up three problems and write these problems in the space below.

The easy problem
The moderately difficult problem
The difficult problem

The Pizza Ratio Problem

Here are some children and pizzas. 7 girls share 2 pizzas equally and 3 boys share 1 pizza equally.

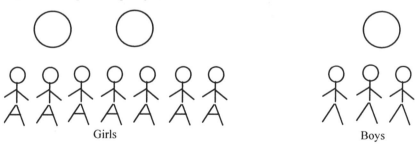

Girls   Boys

A. Does each girl get the same amount as each boy?
   Explain or show how you found your answer.
B. If each girl does not get the same amount as each boy, who gets more?
   Explain or show how you found your answer.

The Hats Averaging Problem

Angela is selling hats for the Mathematics Club. This picture shows the number of hats Angela sold during the first three weeks.

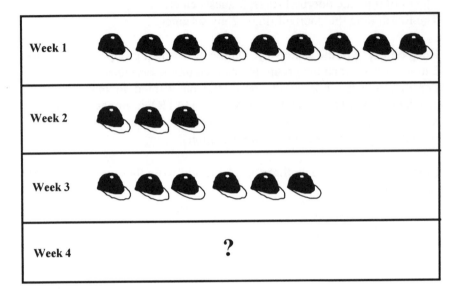

How many hats must Angela sell in Week 4 so that the <u>average</u> number of hats sold is 7?

Show how you found your answer.

Chapter 4

An Examination of Coherence in a Chinese Mathematics Classroom

WANG Tao   MURPHY John

Analyzing discourse in a model Chinese mathematics classroom, we develop the concept of coherence to describe the classroom's most salient features. Coherence refers to the role of unity or connectedness of speech and behavior in the creation of meaningful discourse. Drawing on cross-cultural studies of classroom practices, we examine the instructional, psychological, and social dimensions of coherence in the classroom. We find that, unlike American classrooms, the Chinese classroom is characterized by coherence in each of the three dimensions. The positive pedagogic effects of coherence are discussed and possible negative effects are mentioned.

Key words: cross-cultural discourse analysis, teaching mathematics, coherence

Coherence refers to the role of unity or connectedness of speech and behavior in the creation of meaningful discourse. In classroom discourse, coherence can describe the structure of instructional topics as well as classroom behavior and social values. For example, when a teacher points to thematic or logical connections between a new topic and earlier material, the teacher hopes to enhance student understanding through developing a coherent presentation. When a teacher works to establish daily routines as the school year begins, she is building a coherent set of behavioral expectations for the students. And when the classroom culture is supported by the values and expectations of the broader culture, the teacher has a strong instructional platform from which to work. Because coherence has these instructional, social/psychological, and cultural dimensions, it is a fundamental unit for the analysis of classroom environments. In this chapter we explore these features of coherence in the Chinese mathematics classroom through an examination of classroom discourse. The data we use are from comparative studies of teaching mathematics; discourse examples are usually drawn from a model lesson given in a Shanghai elementary school.[1]

1 Instructional Coherence

Discourse is not a sequence of arbitrary utterances, each with its own topic. Rather, the topics are related to each other, making discourses meaningful (van Dijk, 1997). Discourse coherence reflects the degree of relatedness of topics which affects listeners' understanding (Dore, 1985). A coherent story, for example, with thematically related events is easier for the reader or listener to comprehend. Similarly, students can understand a lesson with highly interrelated events in a coherent way (Fernandez, Yoshida, & Stigler, 1992; Stevenson & Stigler, 1992). Compared to most American lessons, Chinese mathematics lessons often develop in a more coherent way (Stevenson & Stigler, 1992). In this section, we analyze how mathematics is taught in Chinese classrooms in a coherent way.

The thematic coherence can be analyzed on two different levels: within lessons and across lessons. Within lessons, we analyze how mathematic topics or activities within a lesson relate to each other. Across lessons, we analyze how mathematic topics in a series of lessons relate to each other. Given that most current studies of mathematics classroom discourse are limited to analyzing individual lessons, the across lesson coherence is not yet clear (Wang, 2003). In the sections that follow, we analyze the coherence within a lesson.

Researchers (Fernandez et al., 1992; Stevenson & Stigler, 1992) have investigated coherence of activities from two aspects: the coherence of the content in lesson plan activities and the discourse transitions explicating the relationship between activities.

---

[1] The videotape of the class, Area of triangle with equal base and equal height, is from the Institute of General Education, Shanghai Academy of Educational Sciences [上海市教育科学研究院普通教育研究所] (1999).

To make the class instruction coherent, the activities in the lesson should be related to each other, focusing on one or two main topics. Given that a lesson with fewer mathematical topics might be more coherent than one with multiple topics, Stigler and Perry (1990) compared the number of topics included in American (in Chicago) and Chinese (in Taipei) fifth-grade classroom activities. They segmented classroom flow into 5-minute segments (the median length of segments with on-going instruction) and counted the number of topics included in each segment. They found that 55% of all segments in Taipei classrooms focused on only one topic compared to only 17% of the segments in Chicago. On the macro level, researchers (Grow-Maienza, Hahn, & Joo, 2001; Ma, 1999; Stevenson & Stigler, 1992; Stigler & Hiebert, 1999) found that Chinese teachers tended to devote an entire 40-minute class to the solution of only one mathematics problem. In such a lesson, a single mathematic topic was discussed from multiple perspectives. For example, Ma (1999) reported that in Chinese primary classrooms, students are often encouraged to solve one mathematics problem several ways (一題多解). The one-topic design in Chinese classrooms helps teachers organize the activities around this one clear mathematic topic. In our model class video, the teacher conducted the following activities to introduce the new subject matter concerned with the area of equal-base-equal-height (EBEH) triangles. Six activities were conducted in the following sequence (see Table 1).

Table 1
The Activities of the Instructional Phase in the Open-Class

Review		Teaching new content		Practicing	
Activity 1	Activity 2	Activity 3	Activity 4	Activity 5	Activity 6
Review formula of triangle	Practice to calculate areas of triangles with given base and height	Observe 3 triangles and discuss the relationship of their areas (see Figure 1)	Rearrange and discussion (see Figure 2)	Finding out EBEH triangles among 5 triangles	Drawing two EBEH triangles in different shapes

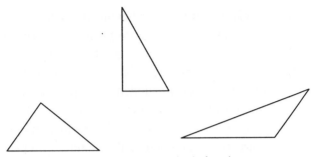

Figure 1. The presentation of three triangles before the rearrangement

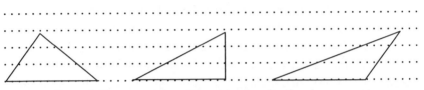

Figure 2. The presentation of three triangles after the rearrangement

The relationships among these activities are significant. First, all six activities relate to the new knowledge, namely 'the areas of EBEH triangles are equal'. The first two activities in the review phase highlight the formula for calculating the triangle's area, which is the theoretical tool for understanding the new knowledge. Based on this formula, Activities 3 and 4 help the students understand that the areas of the three different EBEH triangles are equal because they have equal base length and equal height. With this new knowledge, Activities 5 and 6 encourage the learner to apply the knowledge in solving new problems.

In general, the activities in the lesson are well organized to serve the main theme. The well-related topics in the six activities facilitate student understanding of the new knowledge. Given that inferring the relationships among topics of different activities depends on individual abilities (G. Brown & Yule, 1983), some times even the well-organized nature of activities does not insure that students will grasp the relationships between activities, especially when the relatedness of activities is not explicit enough for young learners. In these occasions, the coherence of activities should be explicitly developed in classroom discourse. One way that teachers can use language to enhance the coherence of a lesson is to use transitional discourse to talk explicitly about the main goal(s) of the lesson and the interrelationship of the activities and the main goal(s). Without this dimension of coherence created through transitional discourse, students might experience some unnecessary difficulties in comprehending the lesson. Stevenson and Stigler (1992) gave the following example of an American first grade lesson to illustrate the importance of the using transitional discourse.

> Ok, open your workbooks to page 12. I want you to measure your desk in pencils, find out how many pencils it takes to go across you desk, and write the answer on the line in your workbooks. [Children carry out instructions.] Ok, the next line says to use green crayons, but we don't have green crayons so we are going to use blue crayons. Raise your hand if you don't have a blue crayon. [Teacher takes approximately 10 minutes to pass out blue crayons to students who raise their hands...] Now write the number of blue crayons next to the line that says green crayons. [Teacher then moves on to the third segment.] Ok, now take out your centimeter ruler and measure the number of centimeters across you desk and write the number on the line in your workbooks. (p. 349)

Sitting in such a classroom, even an advanced first-grade child might find it difficult to make sense of the relationship of the three activities— measuring the desk with a pencil, crayon, and centimeter ruler. There was no discussion of how each exercise helps students understand why standard units are important. A transition between the three activities would make the relationship between the activities more coherent. For example, before the activity of measuring the desk with centimeter rulers, the teacher could discuss with the whole class the difficulty of comparing the lengths of desks with different units (pencils and crayons). She could then organize the class to use a tool with a standard unit to overcome this difficulty. Through these kinds of transitions, the students could be helped to understand the implicit connections between the activities and the meaning of mathematical knowledge being introduced.

In the model class, the teacher used the following transitional statements.

Activity 1—Activity 2: (after a student recited the formula correctly)

Teacher: Very good. Can you use this formula to get the area of a triangle?

Students (in chorus): Yes.

Teacher: Open your exercise book, look at the pictures...calculate the area of the triangles. Start.

Activity 2—Activity 3: (after checking the answers one by one in whole class)

Teacher: This is the knowledge we learned in the pervious lessons [how to calculate the area of a triangle]. From now on, today, we will continue to study the area of triangles. Please take out the three triangles in your exercise book.

Activity 5—Activity 6: (after students correctly pair up all the equal-base-equal-height triangles)

Teacher: Just now we learned that the areas of equal-base-equal-height triangles are equal. Then, now, it is time (for you) to draw two equal-base-equal-height triangles in different shapes on your dotted paper.

The teacher uses language to connect the well-structured activities explicitly. In this way, the student can easily organize the knowledge coherently. Interestingly, the teacher does not use explicit language to connect Activities 3 and 4, and Activities 4 and 5. Unlike the situation in the above American lesson example, the lack of language to connect these activities might not necessarily affect the discourse coherence. This is because these activities are themselves well connected. In Activity 3, the students observe 3 triangles (see Figure 1) and discuss the relationship of their areas. After the whole class reaches the consensus that the areas of the three triangles are not equal, the teacher asks students to rearrange the triangles (see Figure 2). Given that Activities 4 and 5 are also discussions of the areas of the three triangles, the connection of the two activities to the earlier ones is clear. It seems likely that the teacher does not explicitly help students connect the two activities because the teacher wants to leave space for students to explore on their own the relationship of the three triangles in the new context (after rearrangement). In the real class, the teacher gives a very short sentence to direct student attention.

T: Look at this (pointing to Figure 2), what will you find?

The lack of explicit transitions from Activity 4 to Activity 5 has a similar pedagogic explanation. Right after discussing with the students the main new content (Activity 4), the relationship between EBEH triangles, the teacher asks students to pair up EBEH triangles in a new task. The new knowledge of EBEH triangles is the common theme of the two activities. The lack of connecting language in this episode makes the task mathematically more challenging because the students have to make use of the mathematical knowledge (what are EBEH triangles?) just learned in the new task by themselves.

In the model class, sometimes the explicit discussion was extended to connect knowledge obtained in adjacent lessons as, for example, in the following discourse.

T: In the previous lesson, when we calculate the area of a triangle, we must know its...
Students (in chorus): Base and height.
T: But in today's lesson, as we have known that for the equal-base-equal-height triangles their areas are equal, we can get the area of a triangle without knowing its base and height. Right?
Students (in chorus): Right.

In this excerpt, the teacher highlights the connection between the old knowledge and new knowledge by explaining the difference of the two approaches used in this class and the previous class; that is, "we can get the area of a triangle without knowing its base and height." This transitional discourse is necessary because the relationship between the new knowledge and the old knowledge might be not explicit for a fifth grade student.

Various cultural explanations might explain why Asian and American teachers prepare the lesson plan and teach the class in such different ways in terms of the coherence of the lesson. Three related factors of the culture of mathematics pedagogy provide insights into the instructional coherence in Chinese classroom. The three factors are teacher beliefs about the nature of mathematical knowledge and teaching mathematical knowledge, teacher's mathematical preparation, and availability of a supportive environment.

A teacher's teaching behavior is largely underpinned by his or her belief about knowledge and how it is taught (Clarke, 1996). Stigler and Hiebert (1999) call these implicit belief "scripts." They believe that the scripts explain why the lessons within a country followed distinctive patterns because the lessons were designed and taught by teachers who share the same scripts. Chinese teachers, therefore, teach mathematics in a coherent way because they share the implicit belief that mathematics is a set of relationships between concepts, facts, and procedures.

If teachers want to teach mathematics in a coherent way, their mathematical knowledge should be coherently organized. Ma's (1999) remarkable work provides a clear picture of how Chinese primary school teachers are equipped with coherent mathematics knowledge. Using a questionnaire developed by Teacher Education and Learning to Teach Study[2], Ma interviewed 23 American primary school teachers who were considered "better than average" and 72 Chinese teachers from 5 schools ranged from very high to very low quality. Ma found that unlike American teachers who tend to view mathematics knowledge in a "piece-by-piece" way, Chinese teachers often view a piece of knowledge as part of a larger context of knowledge. Some of the pieces are key to the target knowledge. Ma called this kind of knowledge a knowledge package. Correspondingly Chinese teachers see mathematical topics "group-by-group." For example, Ma (1999, p. 19) used the following diagram to illustrate a knowledge package shared by Chinese teachers in teaching subtraction with regrouping of large numbers.

Ma argued that the Chinese teachers organized their mathematics knowledge in this coherent way because it reflects their understanding of the mathematics topics. This mathematics knowledge of teachers is

[2] The study uses questions of this form: Look at these problems ($52 - 25 =$, $91 - 79 =$, etc.). How would you approach these problems if you were teaching second grade? (Ma, 1999, p. 1)

pedagogical content knowledge, which is defined by Shulman (1986) as "the way of representing and formulating the subject that makes it comprehensible to others." (p. 9)

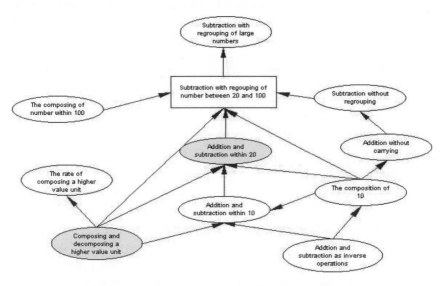

Figure 3. A knowledge package for subtraction with regrouping

In this example, Ma shows that the target knowledge (subtraction, with regrouping, of large numbers) is directly connected with one piece of old knowledge (subtraction with regrouping of numbers between 20 and 100), which is further underpinned by other knowledge pieces. Therefore, Ma argues, for a Chinese teacher, teaching the connections between different pieces of knowledge is important.

In the model lesson, although the teacher does not show a complex knowledge system in teaching the new content (The areas of EBEH triangles are equal), she does put an emphasis on the connection between the new content and what they have learned in the previous lessons (the formula of the area of triangles). The class begins with reviewing and practicing the formula (Activities 1 and 2). After regrouping the three triangles (Activity 4), the teacher guides the students to explore the relationship between the heights and base lines of the three triangles. It is clear that she was trying to help students infer the targeting content from old knowledge. The emphasis is on the process of connecting different pieces of knowledge.

Ma's work not only provides convincing data that Chinese teachers have a more coherent mathematics knowledge than American teachers, but more importantly, it provides insight into the relationship between a teacher's belief, subject knowledge, and the pedagogy she adopts.

In order to obtain coherent knowledge, a teacher also needs a supportive teaching environment. Indeed, in China, teachers are encouraged to prepare lessons in a coherent way. Their environment is full of various supporting resources which help teachers plan and conduct coherent lessons. For example, a detailed teachers' guideline book, a lesson plan by an experienced teacher, and discussions with colleagues in a 'teaching group' (教研组) on a specific activity design are always accessible to teachers for preparing their lessons. Model lessons in China provided by experienced teachers demonstrate how a coherent lesson plan is realized in classroom settings.

In contrast, American teachers do not always enjoy such rich resources in their environment. Their teaching is quite isolated. They rarely have the opportunity to observe other teachers because teaching in U.S. is considered a private, not a public, activity (Stigler & Hiebert, 1999, p. 123). The isolation makes it more difficult for U.S. teachers to plan and conduct a coherent lesson.

Another logistic factor that aids a Chinese teacher in the preparation of the mathematics lesson in a coherent way is that Chinese mathematics teachers usually teach only mathematics. American elementary school teachers teach all subjects. According to Stevenson and Stigler (1992), teachers in Beijing and Taipei spent an average of 9.7 and 9.1 hours per day, respectively in their schools. However, a Chinese teacher teaches less than three hours per day. The rest of the six hours in school are mainly used to read students' homework and to prepare lessons with other colleagues. Therefore, they have enough time and energy to prepare coherent mathematics lessons in the school with colleagues.

2 Social and Psychological Coherence in the Classroom

On entering a Chinese mathematics classroom, a teacher can assume that two important cultural scripts are in play. First, the student respects the authority of the teacher. And secondly, the student tends to have an inter-dependent self-construal. The Chinese teacher often establishes acceptable classroom behavior patterns that build on and reinforce these two scripts. As a result of this match, or coherence, between the culture of the classroom and that of the larger society, teaching in general is more effective.[3] An analysis of classroom discourse can reveal this coherence between the classroom structure and these cultural scripts.

The relationship between teacher and student, the teacher's authority and students' responsibility in the in the education process, is made clear in the opening ritual. Classroom rituals create a comfortable set of expectations of what is to come; they build coherence from day to day. Here, for example, is how the model class begins:

The teacher enters, stands behind the podium looking at the whole class for a couple of seconds and, as the noise drops off, says,

> Teacher: Class begins. (上课)
> Student monitor: Stand at attention. (起立).
> Teacher: Good morning, students. (同学们好)
> Students (in chorus): Good morning, teacher. (老师好）
> Teacher: Sit down please. (请坐)
> (Students sit down).

In terms of classroom management, this formal beginning serves to focus the attention of the large class, encouraging each student to be ready for the lesson. But this small ritual is also the cue for participants to assume their roles of teacher and student with their respective responsibilities in the classroom discourse. Both the teacher's imperative tone as she announces that class begins and the use of a student monitor to direct the students, signal the natural hierarchy in the classroom. The

---

[3] For problems resulting from a mismatch of classroom and student's culture, see Suina and Smolkin, 1994.

teacher's authority is also evident in the nature of the opening statement. The authority expressed by 上课 (class begins) is formidable because the statement is abstract. It is abstract because there is no personal agent expressed. This relationship between authority and its abstract expression may also be seen in the familiar scene of a parent admonishing a child. The parent who says to the child, 'I don't want you to do that!', is expressing his personal authority primarily because he uses the pronoun "I". The parent who uses the abstract statement 'Stop that!', with no pronoun, assumes a larger authority as the transmitter of society's sanctions. Similarly, 'class begins' is abstract; there is no actor or agent, as there is, for example, in the sentence 'let's begin, class'. Instead, 'class begins' is an uncaused act, an event which the teacher does not initiate so much as announce as happening (Christie, 2002, p.166). This opening exchange and a similar closing sequence frame the instructional space. They function to create a ritualized classroom environment in which there is daily recognition of the respect due the teacher and the teacher's authority.

Rituals that reinforce the authority of the teacher and the subservience of the student have a long tradition in China. Similar relationships are described in 'Duties of the student', Chapter 59 of Kuan Tzu, 645 B.C.E., one of the earliest texts on education (Mair, 1994). This ancient text describes in some detail how a student shows respect for the teacher as he performs his academic and household duties. For example,

> After the students sweep the floor in front of the teaching mat and wash their hands, they conduct themselves in a respectful manner.... The teacher then seats himself, and the students in going out or coming in are as respectful as if they were greeting guests. They sit in a dignified manner facing the master, their features composed and never changing. (pp. 27-28)

Although details of teacher and student responsibilities have changed over the centuries, there remains a connection between the tradition exemplified by this ancient text, and the social and educational assumptions that form the modern Chinese circumstances of learning.

The second cultural script that shapes the classroom dynamic is the dominance of the inter-dependent self-construal. The growing literature on culture and self-concepts explores the idea that while some cultures are predominantly collectivist, others are more individualistic. Self-concepts common to a culture will reflect this social variation and will vary between inter-dependent and independent selves. 'Inter-dependent self construal' is a term used by Markus and Kitayama (1991) in a series of articles on cultural variation of self-concepts. They find that the independent self is autonomous and self-contained, focused on his own individualizing traits, such as intelligence and self esteem. In social situations the independent self will seek to change others in order to meet her own needs (Weisz & Blackburn, 1984). The interdependent self, on the other hand, is 'socio-centric' (Shweder, 1991); the elements of the self—thoughts, feelings, social actions, are meaningful primarily in connection to others. In social situations the interdependent self makes adjustments in order to fit harmoniously within relationships.

In the Chinese classroom, a variety of discourse patterns contribute to or reinforce the students' interdependent self-construal. Characteristic features of Chinese classroom discourse, which relate to interdependent learning, are: infrequent use of personal names, choral responses, and the public correction of mistakes.

It is not uncommon for mathematics teachers to correct student mistakes. The Chinese teacher not only makes the correction, but often dwells on the mistake, exploring the reasoning that resulted in the error. For example, in the model class,

T: Tell me why are the areas of the two triangles are equal?
S1: Because AD is their common height...
T: Wait a second. AD is their height? (facing to the whole class)
Do you agree?
Ss (in choral): No.
T: Why?
(several students raise their hands)
T: (pointing to one student) You.
S2: Because there is no vertical mark there.

T: Yes. (To S1) Be careful, AD looks like a height. But we can not rely on our instinct sense. If it is the height, it must have a vertical mark. (To the whole class) Are you all clear about this point?

Ss (in choral): Yes.

Stevenson and Stigler (1992) pointed that "for Americans, errors tend to be interpreted as an indication of failure in learning the lesson. For Chinese and Japanese, they are an index of what still needs to be learned (p. 192)." In Chinese culture, failure has value; it is recognized as a necessary element in achievement. The inseparable relationship is well reflected in a popular Chinese idiom, *shi bai shi cheng gong zhi mu* (失败是成功之母, Failure is the mother of success). Therefore, the Chinese teacher tends to believe that students should learn from their failures. Chinese teachers view the errors from individual students as so valuable that they often discuss them publicly to benefit all the students in the classroom.

American teachers, by contrast, were rarely found to treat students' errors in this way. For an independent self construal, errors can reflect not a lack of knowledge but a lack of ability; public discussion can cause embarrassment and loss of self-esteem. Therefore, Stevenson and Stigler (1992) argued, the American teachers feel uncomfortable with such situations and strive to avoid them.

In cross-cultural classroom observations, Stevenson and Stigler (1992) found that, compared with American children, Asian children showed a "relatively calm acceptance of a negative feedback on their errors in public" (p. 192). Why does this apparent "face-threatening act" (FTA) (P. Brown & Levinson, 1987, p. 60) not affect Chinese children as severely as it does American students? From a cultural perspective, Chinese students share with their teachers the same cultural value of learning from failure, and interpret the so-called "FTA" as not face-threatening. Thus, they accept it without embarrassment. From a sociological perspective, the students accept the FTA because of their teachers' high authority. Indeed, Chinese teachers are found to be more authoritarian than American teachers (Ho, 2001). And from a psychological perspective, the need of the independent self for self-enhancement is challenged by the public discussion, whereas the need of the interdependent self to seek harmonious relationships through self-effacement is not (Kitayama & Markus, 1995).

Seemingly inconsequential discourse features, such as the infrequent use of personal names in the classroom, and choral response gain significance in the context of the interdependent self-construal. In a Chinese classroom, the interdependent learner remains anonymous and self-effacing (Tang, 1996). For example, in the model class, the teacher on twelve occasions requested individuals to answer questions. In no case was the students' name used. The typical discourse example is:

> T: In the previous lessons, we have learned about the area of triangles, who can try to say if we want to get the area of a triangle, we must know which two conditions?
> (Most of the students raise their hands)
> T: (pointing to one student) You.

In the model class more than half of the student responses are choral responses. In these choral responses, the group voice is favored over the individual voice. The frequent use of choral response reinforces the student's identification with the group, a group of interdependent learners.

3 Conclusion

Coherence is a basic feature of successful communication in the classroom. We have shown the strength of the Chinese mathematics classroom in each of the dimensions of coherence: instructional, social and psychological. Further study is needed to determine what all the effects of coherence are and how they work. We have discussed positive pedagogic effects of coherence. Strong coherence in the lesson plan enhances learning. Social coherence (a match between school culture and the culture the child brings to school) provides a strong platform for teaching.

Coherence may also have negative effects. Two effects of coherence are the increased clarity of exposition and the reduction of ambiguity. This has long been a goal of teachers. Han Yu (768-824), for example, wrote, "A teacher is the one who passes on correct principles, teaches skills, and explains uncertainties" (as cited in Cleverley, 1991). One effect of the profound coherence in the Chinese mathematics classroom is that the consequent reduction of ambiguity becomes a style of thinking. And as coherence forms a style of thinking, it reduces ambiguity tolerance, a condition for creativity (Lubart, 1999; Mills, 1959). If the reform of mathematics teaching is concerned with issues of creativity, perhaps the complex issues surrounding coherence should be re-examined first.

References

Brown, G., & Yule, G. (1983). *Discourse analysis*. London: Cambridge University Press.

Brown, P., & Levinson, S. (1987). *Politeness: Some universals in language usage*. Cambridge, UK: Cambridge University Press.

Christie, F. (2002). *Classroom discourse analysis*. New York: Continuum.

Clarke, P. (1996). *Cultural models of teacher thinking and teaching.* Unpublished Qualifying Paper, Harvard University, Cambridge.

Cleverley, J. (1991). *The schooling of China*. North Sydney: Allen & Unwin.

Dore, J. (1985). Children's conversations. In T. A. van Dijk (Ed.), *Handbook of discourse analysis* (Vol. 3, pp. 47-65). New York: Academic Press.

Fernandez, C., Yoshida, M., & Stigler, J. W. (1992). Learning mathematics from classroom instruction: On relating lessons to pupils' interpretations. *The Journal of the Learning Science, 2*(4), 333-365.

Grow-Maienza, J., Hahn, D.-D., & Joo, C.-A. (2001). Mathematics instruction in Korean primary schools structures, processes, and a linguistic analysis of questioning. *Journal of Educational Psychology, 93*(2), 363-376.

Ho, I. T. (2001). Are Chinese teachers authoritarian? In D. A. Watkins & J. B. Biggs (Eds.), *Teaching the Chinese learner: Psychological and pedagogical perspectives* (pp. 99-114). Hong Kong, China: Comparative Education Research Centre, The University of Hong Kong.

Institute of General Education, Shanghai Academy of Educational Sciences. (1999). *An*

Open Lesson: Area of triangle with equal base and equal height [In Chinese 一堂公开课: 等底等高三角形的面积].

Kitayama, S., & Markus, H. R. (1995). Culture and self: Implications for internationalizing psychology. In N. R. Goldberger & J. B. Veroff (Eds.), *Culture and psychology* (pp. 366-383). New York: New York Univeristy Press.

Lubart, T. (1999). Creativity across cultures. In R. J. Sternberg (Ed.), *Handbook of Creativity* (pp. 339-350). Cambridge: Cambridge University Press.

Ma, L. (1999). *Knowing and teaching elementary mathematics.* Mahwah, NJ: Lawrence Erlbaum Associates.

Mair, V. (1994). Attributed to Kuan Chung. In V. Mair (Ed.), *The Columbia anthology of traditional Chinese literature* (pp. 17-30). New York: Columbia University Press.

Markus, H. R., & Kitayama, S. (1991). Culture and self: Implications for cognition, emotion and motivation. *Psychological Review, 98*(2), 224-253.

Mills, C. W. (1959). *The sociological imagination.* New York: Oxford University Press.

Shulman, L. (1986). Those who understand: Knowledge growth in teaching. *Educational Researcher, 15*(2), 4-14.

Shweder, R. A. (1991). *Thinking through cultures.* Cambridge, MA: Harvard University Press.

Stevenson, H. W., & Stigler, J. W. (1992). *The learning gap.* New York: Simon & Schuster.

Stigler, J. W., & Hiebert, J. (1999). *The teaching gap.* New York: The Free Press.

Stigler, J. W., & Perry, M. (1990). Mathematics learning in Japanese, Chinese, and American classrooms. In J. W. Stigler, R. A. Shweder, & G. Herdt (Ed.), *Cultural Psychology* (pp. 328-353). Cambridge, MA: Cambridge University Press.

Suina, J. & Smolkin, L. (1994) From natal culture to school culture to dominant society culture: Supporting transitions for Pueblo Indian students. In P. Greenfield & R. Cocking (Eds.), *Cross-cultural roots of minority child development* (pp.115-130). Hillsdale, NJ: Lawrence Erlbaum Associates, Publishers.

Tang, C. (1996). Collaborative learning: The latent dimension in Chinese students' learning. In D. A. Watkins & J. B. Biggs (Eds.), *The Chinese learner: Cultural, psychological and contextual influences* (pp. 183-204). Hongkong, China: Comparative Education Research Centre, The University of Hong Kong; Melbourne, Australia: Australian Council for Education Research.

van Dijk, T. A. (1997). The study of discourse. In T. A. van Dijk (Ed.), *Discourse as structure and process* (Vol. 1, pp. 1-34). Thousand Oaks, CA: SAGE Publications.

Wang, T. (2003). *Culture and mathematics classroom discourse: A comparative perspective.* Unpublished qualifying paper, available through Gutman Library, Harvard University, Cambridge, MA.

Weisz, R., & Blackburn, T. C. (1984). Standing out and standing in. *American Psychologist, 39*(9), 955-969.

Chapter 5

A Chinese Cultural Model of Learning

LI Jin

Cultural beliefs about learning are an integral part of learners' learning beliefs that guide their learning behavior. Based on recent research, this chapter discusses four key dimensions of Chinese beliefs: (1) purposes, which emphasizes lifelong moral self-perfection; (2) processes, which focus on learning virtues of resolve, diligence, enduring hardship, perseverance, and concentration; (3) achievement standards, which aim at breadth and depth of knowledge, application, and the integration of knowledge and moral character; and (4) affect, which involves commitment, passion, respect, humility, and shame/guilt. Chinese beliefs are also presented in reference to US beliefs in order to highlight cultural variation. It is argued that cultural beliefs about learning are important to consider in research on human learning.

Key words: Chinese learning beliefs, cultural differences, moral self-perfection, learning virtues

1 Introduction

Ever since Kevin was a toddler, he has had what ordinary people would call a "gift" in math. He would spend all day playing with plastic numbers and looking at picture books with numbers in them. At two and half, his grandmother showed him that $1 + 1 = 2$. That day he figured out the rest of the pluses within ten numbers. Kevin knew and enjoyed this level of math at an age when most human children are just beginning to count objects. He moved on to be on every year's math honor roll in all the schools he has attended. Last year, as one of the four highest achieving math students, he represented his state to participate in the most celebrated middle school math competition of the United States. Whenever people marvel at Kevin's math skills, his European-American father would gratefully accept his talent by saying "Thank you, he is great, and I am proud of him". However, whenever his Chinese mother encounters such praises, she will reliably reply that "his talent means nothing if he doesn't work hard".

These rather casual remarks frequently heard in parents' responses to praises of their children turned out to be far from being casual. They reflect fundamental orientations of what I term "cultural beliefs about learning". Even though much of learning must be carried out by the individual learner, involving his or her mind, motivation, general or subject-specific strategies, learning viewed from a sociocultural perspective is far more than an individual process. To the extent to which all children are born into and raised in at least one culture (with an increasing number of children living in more than one culture in today's world), they are bound to be influenced by their culture's value system regarding learning. The views children construct about learning may crucially shape how they approach, engage in, and ultimately achieve learning.

In recent decades, an increasing number of researchers have recognized the significant role contextual factors play in children's learning, even in arguably the most abstract, rule-governed domain of math learning (Burton & Morgan, 2000; N. Y. Wong, Marton, K. M. Wong, & Lam, 2002). In support of this new line of research, I present in this chapter an argument that cultural beliefs about learning are an essential part of the general make-up of any learner's beliefs about learning, and they therefore apply to math learning as well. However, there is insufficient research on this important topic. To proceed with this argument, I begin by reviewing relevant research first. I then discuss in some detail Chinese beliefs about learning in general and my own work in particular. In order to clarify Chinese beliefs, I also refer to Western beliefs from a comparative perspective. In addition, I present some developmental evidence to show that children begin to develop culturally based beliefs about learning early on, and these beliefs guide their learning and achievement. I conclude by addressing relevant deficiencies in traditional research and how alternative approaches may be needed to broaden our understanding of learning across cultures.

2 Review of Relevant Research

2.1 *Western and Asian learning*

Since the 1980s, much cross-cultural research has focused on comparing Western and Asian children's school learning and achievement. Asian children have often been documented to achieve higher than their Western peers, particularly in math and science (Harmon et al., 1997; Kwok & Lytton, 1996; Stevenson & Stigler, 1992; Watkins & Biggs, 1996), although they do not show superior performance on some math tasks (see Cai & Cifarelli, this volume). In presenting their summary empirical findings, Stevenson and Stigler (1992) introduced the term "learning gap" to capture these achievement differences. To explain this "learning gap", researchers have identified a number of key contributing factors. It has been shown that Asian children attend school for a longer period and do more school work (C. Chen & Stevenson, 1989). Their pedagogical practice is more effective (Hess & Azuma, 1991; Lewis, 1995; Matsushita, 1994; Stigler & Hiebert, 1999). Asian parents hold higher expectations and are more involved in their children's education (Au & Harackiewicz, 1986; Shon & Ja, 1982; Yao, 1985). Asian children's motivation for socioeconomic advancement through education leads them to study harder (Salili, Chiu, & S. Lai, 2001; Sue & Okazaki, 1990). Finally, Asian belief in effort (vs. Western belief in ability) has been argued to be the most significant explanation for their achievement (Hau & Salili, 1991; Holloway, 1988; Stevenson & Stigler, 1992).

Despite this extensive knowledge, some gaps in research remain, preventing us from achieving a better understanding of learners from different cultures. Four deficiencies loom particularly large. First, research as a whole tends to focus on the end results of learning, that is, achievement and then to attribute it to a single, but frequently dichotomous, concept such as ability versus effort, success versus failure, intrinsic versus extrinsic motivation, and individualist versus collectivist goals (Dweck, 1999; Lepper, 1981; Triandis, 1995; Yu & Yang, 1994). Research conducted within these frameworks seldom moves beyond these set notions of learning and achievement. Yet, as will be shown, these frames, despite their usefulness, are limited and limiting when learners across cultures are under study.

Second, research tends to privilege cognitive processes in learning over other human capacities and functioning (Dai & Sternberg, 2004) such as the purposive, the social/moral, the affective, and self/identity factors. For example, if a child does not like math, does not regard math as important, or as Steele (1997) showed, does not identify him/herself with the domain of math learning, his or her cognitive ability may not suffice in motivating and helping him/her to learn the subject. These non-cognitive (referred to as "extra-cognitive" by Shavinina and Ferrari [2004]) processes may prove to be indispensable in theorizing and empirical research on learning across cultures.

Third, much research is devoted to the structure of school and organizational factors. These sociological dimensions are certainly important, but they do not explain people's beliefs and behavior fully. In fact, the overt structural elements may not reveal much of the internal psychological workings of the learner. After all, modern Chinese educational system was adopted from the West around the turn of the 20th century. The present-day school structure and curriculum, especially in math and science, resemble each other more than they differ from each other (J. Chen, 1979; National Center for Education Development Research [NCEDR], 2001). In increasingly more regions of China, children now begin learning English in elementary school. What is more puzzling, according to observations by both outsiders and Chinese educators themselves, is that the Chinese educational system largely consists of old fashioned teaching and learning. On the one hand, pedagogy is teacher-centered, authoritarian with a centralized curriculum (implying inflexibility and lack of attention to individual children's learning needs). On the other hand, students are docile, obedient, and uncritical who learn by rote, lack intrinsic motivation, and aim only for exams (Gardner, 1989; Ginsberg, 1992; Ouyang, 2000). In other words, every thing known about good educational practice is violated in the Chinese educational system. Yet, time and again, Chinese learners achieve well (and continue to do so when they come to the West for advanced studies) no matter how they are assessed (Harmon et al., 1997); they frequently outperform their peers from Western progressive and creative educational systems. This stark contrast has led keen observers of Chinese learning such as Watkins and Biggs (1996) to regard the whole phenomenon a paradox begging for a better explanation. Indeed, how could such an educational system with such learners produce any meaningful achievement? The full answer is unlikely to lie in the educational system itself. People's beliefs and associated behavior as well as the development of these beliefs and behaviors need also to be studied.

Fourth, the greatest impediment of all is the field's persistent reliance on Western concepts without attending to indigenous or emic cultural meanings and their psychological manifestation in learning (Gao & Watkins, 2001; Watkins, 2000). The concepts mentioned in my discussion of the first deficiency are some examples that are often applied to Chinese learners. This kind of blind application of Western concepts to children in a very different culture could pose serious validity problems. The aforementioned paradox may well be a result of this uncritical importation of Western concepts and theories.

To illustrate the severity of the problem, I review two particular sets of Western concepts that have recently been investigated empirically. The first is a study by Iyengar and Lepper (1999) examining Asian- and Euro-American school children's intrinsic versus extrinsic motivation for learning and achievement. Their specific focus was on the notion of personal autonomy and choice as a core component of intrinsic motivation and choice made by others as a form of extrinsic motivation. It has long been assumed that personal autonomy and choice are conducive to learning and performance whereas lack of such personal freedom is detrimental (Conti, Amabile, & Pollack, 1995; de Charms, 1968; Deci & Ryan, 1985; Hennessey & Amabile, 1998; Lepper, 1981). However, these researchers demonstrated that whereas this assumption held true for Euro-American children, it did not hold true for their Asian-American counterparts. The former enjoyed learning and performed better when given personal choices (of what to learn and how to learn it), but the latter enjoyed the learning just as much and did better when their task was chosen by significant others (e.g., mothers or trusted peers).

The second study is an investigation by Kim (2002) on the belief in and effect of speaking versus not speaking on thinking and task performance among Euro- and Asian-American college students. It has also been a long-standing Western assumption that speaking promotes thinking and learning whereas not speaking impedes them. Asian learners are generally observed to be quiet in classrooms and are reluctant to speak in any public forum (Duncan & Paulhus, 1998; Kim & Markus, 2002; Tweed & Lehman, 2002; Watkins, 2000; Winner, 1989). Kim found that whereas Euro-American students were much more likely to believe in the causal effect of speaking on thinking and task performance, their Asian-American peers were much less likely. Moreover, objective measures of how each group functioned with speaking showed that speaking did not interfere with Euro-American students' performance, but it did with that of Asian-American students.

These studies illustrate how some of the long-held Western assumptions about processes, motivation, efficacy, and effectiveness of learning cannot be readily applied to studying learners in very different cultures. The reason is quite simple: these concepts and theories were developed by Western people to study Western people based on Western cultural norms and values. Given what we know about significant differences in many aspects of human psychology across cultures, it is perplexing why Western concepts still assume unquestionable validity and potency in much cross-cultural research on learning. If our purpose is to understand learners in different cultures, we stand to benefit more from heeding learners' own thoughts, feelings, and behaviors as they are developed in their respective cultural contexts.

2.2 Chinese beliefs about learning

Recently, a number of researchers have recognized the need to go beyond the limitations discussed previously to investigate cultural meanings that may shape Chinese learners' thoughts, feelings, and behaviors. Important findings in two key areas emerged: cultural beliefs about learning and the learning (and teaching) process itself.

With regard to cultural beliefs, Lee (1996) presented a historical account of core Confucian values regarding learning and argued for their enduring impact on Chinese learners today. Accordingly, most essential is the Confucian belief in human self-perfection pursued as the highest purpose of life through personal commitment to learning. This belief is also linked to other beliefs such as one's social contributions in the form of meritorious service and practical concerns for honoring their families as well as enhancing their own social status and mobility. In support of Lee's argument, Cheng (1996) collected data on people's beliefs about learning in a comprehensive ethnographic study on one Chinese province's primary education. He concluded that Chinese parents, whether well off or destitute, send their children to school not to learn literacy and numeracy skills, but to become a person who is knowledgeable of the world, able to function well in social relations, and most important of all, morally cultivated. Similarly, Ran's (2001) recent qualitative research examined how Chinese parents in Britain and British teachers clashed on the purpose of learning. Whereas British teachers focused on acknowledging and expressing satisfaction with Chinese children's apparent high achievement, Chinese parents were discontented, emphasizing more demanding learning materials and their children's continuous effort to self-improve regardless of their accomplishments.

Related to these studies, some scholars have examined teaching in Chinese culture and revealed converging beliefs about purposes of learning. Jin and Cortazzi (1998) found that the image of a good teacher as described by British students is one who is able to arouse students' interest, explain clearly, use effective instructional methods, and organize activities. However, the image of a good teacher offered by their Chinese peers is one who has deep knowledge, is able to answer questions, and is a good moral model. Similarly, Gao and Watkins (2001) found, with both qualitative and quantitative methods, that Chinese science teachers emphasize cultivating students' adaptive attitudes toward learning and moral guidance. These researchers stated that these beliefs are rarely emphasized by Western science teachers, a finding also echoed by Western scholars on moral development and education (Damon, 2003).

With regard to the learning process itself, the influential volume *The Chinese Learner* by Watkins and Biggs (1996) assembled a group of scholars who offered intriguing research results. For example, Marton, Dall'Alba, and Tse (1996) investigated the topic of rote learning and memorization, a Chinese style of learning that has received much criticism from the West as well as from Chinese educators themselves. However, it turned out that Chinese rote learning is not the end in itself but is used as a strategy for achieving deeper understanding. Pratt, Kelly, and K. M. Wong (1999) also came to the same conclusion in a separate study. In a related study comparing British and Chinese students' use of memorization/repetition, Dahlin and Watkins (2000) further found significant cultural differences. Whereas British students used repetition to check if they really remembered something, Chinese students used it to create "deep impressions" to lay a foundation for developing understanding. Moreover, British students viewed understanding as a process of sudden insight, but Chinese students believed understanding to be a long process that requires extensive mental effort.

In exploring perceptions of effective teaching by Hong Kong college students and faculty (both Chinese and Western expatriate), Pratt et al. (1999) found that Chinese students and faculty held different views of learning from that of Western teachers. Western teachers often characterized Chinese students "as not knowing how to think, having only short term goals..., wanting to be spoon-fed, needing too much structure...., taking a quiet, receptive, and deferential attitude during class, and lack of challenge or questioning of the authority.... " (p. 250). However, Chinese students believed that learning is a gradual process that requires tremendous dedication and methodical steps (similar to Japanese learning and teaching style [Hess & Azuma, 1991]). Generally they engage in four distinct steps to accomplish any learning task. Upon encountering new materials, Chinese students initially commit the material to memory; next they seek to understand the intention, style, and meaning of the material. They then try to apply their understanding to situations that call for use of such knowledge, and finally they enter a deeper level of questioning and modification of the original material. Whereas the last step in their approach is verbally interactive by nature, the first three steps may call for more solitary learning and contemplation (which is an important aspect of Chinese intellectual tradition [de Bary, 1983]). Clearly, this style is not bound by the immediate verbal exchange at the moment but can extend over a period of days, weeks, months, and in some cases even several years (as a doctoral student may publish a paper to challenge his or her mentor's ideas with which the student disagreed several years earlier)! Additionally, as Kim (2002) has shown, Asian students not only do not believe that speaking promotes thinking as do Western students; they believe in the opposite: speaking interferes with thinking. This corroborates with the observation by Pratt et al. (1999) that Chinese students often feel frustrated and bewildered when they are confronted with a Western teacher "whose expectations and forms of assessment thrust them immediately to the far end of this chain (questioning and analysis)" (p. 253).

The research efforts by the above scholars have greatly enhanced our understanding of Chinese learners. Notably, all of these studies were conducted with qualitative methods, which were designed to uncover valid cultural meanings from emic views without preconceived notions of learning, teaching, and achievement from the West. This new line of inquiry has indeed provided promising directions for further research. In what follows, I present research that I have conducted in the area of Chinese learning beliefs.

3 My Further Exploration: Chinese Cultural Model of Learning

In joining these researchers, I explored the topic from an emic perspective, that is, conceptions of learning as defined, experienced, and pursued by Chinese learners themselves. The particular approach I adopted was "cultural meaning systems" or "cultural models" (D'Andrade, 1995; Harkness & Super, 1999; Quinn & Holland, 1987; Shweder, 1991) of learning. Anthropologists have long advocated for this approach to study belief systems in cultures. Accordingly, "cultural models" refer to culturally constructed and shared domains of knowledge that serve to structure and constrain people's experiences, "supplying interpretations" of and "inferences" about those experiences and "goals for action" (Quinn & Holland, 1987, p. 6) in a given culture. Moreover, cultural models of a given domain have what D'Andrade (1992) termed "directive force" that serves to motivate people to action and to guide their behaviors toward obtaining their goals. Learning is one such cultural meaning system that can be examined as a whole instead of a few isolated variables at a time.

To explore the Chinese cultural model of learning, I conducted two studies both of which were also replicated with US students (therefore I discuss them both here in order to situate the Chinese model in a larger research context). Prototype methods were used (D'Andrade, 1995; Rosch, 1975; Shaver, Schwartz, Kirson, & O'Connor, 1987). First, I (Li, 2001, 2003a; Li & Fischer, 2004) asked 23 Chinese and 23 US middle class Euro-America (the term "US" is used for convenience hereafter) college students to free-associate the Chinese term *xue xi* (学习) and its English term "learn/learning" respectively. These terms were determined to be the closest equivalents in meaning through word frequencies and a cross-translation procedure (see Li, 2003a for more detail). I initially collected nearly 500 terms from each culture. By using a rating procedure (60 participants in each culture) for relevance to learning, I obtained 225 Chinese and 205 English terms as the core list for each culture, respectively. These core items were then given to 100 college students in their own culture to sort, based on similarity in meaning, into groups. With cluster analyses, the sorted groups finally resulted in each culture's conceptual map of learning as shown in Figures 1 and 2.

Although these maps contain much detailed information, it suffices to highlight the most relevant features to this chapter. The Chinese map (Figure 1) displays desirable versus undesirable approaches to learning with a clear statement of preference/value. The majority of terms fall on the desirable side, which contains two further distinctions: seeking knowledge (with heightened personal agency) and achievement categories and standards. Based on the assumption of prototype methods, a greater number of items indicate greater awareness/emphasis of the conceptions in that culture (Li, 2003a; Shaver et al., 1987). Under seeking knowledge, the most significant groups are (1) heart and mind for wanting to learn which includes, in Chinese, *hao xue xin*, (好学心) (a) lifelong pursuit, (b) a set of learning virtues (diligence, endurance of hardship, steadfast perseverance, and concentration), (c) humility, and (d) desire; (2) purpose of learning containing three essential idea: (a) learning as an end in itself, (b) status, and (c) contributions to society. Under achievement there is one significant dimension: kinds of

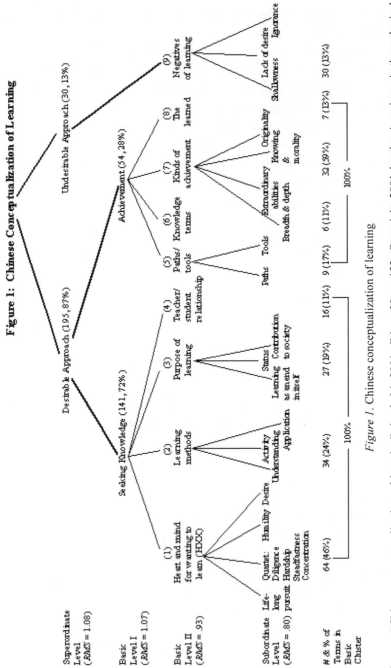

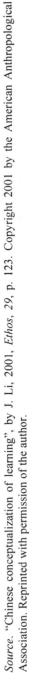

Figure 1. Chinese conceptualization of learning

Source. "Chinese conceptualization of learning", by J. Li, 2001, *Ethos*, 29, p. 123. Copyright 2001 by the American Anthropological Association. Reprinted with permission of the author.

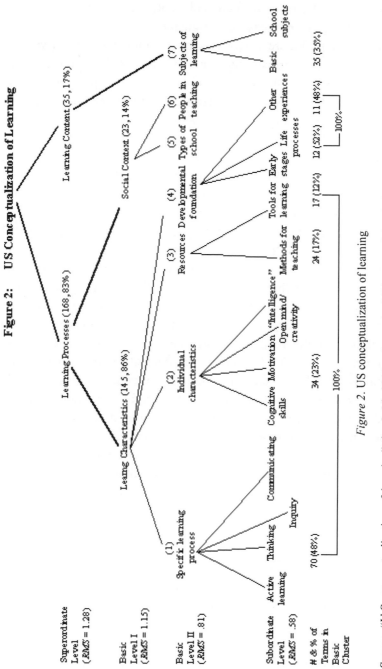

Figure 2. US conceptualization of learning

achievement emphasizing breadth and depth of knowledge, abilities, unity of knowing and morality, and originality.

The US map (Figure 2) focuses on learning processes (with the majority of terms) on one side and learning content (with fewer terms) on another. Compared to the Chinese map, the US map displays more neutral terms instead of value laden terms. Within the learning processes, a great many more terms fall within learner characteristics than within social context. The two most significant dimensions of these learner characteristics are as follows: (1) specific learning processes elaborating on (a) active learning, (b) thinking, (c) inquiry, and (c) communicating and (2) individual characteristics stressing (a) cognitive skills, (b) motivation, (c) open mind, and (d) intelligence.

In the second study, I (Li, 2002a; Li & Fischer, 2004) asked 62 Chinese and 65 US college students to describe their ideal learners in order to obtain a fuller account of cultural learning images than the language expressions that I analyzed in my first study. I probed four specific dimensions: (1) thinking on the nature of knowledge, purposes and processes of learning, and views of intelligence and excellence, (2) understanding of the relationship between learning and one's moral development, (3) learning behaviors in routine situations such as facing high achievement, high intelligence, failure, not understanding concepts, inability to learn despite effort, and boredom, and (4) emotional patterns associated with good or poor learning. The written descriptions of each of these dimensions were analyzed both qualitatively quantitatively (Li, 2002a). These procedures yielded four profiles corresponding to the four probed dimensions of the ideal learner for each culture.[1]

The basic findings from the two studies converge to two comprehensive models of the two cultures. Table 1 summarizes the components and dimensions of these two different belief systems. There are four large common component headings across the two cultures: purpose, process, achievement, and affect. The specific items within each component were decided on the frequency of the number of each culture's respondents who referred to these ideas as well as the presence

---

[1] The Chinese data have been fully analyzed and published, but the US data are still being analyzed. The presentation of the US data is based on preliminary analysis.

of these components on the two cultural maps of learning beliefs as derived from learning related terms. Purpose contains beliefs about personal meanings, significance, and value people attach to learning. Process includes conceptions regarding how learning takes place, what enables a person to learn, what preferred activities are, what course of action to take, and so forth. Achievement refers to views of what counts as worthy levels of achievement and the standards people strive for. Finally, affect encompasses emotional and attitudinal aspects that exist and function dynamically in the various components and their relations. Affect also includes both positive and negative valences that serve either to promote or discourage learning. Below I discuss the components of the Chinese cultural model and only use the US components as a comparative reference.

3.1 *Purpose of learning*

Four main purposes emerged from the data: (1) Perfect oneself morally, (2) acquire knowledge/skills for self, (3) contribute to society, and (4) obtain social respect/mobility (Table 1). The first, the most significant, sees the purpose of learning as a need to perfect oneself morally. This purpose is deeply influenced by Confucian teaching of *ren* (仁), a lifelong striving to become the most genuine, sincere, and humane person one can become (de Bary, 1983; Tu, 1979). *Ren* is regarded as the highest purpose of human lives. However, a person is not born but *learns* to become *ren*. Therefore, the most important purpose of learning is to engage in this process of one's own moral development. Such learning is called the "great learning," as opposed to narrowly defined skill learning (Lee, 1996; Li, 2002a). Indeed, this purpose has also been found by various researchers reviewed previously.

The second purpose is acquiring knowledge and skills for oneself, emphasizing mastery of knowledge. For Chinese model learners, knowledge and skill are also needed for their survival, self-sufficiency, and successful careers. Similarly, these skills are seen as enabling and empowering them to solve problems, maintain satisfying social relations, and reach their personal goals.

Table 1

Components and Dimensions of Chinese and US Beliefs about Learning

Chinese	US
Purpose of Learning	
Perfect oneself morally	Cultivate the mind/understand the world
Acquire knowledge/skills for self	Develop one's ability/skill
Contribute to society	Reach personal goals
Obtain social respect/mobility	
Process of Learning	
Resolve	Active learning
Diligence	Thinking
Endurance of hardship	Inquiry
Perseverance	Task management
Concentration	Communication
(Virtue-oriented)	(Task-oriented)
Kinds of Achievement	
Breadth-depth/mastery of knowledge	Understanding of essentials/expertise
Application of knowledge	Personal insights/creative problem
Unity of knowledge and moral character	solving
	Being the best one can be
Affect	
Positive	
Commitment ("establish one's will")	Curiosity/interest/motivation
Love/passion/thirst (may not favor	Intrinsic enjoyment
intrinsic source, but cultivated affect,	
incl. personal, social, spiritual, or	
moral)	
Respect	Challenging attitudes
Humility for achievement	Pride for achievement
Negative	
Lack of desire	Indifference/boredom
Arrogance	Extrinsic motivation
Shame/guilt for failure	Low self-esteem for failure

The third purpose is contributing to society, which has been a consistent call of the Confucian learning model that inspires Chinese learners. This call functions not only to validate individuals' self-perfection and their pursuit of knowledge, but also to bind it to a higher moral and social obligation. Learning, thus, is no longer delineated as an individual and personal matter; it is also linked to society and the commonwealth of which one is a part (Cheng, 1996; Li, 2002a; Wu & C. Lai, 1992).

The fourth purpose is obtaining social respect/mobility. As Lee (1996) stated, Chinese people pursue learning also for practical purposes. On the one hand, this is due to the historical influence of the Civil Service Examination that lasted from the 7th century to the beginning of the 20th century. In this system, scholars from all walks of life, irrespective of their social strata, were selected for their superior moral character and knowledge to serve the royal government. Those who succeeded in the examination gained respect, social mobility, and power not just for themselves but also for their kin. On the other hand, the present educational systems in Chinese regions continue to rely on examinations for selecting academically more able students to attend highly competitive higher education. High achievement is tantamount to better jobs and social mobility. Not unlike the Civil Service Examination, a better economic and social future combined with honor and respect can have lasting motivating impact.

These Chinese purposes are inherently related. The first three have been explicitly part of Confucian beliefs about learning and are actively promoted by families, communities, schools, and society at large (Cheng, 1996; Gao & Watkins, 2001; Lee, 1996; Yu & Yang, 1994). However, Chinese people do not view the fourth purpose as contradictory to the first three more "lofty" goals because a person is believed to need all of them in order to lead a fuller life.

Compared to the Chinese purposes, the US model's most important purpose is developing the mind and understanding the world, which is cognitive in nature. These references cover a wide range of mental functioning and inquiry, such as critical reasoning and scientific discovery, to which few Chinese respondents referred. Even though some US respondents also mentioned self-fulfillment and self-actualization, they more often emphasized being one's best through learning academic subjects rather than cultivating themselves morally as defined in Confucian terms. The second US purpose is also reminiscent of the Chinese acquisition/mastery of skill for self. However, whereas the Chinese model stresses more mastery of knowledge, the US model elaborates more on developing one's ability. Many US model learners also harbored moral purposes such as relieving suffering and helping others, but this purpose was not as strongly and prevalently expressed as by their Chinese peers. Finally, while in the US model reaching personal goals may have contained practical purposes such as careers and social mobility, it emphasized personal excellence more than social respect and honor associated with achievement.

3.2 *Process of learning*

When Chinese respondents were asked to describe how their model learners learn (i.e., what they do, how they behaved when they encountered difficulties, failure, etc.), they surprisingly did not describe much that would be considered typical learning tasks and processes (e.g., reading and solving problems as mostly described by US respondents). Instead, they wrote extensively about what I (Li, 2003a, 2003b, in press) termed "learning virtues", which were also found as central notions of Chinese learning beliefs in my lexicon study (see "quartet" in Figure 1). The term "learning virtues" was used because these aspects emphasize a morally good and desirable dispositional quality that underlies personal agency, action, even the use of learning strategies that are integral parts of the learning process. Five such virtues emerged.

The first is the notion of resolve (*fen,* 奋, or *fa fen,* 发奋). This concept specifies the determination the learner makes to come to a course of action and the high degree to which he or she is prepared to follow through his or her commitment. *Fen* is believed necessary to ensure one's clarification of desire or goal; the course of action one must take to realize one's desire and goal; and a way to hold oneself accountable for one's own temptation to stray from the course of action, or simply to give up in the face of obstacles. Frequently, upon making the resolve, the person shares his or her *fen* with his or her family or close friends who serve as witnesses. Such witnesses are invited to monitor, to watch for, and even to demand consistency between one's resolve and follow-up action.

The second virtue is diligence (*qin,* 勤), which refers to frequent studying behavior. The emphasis falls on much learning and much time spent on learning. If one is required to act in a manner that requires personal resolve, diligence is the immediate measure and manifestation of resolve. Therefore, resolve and diligence go hand in hand, thus the combined term in Chinese *qin fen*, 勤奋. However, psychologically there are two steps even though behaviorally only diligence is observable. Diligence is also believed necessary because frequent learning ensures familiarity, which in turn opens opportunities for mastery (Li, 2001).

The third virtue is endurance of hardship (*ke ku*, 刻苦), which focuses on facing and overcoming difficulties and obstacles one is bound to encounter in learning. Respondents referred to three kinds of difficulties: (1) physical drudgery and poverty, (2) difficult knowledge and learning tasks, (3) lack of natural ability. First, physical drudgery and poverty are considered hardships because they have been an unavoidable living condition throughout Chinese history. Despite recent improved living standards, physical labor and poverty remain the harsh reality for many. Difficulty in understanding particular academic concepts is a routine encounter for any learner. Respondents were also very clear about individual differences in their natural capacity and acknowledged the impact of such differences on people's learning. However, there was also consensus that these obstacles are not reasons for not learning. Instead, one needs to develop the virtue of endurance of hardship, which is believed to enable the learner to face and combat these hardships.

The fourth virtue is perseverance (*heng xin*, 恒心) that addresses a general attitude toward learning and behavioral tendency in a person's life course. Perseverance is believed important because there is no shortcut to learning. Knowledge does not come about overnight, but through a bit-by-bit, accumulative process over a long period of time, a process fraught with obstacles and distractions. Perseverance is believed potent in helping a person stay on the course from the beginning to the very end no matter how long it takes. It is a virtue required to achieve any serious learning (Huang & H. J. Peng, 1992; Lee, 1996; Liu, 1973).

The final virtue is concentration (*zhuan xin*, 专心). Concentration reminds one of the concept of "being engrossed in something" that can refer to specific tasks. However, concentration in Chinese is used more often to describe a general learning disposition, not necessarily linked to specific tasks. Concentration emphasizes studying with consistent focus and dedication without ever swerving from it. It also includes earnestness, patience, carefulness, and thoroughness of learning. Concentration as an essential disposition of the learner is believed to allow the full engagement of one's mind and heart in study. Without such engagement, there would be no true understanding, no mastery, let alone application of knowledge (Li, 2002b).

These five learning virtues form a coherent whole in the learning process. They all presume a desire to learn because, without it, these learning processes and behaviors cannot be sustained. Without resolve and its resultant commitment, diligence, endurance of hardship, and persistence may be limited to sheer situational factors. Likewise, if concentration can be halted by "hardship" or if one lacks perseverance, one's resolve may be aborted half-way.

Compared to the Chinese virtue-oriented notions, the US notions are more task-oriented. They emphasize active learning activities, many specific processes of thinking (e.g., logic and analysis), scientific inquiry into the unknown world, task management skills, and communication (e.g., discussion, debate, and self-expression). The two cultures' differ greatly in this component. Even though some Chinese respondents also revealed these US notions, they mentioned those categories far less often. Similarly, whereas US respondents also acknowledged their model learners' hard work and persistence, their reference to these learning virtues was also less consistent.

3.3 *Kinds of achievement*

There were three general kinds of achievement for which Chinese model learners aimed and against which they are measured. The first one is depth and breadth and/or mastery of knowledge. Whereas breadth refers to one's extensive knowledge of different disciplines, depth concerns one's deep understanding of a subject or genuine scholarship. Moreover, the integration of breadth and depth is also emphasized. The notion of mastery may not highlight breadth and depth, it nevertheless stresses ownership of knowledge, and by implication the broader and deeper such ownership, the better. This achievement standard seems sensible considering that the ultimate goal is self-perfection, which is open-ended and lifelong in nature. Pursuing knowledge for a life's course could make breadth and depth and related mastery obtainable even though knowledge is boundless.

The second standard is application of knowledge. Although this idea is reminiscent of the US personal problem solving, the Chinese emphasis falls on the *use* of what one has learned in real life situations. The conceptual distinction lies in book knowledge versus knowledge in use. Whether such use is personal or social in origin matters less. This standard thus includes application of knowledge that may not be deemed as creative in any sense (e.g., use math to verify a store transaction), personal creative problem solving and insight (similar to the US standard), and genuine advancement of one's field or historical impact of the whole society.

The third standard is unity of knowledge and moral character. Consistent with the purposes of moral self-perfection, acquisition of knowledge for self, and contribution to society, achieving the unity of the cognitive/intellectual with the moral is only natural.

As alluded to previously, these achievement standards are inherently related to each other. Acquisition of depth and breadth of knowledge can enable the person to better apply such knowledge, which in turn can broaden and deepen one's knowledge further. So long as the learner also continues to self-perfect morally, he or she will likely continue to seek breadth and depth of learning, which loops back to his or her ability to use his or her knowledge in life.

Compared to the Chinese model, US achievement standards center around understanding essentials of the subject and acquiring expertise. Personal insights, creativity, achieving the best one can be are also emphasized. All of these standards seem to highlight the individual's brilliance and achievement.

3.4 *Affect*

Chinese affect shows both positive and negative types as does the US model. Four most commonly mentioned positive affects were found: (1) commitment, (2) love, passion, and thirst for learning, and (3) respect, and (4) humility. Two negative affects are for purposes and learning processes: (1) lack of desire and (2) arrogance. For lack of achievement, there is also only one general negative affect of shame and guilt.

The notion of commitment, *li zhi* (立志, "establish one's will") in Chinese, is part of one's learning purpose. This concept aims at helping the learner, often during secondary school, to start pondering his or her life's purposes in order to come to a clear personal vision (*zhi xiang*, 志向 or *bao fu*, 抱负). This process is deliberately designed and practiced to lead the learner to imagine or envision something greater than his or her current (temporal sense) and own (individual sense) life. It is orienting oneself in learning toward one's future (parents and teachers frequently engage adolescent children in this discussion). In doing so, Chinese learners believe that they will not only find a more specific path to focus on (e.g., I want to be a scientist making important discoveries to benefit mankind) but also know to what path to attach their energy, dedication, emotion, and action (e.g., therefore I will study math and science hard). Therefore, the process of "establish one's will" is a spiritually uplifting and emotionally positive process.

Notice that "establish one's will" is not to be confused with career goal setting, although it may coincide with it; it is searching for an inspirational purpose in the large framework of the four purposes discussed earlier in order to channel one's lifelong learning.

Some US respondents also touched on personal ambitions. However, such cases were not described consistently as a deliberate and socially orchestrated process where the learner is guided to search for a purpose and to establish commitment to reaching that goal for life.

Love, passion, and thirst were described similarly as enjoyment among US model learners for both purposes and processes of learning. However, a significant difference lies in the source of such affect between the two cultures' models. Whereas for the US learners, intrinsic enjoyment, curiosity, and motivation were described as essential, this intrinsic source was not emphasized by Chinese respondents. In fact, many of the respondents acknowledged that their model learners were initially not motivated to learn in young age, but they developed love and passion once they realized the importance of learning for their lives or once their parents and teachers guided them into the process. Deliberate cultivation of love and passion by oneself and one's social world parallels the recent work on intrinsic motivation as less essential for Asian-American children for school learning (Iyengar & Lepper, 1999).

Respect is another distinct affect that Chinese model learners express toward knowledge and teachers in the form of humility. Because learning in the Confucian persuasion is not limited to academic learning but more importantly social and moral learning, respect toward knowledge and teachers, who ideally embody the self-perfecting process (Gao & Watkins, 2001; Jin & Cortazzi, 1998), is sensible and expected. However, this general attitude of respect among Asian learners has been taken as a sign of obedience and lack of critical thinking (Keats, 1982; Pratt et al., 1999; Tweed & Lehman, 2002). This is a persistent misunderstanding (Inagaki, Hatano, & Morita, 1998; Li, 2003b). Asian learners' deference toward teachers does not stem from their fear or blind acceptance of authority but from their deep sense of humility. Instead of treating humility as a personal weakness, they regard it a personal strength and courage because those who are humble are willing to self-examine, admit their inadequacies, and self-improve. Humility also leads one to want to learn from anyone. Therefore, respect and humility go hand in hand. In these processes, one's ego or self-esteem generated by lack of competence is not seriously threatened and in need of protection as may be the case among some US learners (Brickman & Bulman, 1977; Ruble, Eisenberg, & Higgins, 1994). Chinese learners believe that one can always self-improve so long as one learns humbly and respectfully from others (Li & Q. Wang, in press).

As alluded to earlier, Chinese learners' respect and humility may be very different from US learners' challenging attitude, especially in the form of immediate verbal exchange in the midst of a discussion. It was generally the case that Chinese respondents made few references to such challenging attitudes toward teachers and experts even though their model learners did engage in discussions and debates with their peers. However, this does not mean that Chinese learners do not challenge. In fact, many respondents wrote that challenging old knowledge or advancing new knowledge is an important goal for learners in the end. But one is reluctant to engage in challenges until one has thoroughly understood the knowledge in question or mastered one's field. This finding concurs with the finding by Pratt et al. (1999).

For achievement, Chinese learners generally do not display pride although they may be happy themselves (Li, 2002a). This tendency is different from their US peers who usually feel proud of themselves and like to share their joy with others (Mascolo, Fischer, & Li, 2003). Chinese model learners were described as feeling a need to remain humble. Related to the forgoing discussion of respect and humility, the need to be humble stems from the same recognition that learning is a lifelong journey. Although others may acknowledge one's achievement publicly, focusing on celebration for *oneself* may be perceived as a negative tendency that pulls one away from further self-perfection (Li & Q. Wang, in press).

The two negative affects associated with purpose and processes of learning are lack of desire and arrogance. The former shows some affinity to the US indifference and boredom. Lack of desire is the opposite of a heart and mind for wanting to learn (Li, 2001). Many Chinese learning related words and phrases refer to this state as lying at the heart of any motivational problem.

Arrogance is also an affect that refers to complacency and hubris, which is the opposite of humility. Learners who achieve highly are believed to be vulnerable to this inflated sense of oneself. Given the importance of humility in Chinese learning beliefs, there is little wonder why pride/arrogance is a great concern among learners (Li, 2002a).

Similar to their US peers, Chinese model learners were described to feel a number of related negative emotions such as sadness and pain when they experience failure. The most frequently revealed emotions are shame and guilt both for themselves as well as their families. Shame is a powerful and prevalent emotion in Chinese culture (Li, 2002a; Li, L. Wang, & Fischer, in press). Even though shame in Chinese culture is an emotion of disgrace or humiliation as in most cultures, it is also a moral discretion and sensibility that people desire to develop (Fung, 1999; Fung & E. C.-H. Chen, 2001). Thus, the meanings of shame and guilt shade into each other. Together they function to direct people into self-examination in social situations in order to recognize their own wrong doings as well as to motivate people to improve themselves. Compared to the Chinese model, the US contained few references to shame/guilt but instead referred to low self-esteem.

3.5 *Learners' own beliefs and developmental evidence*

The forgoing research provides descriptions of a Chinese learning model at the *cultural* level, which is not to be taken as a model of individuals. The question remains: Do ordinary Chinese learners themselves share these beliefs? In order to explore this essential question, my colleagues and I (Li, 2004a; Li & Yue, in press) have conducted two further studies, and our answer is a yes, although individuals' beliefs reflecting their cultural beliefs may vary in degree and configuration depending on their personal characteristics and socialization experiences. We asked 1800 students in 5th though 11th grade across six regions of China to respond to an open-ended questionnaire in writing on how they themselves viewed the nature of knowledge, their purposes of learning, origin of intelligence and excellence of learning, their moral aspirations and whether learning had anything to do their own moral development, how they actually learned, and how they would respond to good versus poor learning emotionally.

An analysis of a random set of 187 adolescents' data revealed by and large similar purposes and learning virtues as those at the cultural level (Li & Yue, in press). Differences appeared to lie in the more fine-grained details of each purpose but not the basic categories. For example, within the purpose of moral self-perfection, adolescents referred also to finer distinctions of forging their moral character, finding meaning in life, and obtaining wisdom through learning. Regarding skill acquisition and mastery, they differentiated developing their ability and competence, expanding their horizons, and mastering knowledge. Learning virtues practically converged with those at the cultural level.

To trace developmental origins of these beliefs, I (Li, 2004b, in press) conducted an additional study to examine Chinese and US preschool children's beliefs about learning. Children were told story beginnings and asked to complete the stories, again by using methods of free narratives. One set of stories depicted a protagonist child who liked to go to school and one who did not. Another set of stories showed a diligent, bird who tried hard to learn how to fly and succeeded whereas a bear who tried to learn how to catch fish but gave up in the end. The first set of stories was designed to elicit children's perceptions of the purposes of school learning. The second set of stories focused on children's construals of what is involved in the learning process.

Results showed that consistent with their cultural model, Chinese children mentioned moral self-improving purposes, mastery of knowledge, social contribution, and social respect/economic reward more than US children (who mentioned smartness, literacy, friendship, play purposes more. With regard to their construals of the learning process, Chinese children again referred to learning virtues of diligence, persistence, and concentration more than their US peers. By contrast, US children named more ability, attempting the task, and creative use of strategies than Chinese children. Moreover, these trends became more consistent as children's age increased. Thus, from both data on learners themselves and development, it appears that cultural models of learning do influence their members' beliefs, al though caution should be exercised about these findings' generalizibility to the two cultures' populations because most children studied were from college educated, middle-class backgrounds.

3.6 *Summary of research findings*

Based on the forgoing findings and analyses, Chinese beliefs center around a set of purposes that focus on perfecting oneself morally, acquiring knowledge and skill for oneself, contributing to society, and obtaining social respect/mobility (unlike Western beliefs that elaborate on the mind, its processes, understanding of the world, and personal excellence). Embedded in these purposes are commitment and passion, which may or may not be intrinsic in origin as understood in the West. To pursue those purposes of learning, one needs to develop the so-called learning virtues of resolve, diligence, endurance of hardship, perseverance, and concentration. These virtues are seen as more essential than actual learning activities such as reading or doing research. Chinese learners believe that once the learning virtues are there, one can apply them to all learning activities and processes. These purposes and virtues are coalesced with four strong affects: (1) commitment, (2) love and passion for learning, (3) respect for teaching authority, which does not mean obedience and blind acceptance of what is taught, but personal trust and sincerity toward teachers, and (4) humility, which does not mean weakness but personal courage for self-reflection and self-improvement. Such learning aims at breadth and depth or mastery of knowledge, application to real life situations, and unity of one's knowledge and moral character. When learners achieve learning, they remain humble; they also watch out for signs of complacency and arrogance in order to continue self-perfecting. When encountering failure and setbacks, they feel shame and guilt not only themselves but also in reference to those who nurtured them. These emotions, surprisingly, may not lead them to give up, but may motivate them to self-improve further. So long as they still hold their ultimate purposes and believe in the power of their learning virtues, they may derive happiness and satisfaction from the process itself rather than reaching the end of their journey.

4 Conclusion

In this chapter I presented a Chinese cultural learning model that may serve as a general belief system that guides Chinese children's learning, including mathematics learning. In the introduction, I addressed four deficiencies in traditional research on human learning across cultures. First is the focus on comparing the end results of learning and reliance on set but often also dichotomous concepts of learning from the West. Even though the learning model reviewed in this chapter also refers to achievement standards, its emphasis is not on the end results but on the purposes and processes of learning.

Moreover, this Chinese learning model shows few if any dichotomous concepts. Individual concepts such as ability, effort, success, and failure did emerge. Yet, they were never expressed as opposites, but viewed instead in dialectical relationships (K. Peng & Nisbett, 1999) that function jointly and dynamically in people's learning. For example, Chinese learners did not believe that superior inherent ability lead to good learning without the learning virtues. Likewise, failure and success are never ends themselves but only markers for orienting oneself in further learning. This belief is aptly expressed by many respondents as "failure is the mother of success". Neither does the concept of motivation hinge on intrinsic versus extrinsic source. Children who lacked intrinsic motivation were believed to be able to develop passion and love for learning, depending on their development, experience, and supporting environment. Finally, both individualist and collectivist goals, such as moral self-perfection, personal skills, and contribution to society, co-existed, informed, and fulfilled each other rather than standing in contradiction.

The second deficiency in research is the privilege that cognitive processes in learning assume, as if cognition is all that matters in learning. Much recent research shows that human psychological functioning rarely if at all involves only cognition in any domain, let alone the highly complex domain of learning. As discussed earlier, the Chinese learning model indicates that the purposive, the social/moral, the affective, and self/identity factors are intertwined and are all present, interacting dynamically to produce learning behavior. Thus, research on children's learning must consider all of these factors.

As a third limitation, much traditional research emphasizes the structural factors of school, which alone do not explain children's learning processes and results fully. In fact, much misunderstanding and stereotyping have resulted from the assumption that educational system and structural factors alone can reveal and determine how children learn and achieve. These misunderstandings and stereotypes were born because the perspectives of teachers and children were neglected. As the data presented in this chapter showed, research has much to gain by studying individual learners' beliefs and behaviors in addition to structural elements.

The fourth and the greatest deficiency in research is the field's persistent reliance on Western concepts without attending to indigenous or emic cultural meanings and their psychological manifestation in learning (Gao & Watkins, 2001; Watkins, 2000). The studies reviewed in this chapter offer alternative ways to gather data and to conduct analyses that retain empirical rigor and at the same time examine emic meaning systems of learning in Chinese and Western cultures. As a result, our understanding has been enriched.

Much remains to be studied about culture and learning. Even though individual children have their own cognitive capacities, social and affective orientations, and idiosyncratic learning styles, they are born into and raised in at least one culture. Invariably, they begin developing beliefs about learning early on. What their cultures regard as important purposes, processes, and outcomes will influence their beliefs profoundly. Children growing up in different cultures may hold different outlooks, attitudes, emotions, and achievement standards that may affect their engagement in and ultimate achievement of learning. Yet, the development of culturally based learning beliefs often remains so invisible and gradual that it often evades research attention. Considering how vast a topic learning is, it is surprising how few researchers have heeded beliefs about learning in any culture. The recent research reviewed in this chapter marks the beginning of an important inquiry. It is hoped that this inquiry can shed light not only on learning in general but also on learning in specific domains such as mathematics.

References

Au, T. K. F., & Harackiewicz, J. M. (1986). The effects of perceived parental expectations on Chinese children's mathematics performance. *Merrill-Palmer Quarterly, 32*(4), 383-392.

Brickman, P., & Bulman, R. J. (1977). Pleasure and pain in social comparison. In J. M. Suls & R. L. Miller (Eds.), *Social comparison processes: Theoretical and empirical perspectives* (pp. 149-186). Washington, DC: Hemishpere.

Burton, L., & Morgan, C. (2000). Mathematicians writing. *Journal for Research in Mathematics Education, 31*(4), 429 - 453.

Chen, C., & Stevenson, H. W. (1989). Homework: A cross-cultural examination. *Child Development, 60*(3), 551-561.

Chen, J. (1979). *Recent history of Chinese education* [In Chinese 中国近代教育史]. Beijing: People's Press.

Cheng, K. M. (1996). *The quality of primary education: A case study of Zhejiang Province, China.* Paris: International Institute for Educational Planning.

Conti, R., Amabile, T. M., & Pollack, S. (1995). Enhancing intrinsic motivation, learning, and creativity. *Personality and Social Psychology Bulletin, 21*(9), 1107-1116.

Dahlin, B., & Watkins, D. A. (2000). The role of repetition in the processes of memorizing and understanding: A comparison of the views of Western and Chinese secondary school students in Hong Kong. *British Journal of Educational Psychology, 70*(1), 65-84.

Dai, D. Y., & Sternberg, R. J. (Eds.). (2004). *Motivation, emotion, and cognition: Integrative perspectives on intellectual functioning and development.* Mahwah, NJ: Erlbaum.

Damon, W. (2003). *Noble purpose: The joy of living a meaningful life.* Philadelphia, PA: Templeton Foundation Press.

D'Andrade, R. G. (1992). Schemas and motivation. In R. G. D'Andrade & C. Strauss (Eds.), *Human motives and cultural models* (pp. 23-44). New York: Cambridge University Press.

D'Andrade, R. G. (1995). *The development of cognitive anthropology.* New York: Cambridge University Press.

de Bary, W. T. (1983). *The liberal tradition in China.* New York: Columbia University Press.

de Charms, R. (1968). *Personal causation.* New York: Academic Press.

Deci, E. L., & Ryan, R. M. (1985). *Intrinsic motivation and self-determination in human behavior.* New York: Academic Press.

Duncan, J., & Paulhus, D. L. (1998, August). *Varieties of shyness in Asian- and European-Canadians.* Paper presented at the 106th Annual Convention of the American Psychological Association, San Francisco, CA.

Dweck, C. S. (1999). *Self-theories.* Philadelphia: Psychology Press.

Fung, H. (1999). Becoming a moral child: The socialization of shame among young Chinese children. *Ethos, 27*(2), 180-209.

Fung, H., & Chen, E. C.-H. (2001). Across time and beyond skin: Self and transgression in the everyday socialization of shame among Taiwanese preschool children. *Social Development, 10*(3), 420-437.

Gardner, H. (1989). *To open minds.* New York: Basic Books.

Gao, L., & Watkins, D. A. (2001). Identifying and assessing the conceptions of teaching of secondary school physics teachers in China. *British Journal of Educational Psychology, 71*(3), 443-469.

Ginsberg, E. (1992). Not just a matter of English. *HERDSA News, 14*(1), 6-8.

Harkness, S., & Super, C. M. (1999). From parents' cultural belief systems to behavior: Implications for the development of early intervention programs. In L. Eldering & P. Leseman (Eds.), *Effective early education: Cross-cultural perspectives* (pp. 67-90). New York: Falmer Press.

Harmon, M., Smith, T. A., Martin, M. O., Kelly, D. L., Beaton, A. E., Mullis, I.V. S., et al. (1997). *Performance assessment in IEA's Third International Mathematics and*

Science Study (TIMSS). Chestnut Hill, MA: Boston College, TIMSS International Study Center.

Hau, K. T., & Salili, F. (1991). Structure and semantic differential placement of specific causes: Academic causal attributions by Chinese students in Hong Kong. *International Journal of Psychology, 26*(2), 175-193.

Hennessey, B. A., & Amabile, T. M. (1998). Reward, intrinsic motivation, and creativity. *American Psychologist, 53*(6), 674-675.

Hess, R. D., & Azuma, H. (1991). Cultural support for schooling: Contrasts between Japan and the United States. *Educational Researcher, 20*(9), 2-8.

Holloway, S. D. (1988). Concepts of ability and effort in Japan and the US. *Review of Educational Research, 58*(3), 327-345.

Huang, D. Y., & Peng, H, J. (1992). Three character classic [In Chinese 三字经]. Taipei: Ruisheng.

Inagaki, K., Hatano, G., & Morita, E. (1998). Construction of mathematical knowledge through whole-class discussion. *Learning and Instruction, 8*(6), 503-526.

Iyengar, S. S., & Lepper, M. R. (1999). Rethinking the value of choice: A cultural perspective on intrinsic motivation. *Journal of Personality and Social Psychology, 76*(3), 349-366.

Jin, L., & Cortazzi, M. (1998). Dimensions of dialogue: Large classes in China. *International Journal of Educational Research, 29*(8), 739-791.

Keats, D. M. (1982). Cultural bases of concepts of intelligence: A Chinese versus Australian comparison. In P. Sukontasarp, N. Yongsiri, P. Intasuwan, N. Jotiban, & C. Suvannathat (Eds.), *Proceedings of second Asian workshop on child and adolescent development* (pp. 67-75). Bangkok, Thailand: Behavioral Science Research Institute.

Kim, H. S. (2002). We talk, therefore we think? A Cultural analysis of the effect of talking on thinking. *Journal of Personality and Social Psychology, 83*(4), 828-842.

Kim, H., S. & Markus, H. R. (2002). Freedom of speech and freedom of silence: An analysis of talking as a cultural practice. In R. A. Shweder, M. Minow, & H. R. Markus (Eds.), *Engaging cultural differences: The multicultural challenge in liberal democracies* (pp. 432-452). New York: Russell Sage Foundation.

Kwok, D. C., & Lytton, H. (1996). Perceptions of mathematics ability versus actual mathematics performance: Canadian and Hong Kong Chinese children. *British Journal of Educational Psychology, 66*(2), 209-222.

Lee, W. O. (1996). The cultural context for Chinese learners: Conceptions of learning in the Confucian Tradition. In D. A. Watkins & J. B. Biggs (Eds.), *The Chinese learner* (pp. 45-67). Hong Kong: Comparative Education Research Centre.

Lepper, M. R. (1981). Intrinsic and extrinsic motivation in children: Detrimental effects of superfluous social controls. In W. A. Collins (Ed.), *Aspects of the development of competence: The Minnesota symposium on child psychology* (Vol. 14, pp. 155-214). Hillsdale, NJ: Erlbaum.

Lewis, C. C. (1995). *Educating hearts and minds: Reflections on Japanese preschool and elementary education.* New York: Cambridge University Press.

Li, J. (2001). Chinese conceptualization of learning. *Ethos, 29*(2), 111-137.

Li, J. (2002a). A cultural model of learning: Chinese "heart and mind for wanting to Learn." *Journal of Cross-Cultural Psychology, 33*(3), 248-269.

Li, J. (2002b). Models of learning in different cultures. In J. Bempechat & J. Elliott (Eds.), *Achievement motivation in culture and context: Understanding children's learning experiences, New Directions in Child and Adolescent Development* (pp. 45-63). San Francisco: Jossey-Bass.

Li, J. (2003a). U.S. and Chinese cultural beliefs about learning. *Journal of Educational Psychology, 95*(2), 258-267.

Li, J. (2003b). The core of Confucian learning. *American Psychologist, 58*(2), 146-147.

Li, J. (2004a). "I learn and I grow big:" Chinese preschoolers' purposes for learning. *International Journal of Behavioral Development, 28*(2), 116-128.

Li, J. (2004b). High abilities and excellence: A cultural perspective. In L. V. Shavinina & M. Ferrari (Eds.), *Beyond knowledge: Extracognitive aspects of developing high ability* (pp. 187-208). Mahwah, NJ: Erlbaum.

Li, J. (in press). Learning as a task and a virtue: U.S. and Chinese preschoolers explain learning. *Developmental Psychology.*

Li, J., & Fischer, K. W. (2004). Thoughts and emotions in American and Chinese cultural beliefs about learning. In D. Y. Dai & R. J. Sternberg (Eds.), *Motivation, emotion, and cognition: Integrative perspectives on intellectual functioning.* Mahwah, NJ: Erlbaum.

Li, J., & Wang, Q. (in press). U.S. and Chinese preschool children's perceptions of achievement and their achieving peers. *Social Development.*

Li, J, & Yue, X. (in press). Self in learning among Chinese adolescents. In M. F. Mascolo & J. Li. (Eds.), *Culture and developing selves: Beyond dichotomization. New Directions in Child and Adolescent Development Series.* W. Damon (Series Ed.). San Francisco, CA: Jossey-Bass.

Li, J., Wang, L., & Fischer, K. W. (in press). The organization of the Chinese shame concept. *Cognition and Emotion.*

Liu, Z. (1973). Principles of teacherhood [In Chinese 师道]. Taipei: Chung Hwa.

Marton, F., Dall'Alba, G., & Tse, L. K. (1996). Memorizing and Understanding: The keys to the paradox? In D. A. Watkins & J. B. Biggs (Eds.), *The Chinese learner* (pp. 69-83). Hong Kong: Comparative Education Research Centre.

Mascolo, M. F., Fischer, K. W., & Li, J. (2003). The dynamic construction of emotions in development: A component systems approach. In N. Davidson, K. Scherer, & H. Goldsmith (Eds.), *Handbook of affective science* (pp. 375-408). New York: Oxford University Press.

Matsushita, K. (1994). Acquiring mathematical knowledge through semantic and pragmatic problem solving. *Human Development, 37*(4), 220-232.

National Center for Education Development Research. (2001). *2001 green paper on education in China: Annual report on policies of China's education* [In Chinese 2001 年中国教育绿皮书: 中国教育政策年度分析保告]. Beijing: Educational Science.

Ouyang, H.-H. (2000). One way ticket: A story of an innovative teacher in mainland China. *Anthropology and Education Quarterly, 31*(4), 397-425.

Peng, K., & Nisbett, R. E. (1999). Culture, dialects, and reasoning about contradiction. *American Psychologist, 54*, 741-754.

Pratt, D. D., Kelly, M., & Wong, K. M. (1999). Chinese conceptions of "effective teaching" in Hong Kong: Towards culturally sensitive evaluation of teaching. *International Journal of Lifelong Learning, 18*(4), 241-258.

Quinn, N., & Holland, D. (1987). Introduction. In D. Holland & N. Quinn (Eds.), *Cultural models in language and thought* (pp. 3-40). New York: Cambridge University Press.

Ran, A. (2001). Traveling on parallel tracks: Chinese parents and English teachers. *Educational Research, 43*, 311-328.

Rosch, E. (1975). Cognitive representations of semantic categories. *Journal of Experimental Psychology: General, 104*(5), 192-233.

Ruble, D. N., Eisenberg, R., Higgins, E. T. (1994). Developmental changes in achievement evaluations: Motivational implications of self-other differences. *Child Development, 65*, 1095-1110.

Salili, F., Chiu, C. Y., & Lai, S. (2001). The influence of culture and context on students' achievement orientations. In F. Salili, C. Y. Chiu, & Y. Y. Hong (Eds.), *Student motivation: The culture and context of learning* (pp. 221-247). New York: Plenum.

Shaver, P., Schwartz, J., Kirson, D., & O'Connor, C. (1987). Emotion knowledge: Further exploration of a prototype approach. *Journal of Personality and Social Psychology, 52*(1), 1061-1086.

Shavinina, L. V., & Ferrari, M. (Eds.). (2004). *Beyond knowledge: Extracognitive aspects of developing high ability.* Mahwah, NJ: Erlbaum.

Shon, S. P., & Ja, D. Y. (1982). Asian families. In M. McGoldrick, J. K. Pearce, & J. Giordano (Eds.), *Ethnicity and family therapy* (pp. 134-163). New York: Guildford.

Shweder, R. A. (1991). *Thinking through cultures.* Cambridge, MA: Harvard University Press.

Steele, C. M. (1997). A threat in the air: How stereotypes shape intellectual identity and performance. *American Psychologist, 52*(6), 613-629.

Stevenson, H. W., & Stigler, J. W. (1992). *The learning gap: Why our schools are failing and what we can learn from Japanese and Chinese education?* New York: Simon & Schuster.

Stigler, J. W., & Hiebert, J. (1999). *The teaching gap: Best ideas from the world's teachers for improving education in the classroom.* New York: Free Press.

Sue, S., & Okazaki, S. (1990). Asian-American educational achievements: A phenomenon in search of an explanation. *American Psychologist, 45*(8), 913-920.

Triandis, H. C. (1995). *Individualism and collectivism*. Boulder, CO: Westview.

Tu, W. M. (1979). *Humanity and self-cultivation: Essays in Confucian thought*. Berkeley, CA: Asian Humanities Press.

Tweed, R. G., & Lehman, D. R. (2002). Learning considered within a cultural context: Confucian and Socratic Approaches. *American Psychologist, 57*(2), 89-99.

Watkins, D. A. (2000). Learning and teaching: a cross-cultural perspective. *School Leadership & Management, 20* (2), 161-173.

Watkins, D. A., & Biggs, J. B. (Eds.). (1996). *The Chinese learner: Cultural, psychological, and contextual influences*. Hong Kong: Comparative Education Research Centre.

Winner, E. (1989). How can Chinese children draw so well? *Journal of Aesthetic Education, 23*(1), 65-84.

Wong, N. Y., Marton, F., Wong, K. M., & Lam, C. C. (2002). The lived space of mathematics learning. *Journal of Mathematics Behavior, 21*(1), 25-47.

Wu, S., & Lai, C. (1992). *Complete text of the four books and five classics in modern Chinese* [In Chinese 全译本白话四书五经]. Beijing: International Culture Press.

Yao, E. (1985). A comparison of family characteristics of Asian-American and Anglo-American high achievers. *International Journal of Comparative Sociology, 26*(34), 198-208.

Yu, A. B., & Yang, K. S. (1994). The nature of achievement motivation in collectivist societies. In U. Kim, H. C. Triandis, C. Kagitcibasi, S. C. Choi, & G. Yoon (Eds.), *Individualism and collectivism: Theory, method, and applications* (pp. 239-250). Thousand Oaks, CA: Sage.

Chapter 6

Official Curriculum in Mathematics in Ancient China: How Did Candidates Study for the Examination?

This chapter starts with a brief general account of mathematics education in ancient China, then discusses in detail the official curriculum and the state examination system in mathematics in the Tang Dynasty. In the second part of the chapter some examples of examination questions are re-constructed with "circumstantial evidence" to offer an alternative viewpoint from a traditional one, to argue that study in mathematics in ancient China did not proceed in an examination-oriented, rote-based learning environment. This "animated" historical account may help to shed some light on the comparative study of mathematics education in the East and West.

Key words: mathematics curriculum, state examination system, Tang Dynasty

1 Introduction: The CHC Learner Paradox and the CHC Teacher Paradox

Ever since the early 1990s some educators have begun to pay attention to cultural differences that may affect the learning and teaching of subjects like science and mathematics, which are usually regarded as universal in content (Cai, 1995; Stevenson & Stigler, 1992; Watkins & Biggs, 1996). Interest in this aspect is further reinforced by the results coming out of several international studies sponsored by organizations like the International Association for the Study of Educational Achievement (IEA) or the Organization for Economic Cooperation and Development (OECD). In particular, the learning process of Asian students brought up in the tradition of the Confucian heritage culture (CHC) has become a much discussed issue in the past decade (Leung, 2001; Watkins & Biggs, 1996; Wong, 1998). As a natural consequence, the teaching process of Asian teachers in CHC classrooms has come under review as well (L. Ma, 1999; Stigler & Hiebert, 1999; Watkins & Biggs, 2001). These two closely inter-related issues can be brought into focus in the form of two paradoxes, *viz*

(1) The CHC Learner Paradox: CHC students are perceived as using low-level, rote-based strategies in a classroom environment which should not be conducive to high achievement, yet CHC students report a preference for high-level, meaning-based learning strategies and they achieve significantly better in international assessments!

(2) The CHC Teacher Paradox: Teachers in CHC classrooms produce a positive learning outcome under substandard conditions that Western educators would regard as most unpromising!

In this chapter we look at these issues from a historical angle by investigating the official curriculum in mathematics in ancient China. After giving a brief general account of mathematics education in ancient China, we will confine the discussion to the curriculum of the state university of the Tang Dynasty (唐, 618 – 917), particularly to the state examination system in mathematics in that period. That period is chosen not only because the state examination system in mathematics was in its most established form by then, but because the system in later dynasties was either modeled after it or was no longer in place. A major part of this chapter is spent on the state examination system, because the CHC classroom is usually labeled as dominated by an examination-oriented culture and it is commonly believed that an examination-oriented culture hinders the learning process. But is it really so? By piecing together, from official records in the ancient chronicles, a "rational re-construction" of the state examination in mathematics in the Tang Dynasty — as there is no single extant document on the examination itself — we are prepared to ask questions such as: Is the examination system really that damaging to learning? Is the examination a necessary evil? Or is it beneficial to the learning process to some extent? Was the state examination a mere test on rote learning?

The author borrows heavily from three of his articles (Siu, 1995, 2001; Siu & Volkov, 1999), which happen to be not very readily accessible to teachers and educators in mathematics, so that an edited summarized presentation here may prove useful to shed light on a comparative study of mathematics education in the East and West. The first article, which is the text of a talk given in 1992 on mathematics education in ancient China, should be regarded as a "first approximation" in view of the more in-depth historical study carried out later (in collaboration with the historian of mathematics Alexeï Volkov) in the second article. The third article, which is the text of a talk given in 1998, is more inclined towards the pedagogical aspect and is closest to the main message to be conveyed in this chapter. The author wishes to acknowledge with heartfelt gratitude the permission of Madame Patricia Radelet-de Grave, the editor of the Proceedings of the Third European Summer University held at Louvain-la-Neuve and Leuven in 1998, for him to incorporate parts of his article (Siu, 2001) into Section 4, Section 5 and Section 6 of this chapter.

2 Mathematics Education in Ancient China

Even if it is debatable what constituted a genuine beginning of mathematics in the history of civilization — is it drawing? or counting? or calculation? or argumentation? or reasoning? or proof? — it seems fair to say that mathematics education, at least in its narrower sense of transmission of mathematical skill and knowledge, came into existence alongside mathematics.

In ancient China the school system in its formal setting began in about 2000 B.C. during the latter part of the Xia Dynasty (夏, 21st century B.C. to 16th century B.C.). Run by the state, it was intended as a training ground for youths and children of the aristocracy. The official system became more institutionalized in the Shang Dynasty (商, 16th century B.C. to 1066 B.C.) and the Western Zhou Dynasty (西周, 1066

B.C. to 771 B.C.). The invasion of barbarian hordes in 770 B.C. forced a transfer of the capital, thereby starting the Eastern Zhou Dynasty (东周, 770 B.C. to 256 B.C.) during which the state power of the Zhou Kingdom was waning, resulting in a continual vying for political domination among the many feudal lords. This long period known as the "Spring and Autumn Period" (春秋时代) followed by the "Warring States Period" (战国时代) was to last for five centuries. Beset with conflicts and unrest, it was a stirring and eventful period as well as, ironically, a most stimulating and prosperous period in terms of intellectual development in the history of China. The decline in state-run institutions of learning was more than compensated for by the formation of private academies (not necessarily with a physical setting) around some scholars of fame. In later dynasties such private academics gradually developed into an important part of the education system (with physical setting) under the name of *shu yuan* (书院, an academy of classical learning). 'An academy of classical learning', was originally set up as an official organization in the Tang Dynasty to collect and compile books of learning. The evolvement of 'an academy of classical learning' has been a topic of intensive research. However, as there is hardly any trace of a mathematics curriculum found in documents about these private academics, we will not further dwell on them, but note that this dual system of learning, which comprised state-run institutions and private academies side by side, persisted in China for the next two millennia (G. Chen & Deng, 1997; G. Ding & Q. Liu, 1992; Z.-F. Zhang, 1985; S. Zhao & Xue, 1995).

In the Han Dynasty (汉, 206 B.C. to 220 A.D.), Confucianism was established as the supreme state philosophy. With the emphasis on the study of classics, mathematics was accorded attention after a fashion, because some classics made allusions to mathematical knowledge here and there. Indeed, for the curriculum in higher education, the "Six Arts" (六艺) comprised Rituals (礼), Music (乐), Archery (射), Charioteering (御), History (书) and Arithmetic (数). (In the early days, the subject Arithmetic was intimately tied up with numerology. The latter was referred to as the "internal arithmetic" (内算), while what we understand as mathematics today was referred to as "external arithmetic" (外算) (D. Liu, 1993, p. 71) This sixth Art of Arithmetic was further divided into nine topics, as recorded in the commentary by ZHENG Xuan (郑玄) in the 2nd century, with their titles not too much different from the nine chapter titles of the very famous mathematical classics *jiu zhang suan shu* (九章算术, Nine Chapters on the Mathematical Art), which is believed to have been compiled some time between 100 B.C. and 100 A.D. In 1984, in an Han tomb in Hubei Province, a book written on bamboo strips bearing the title *suan shu shu* (算数书, Book on the Mathematical Art) was discovered (during excavation). The book is dated at around 200 B.C. and its content exhibits a marked resemblance to that of 'Nine Chapters on the Mathematical Art', lending evidence to the belief that the content of 'Nine Chapters on the Mathematical Art' is much older than the book itself (Peng, 2001). In any case, the format of either book became a prototype for all Chinese mathematical classics in the subsequent one-and-a-half millennia. 'Nine Chapters on the Mathematical Art' is a conglomeration of 246 mathematical problems grouped into nine chapters: (1) Survey of land, (2) Millet and rice, (3) Distribution by progressions, (4) Diminishing breadth, (5) Consultation on engineering works, (6) Imperial taxation, (7) Excess and deficiency, (8) Calculating by tabulation, (9) *gou-gu* (勾股, right triangles). In the text a few problems of the same type are given, along with answers, after which a general method (algorithm) follows. It should be noted that the numerical data given in the text are specific rather than special, so they are in fact generic, making the method (algorithm) essentially a general procedure. In the very early edition no further explanation was added to the text, that being perhaps supplied by the teachers. Later editions were appended with commentaries from various authors, which were an indication of serious and assiduous self-study on the part of the author and provided useful aid-to-study for future generations of readers. One of the most notable commentators, LIU Hui (刘徽) of the mid 3rd century, wrote in the preface, "I studied 'Nine Chapters on the Mathematical Art' at an early age and perused it when I got older. I see the separation of the Yin and the Yang and arrive at the root of the mathematical art. In this process of probing I comprehend its meaning. Despite ignorance and incompetence on my part, I dare expose what I understand in these commentaries. Things are related to each other through logical reasoning so that like branches of a tree, diversified as they are, they nevertheless come out of a single trunk. If we elucidated by prose and illustrated by pictures, then we may be able to attain conciseness as well as comprehensiveness, clarity as well as rigor. Looking at a part we will understand the rest." (Siu, 1993, p. 355). This is a clear message of the balanced employment of rigorous argument and heuristic reasoning with an aim of achieving enhanced understanding. For more illustrative examples, readers can consult (Siu, 1993).

Beginning with the Sui Dynasty (隋, 581 – 618), a comprehensive official system of education was established, further consolidated in the Tang Dynasty (唐, 681 – 907) and the Song Dynasty (宋, 960 – 1279). There was a well-planned curriculum, including the syllabus and the adopted textbooks, for each of several chosen disciplines. The institutional setting for these chosen disciplines was documented down to the quota of student enrollment, the number of the teaching and administrative staff, and the criteria for admission. State examinations for these chosen disciplines were held regularly and successful candidates were appointed to official posts according to merit in their performance at examinations. As explained in Section 1 of this chapter, we will confine our attention only to the discipline of mathematics as recorded in chronicles about the official system in the Tang Dynasty. This will be discussed in Sections 3 and 5.

Although the official system of education was furthered consolidated and expanded in the Song Dynasty, in the discipline of mathematics there was, however, a decline, with the exception of a strengthening of curriculum in calendarial reckoning and astronomy/astrology. Subsequently, mathematics was even removed as a subject altogether from the state examinations, and was never reinstated in the next several dynasties. From the beginning of the 17th century onwards, mathematical development in China began to come under foreign influence through large-scale contact with Western mathematics, first during the late Ming Dynasty (明, 1368 – 1644), then during the early Qing Dynasty (清, 1616 – 1911) and again during the final quarter of the Qing Dynasty in the mid 19th century. As Chinese mathematics entered its modern era and gradually fused with a more universal mathematics (universal in the sense that it is practiced and studied along a certain trend and style in countries which play a dominant role in world politics and in cultural influence), mathematics education in China became basically not too different from that of most other (Western) countries (For more references on mathematics education in ancient China, see F. Chen, 2002; S. Ding & Z.-G. Zhang, 1989; Jin, 1990; H. Li, 1994; Y. Li, 1954-55; Lin, 1997; D. Liu, 1993; Z. Ma, H. Wang, Sun, & Y. Wang, 1991; Mei & S. Li, 1992; Siu, 1995; Wu, 1997; Xie & D. Tang, 1995; Yan, 1965; L. Zhao, 1991).

Readers should note that mathematical knowledge was also transmitted in ancient China through channels other than the official school system. In the prefaces to some mathematical classics, references were made to learning from a master or even from a hermit or by self-education. Some historians of science argue that transmission through a religious network might play a considerable part (Needham, 1959; Volkov, 1996). Although the official system did produce tens of thousands of capable "mathocrats" who were employed as officials or imperial astronomers, almost all the eminent mathematicians who left their footprints in the history of mathematics seem to have been nurtured through other channels. An historian of mathematics once listed 50 Chinese mathematicians of fame who flourished between the 4th century B.C. and the end of the 19th century, with only two who can be labeled as educated in the official system (S. R. Guo, 1991).

Before closing this section, let us look at an unusual treatise which contains perhaps the first paper on mathematics education in China. The treatise was *cheng chu tong bian ben mo* (乘除通变本末, alpha and omega of variations on multiplication and division) written by the Song mathematician YANG Hui (杨辉) in 1274. The preface to the first chapter of the book is titled *xi suan gang mu* (习算纲目, A General Outline of Mathematical Studies). It offers a re-organized syllabus of the traditional curriculum accompanied by a time-table of a comprehensive study programme which takes only 260 days. This is comparable to a modern programme of about 1500 hours in secondary school mathematics. (Compare with the 7-year programme in the official system, which will be discussed in Section 3!) It is interesting and instructive to look at a few passages in this book, which explain quite well that rote learning is not to be equated with repetitive learning, and that doing a large number of exercises, is not incompatible with acquiring deep understanding. (The translated texts in the treatise of YANG Hui quoted below are taken from Lam [1977]. See also Zhou [1990].)

"In the *jia* (加, addition) method the number is increased, while in the *jian* (减, subtraction) method a certain number is taken away. Whenever there is addition there is subtraction. One who learns the 'subtraction' method should test the result by applying the 'addition' method to the answer of the problem. This will enable one to understand the method to its origin. Five days are sufficient for revision." (Book I, Chapter 1)

"In knowing the *jiu gui* (九归, tables of division) one will need at least five to seven days to become familiar with the recitation of the forty-four sentences. However if one examines carefully the explanatory notes of the art on 'tables of division' in the *xiang jie suan fa* (详解算法, a detailed analysis of the methods of computation — a lost treatise by YANG Hui), one can then understand the inner meaning of the process and a single day will suffice for committing the tables and their applications to memory. Revise the subject on 'tables of division' for one day." (Book I, Chapter 1)

"Learn a method a day and work on the subject for two months. It is essential to inquire into the origins of the applications of the methods so that they will not be forgotten for a long time." (Book I, Chapter 1)

"The working of a problem is selected from various methods, and the method should suit the problem. In order that a method is to be clearly understood, it should be illustrated by an example. If one meets a problem, its method must be carefully chosen .... If numerical exercises are performed daily, this establishes a quicker insight into analyzing a problem and hence is beneficial to all." (Book I, Chapter 3)

"It is difficult to see the logic and method behind complicated problems. Simple problems are hereby given and elucidated.

Once these are understood, problems, however difficult, will become clear." (Book II)

3 Official Curriculum in Mathematics in the Tang Dynasty

By the time mathematics was established as one of the disciplines of study in the official system in the Tang Dynasty, Chinese mathematics already enjoyed a scholarly tradition with a long history. In the middle of the 7th century, the mathematician LI Chunfeng (李淳风) collated the *suan jing shi shu* (算经十书, Ten Mathematical Manuals) at an Imperial Order, and it was adopted as the official textbook in the School of Mathematics in 656. The 'Ten Mathematical Manuals' comprised ten classics compiled by different authors at different times, listed below roughly in chronological order: (1) *zhou bi suan jing* (周髀算经, The Arithmetical Classic of the Gnomon and the Circular Paths), 100 B.C., (2) 'Nine Chapters on the Mathematical Art' 100 B.C. to 100A.D., (3) *hai dao suan jing* (海岛算经, Sea Island Mathematical Manual), 3rd century, (4) *wu cao suan jing* (五曹算经, Mathematical Manual of the Five Government Departments), 6th century, (5) *sun zi suan jing* (孙子算经, Master Sun's Mathematical Manual), 4th century, (6) *xia hou yang suan jing* (夏侯阳算经, Xia Hou Yang's Mathematical Manual), 5th century, (7) *zhang qiu jian suan jing* (张丘建算经, Zhang Qiu Jian's Mathematical Manual), 5th century, (8) *wu jing suan shu* (五经算术, Arithmetic in the Five Classics), 6th century, (9) *qi gu suan jing* (缉古算经, Continuation of Ancient Mathematics), 7th century, (10) *zhui shu* (缀术, Art of Mending), 5th century. The original text of 'Art of Mending' was lost in about the 10th century. Its role in the 'Ten Mathematical Manuals' was subsequently replaced in the Song Dynasty by *shu shu ji yi* (数术记遗, Memoir on Some Traditions of the Mathematical Art), a book of doubtful 6th century authorship. (The original texts of (1) to (9) can be found in many references, for instance, S. C. Guo [1993].) It is recorded in *xin tang shu* (新唐书, The New History of the Tang Dynasty) and *tang liu dian* (唐六典, The Six Codes of the Tang Dynasty) how these ten books were studied with specified duration. Students were divided into two programs, which for convenience will be denoted by A and B for short in this chapter. Students in Program A studied (1) to (8), *viz* 'Master Sun's Mathematical Manual' and 'Mathematical Manual of the Five Government Departments' for 1 year, 'Nine Chapters on the Mathematical Art' and 'Sea Island Mathematical Manual' for 3 years, 'Zhang Qiu Jian's Mathematical Manual' for 1 year, 'Xia Hou Yang's Mathematical Manual' for 1 year, 'The Arithmetical Classic of the Gnomon and the Circular Paths' and 'Arithmetic in the Five Classics' for 1 year. Students in Program B studied (9) to (10), *viz* 'Art of Mending' for 4 years, and 'Continuation of Ancient Mathematics' for 3 years. In addition to these books, students in each of the two programs must also study two more manuals, *shu shu ji yi* (数术记遗, Memoir on Some Traditions of the Mathematical Art) and *san deng shu* (三等数, Three Hierarchies of Numbers). (The last manual was written not later than the mid 6th century but was lost by the Song Dynasty.) Regular examinations were held throughout the seven years of study, and at the end of each year an annual examination was held. Any student who failed thrice or who had spent nine years at the School of Mathematics would be discontinued. Judging from the age of admission at 14 to 19 years old, we know that a mathematics student would sit for the state examination at around 22 (For a more detailed discussion, see Siu & Volkov, 1999).

Although mathematics was included as one discipline in the official system, it received rather low regard. For instance, it was recorded in 'The New History of the Tang Dynasty' that 2 professors of mathematics and 1 teaching assistant of mathematics were appointed with 15 students admitted each year in each of Program A and Program B, while in the discipline of the classics 5 professors and 5 teaching assistants were appointed with 300 students admitted each year. If the number of the faculty and that of the student enrollment in itself do not bespeak the significance accorded to a discipline, the rank and salary of the faculty would. It was recorded in 'The New History of the Tang Dynasty' that a professor in mathematics was appointed as an official of the lowest rank (grade 30) while a teaching assistant was appointed with no official rank at all. But a professor in classics was appointed as an official of high rank (grade 11) and even a teaching assistant in classics was appointed as an official of only a slightly lower rank (grade 17)!

4 State Examination in the Tang Dynasty

The Chinese term for state examination is *keju* (科舉), which means literally "subject-recommendation", i.e., recommendation of suitable candidates (for taking up official positions) through examinations in different subjects. Some historians date the beginning of the *keju* system to the Sui Dynasty when the emperor convened a state examination by decree. But some historians maintain that it started in 622 when the first Tang emperor decreed that any qualified candidate could sit for the state examination without having to be recommended by a provincial magistrate. As we will soon see, initially the *keju* system was a rather lively and efficient means for searching out and selecting capable persons to serve the country, based on their academic merit rather than their social background or hereditary aristocracy. However, in the long span of near to thirteen centuries of the operation of this system through different dynasties, it degenerated in later centuries into a kind of straitjacket of the mind which bred rote learning and a pedantic mindset. The *keju* system was abolished in 1905 by an imperial edict towards the end of the last imperial dynasty in China, the Qing Dynasty (Franke, 1968; Jin, 1990; H.-F. Liu, 1996; Wu, 1997; Xie & D. Tang, 1995; Yang, Zhu, & H. Zhang, 1992).

"One of China's most significant contributions to the world has been the creation of her system of civil service administration, and of the examinations which from 622 to 1905 served as the core of the system." (Kracke, 1947, p. 103). Indeed, as early as in the beginning of the 17th century, the Jesuit Father, Matteo Ricci, reported with commendation in his journal "the progress the Chinese have made in literature and in the sciences, and of the nature of the academic degrees which they are accustomed to confer" (Ricci, 1615/1953). Voltaire (F.M. Arouet) made a similar observation in the mid 18th century, "The human mind certainly cannot imagine a government better than this one where everything is to be decided by the large tribunals, subordinated to each other, of which the members are received only after several severe examinations. Everything in China regulates itself by these tribunals." (Voltaire, 1756/1878, p. 162). Dr. Sun Yat-Sen, founder of the Republic of China in 1911, said in The *Five-Power Constitution*, "At present, the civil service examination in the (Western) nations is copied largely from England. But when we trace the history further, we find that the civil service of England was copied from China. We have very good reason to believe that the Chinese examination system was the earliest and the most elaborate system in the world." (Teng, 1942-43, p. 267). Dr. Sun even instituted the division of the government structure into five-powers, *viz* the Legislative Yuan, the Executive Yuan, the Judicial Yuan, the Examination Yuan and the Censorate.

Detailed official records of the *keju* system (in the Tang Dynasty) can be found in certain ancient chronicles, among which the main primary sources are:

> *jiu tang shu* (旧唐书, Old History of the Tang Dynasty), 941–945;
>
> *xin tang shu* (新唐书, New History of the Tang Dynasty), 1044–1058;
>
> *tang liu dian* (唐六典, Six Codes of the Tang Dynasty), 738;
>
> *tong dian* (通典, Complete Structure of Government), 770–801;
>
> *tang hui yao* (唐会要, Collection of Important Documents of the Tang Dynasty), 961.

One informative secondary source which contains the main excerpts of relevant interest in the chronicles listed above plus a lot more of interesting information and anecdotes is the *deng ke ji kao* (登科记考, Journal on the Examinations in the Tang Dynasty) compiled by the Qing Scholar XU Song (徐松) in 1838. (Most of the anecdotes given in this section can be found in this book (S. Xu, 1838/1984).) In Western literature one of the earliest works on the state examination system in the Tang Dynasty is that of the famed French sinologist Edouard Biot, who did not seem to have a high regard for the official curriculum. He claimed that "the name of School of Mathematics is too high-sounding for the studies in this elementary establishment" and that the adopted textbooks were "collections of problems which are for the most part elementary and whose solutions are given without proofs" (Biot, 1847/1969, pp. 257, 262). The first comprehensive account in a Western language of the state examination system in the Tang Dynasty, together with a reliable translation of the relevant documents, was provided by Robert des Rotours in 1932 (des Rotours, 1932).

In 'The New History of the Tang Dynasty', a section on recruitment by examinations records that there were two kinds of state examinations: (1) regular examinations held annually in the first or second lunar month for graduates of colleges and universities or for provincial candidates, (2) special examinations held by imperial decree. The second kind depended on the need at the time or on the whim of the emperor, so it covered a wide range of expertise, but could also sound rather strange. In official records, one can find about a hundred of such special examinations. Just to cite a few, there were: examination on "vast erudition and great composition", examination on "deep knowledge of the ancient books and great talents in the art of teaching", examination on "having military plans with foresight and well qualified as a general", examination on "wisdom and good nature, rectitude and righteousness, and speaking honestly and remonstrating insistently", examination on "remarkable understanding of the art of government and suitability for administering people". A most amusing item is examination on "leading an hermetic life at Qiuyuan, not seeking fame", since logically speaking one should be awarded a degree in that if and only if one should not be! (In fact, it was recorded in 'Journal on the Examinations in the Tang Dynasty' that somebody was awarded the degree *in absentia* in 794 as he refused to receive it!) For the first kind there were initially seven subjects: examination on perfect talent, examination on classics, examination on distinguished man of letters, examination on accomplished man of letters, examination on law, examination on calligraphy and examination on mathematics. Examination on perfect talent was soon abolished, while examination on accomplished man of letters became in time the main focus enjoying the highest prestige. It was recorded in 'Complete Structure of Government' that by 752, of a thousand candidates who sat for the annual examination on accomplished man of letters only one or two were awarded the degree, while for instance, successful candidates for the examination on classics numbered in the tens. A source of the time said that one who passed the examination on accomplished man of letters at fifty (perhaps after many repeated attempts) was still regarded as outstanding, while one who passed the examination on classics at thirty was considered too old already! No similar data or remark is found for examination on mathematics, which again serves to indicate that mathematics was accorded a lower prestige among the various subjects, only on a par with calligraphy. This becomes even more apparent when we look at the number of students enrolled at the state university. Tang institutions of higher education were divided into hierarchies. The highest institution was the School for the Sons of the State which accepted only sons of noblemen or officials from a certain rank upward. Next came the National University which accepted a similar crop with the official rank somewhat lowered. Then came the School of Four Gates which accepted, besides sons of officials, also a small number of sons of ordinary citizens. The three Schools of Law, Calligraphy and Mathematics accepted sons of officials of low rank and of ordinary citizens. In the early Tang Dynasty, according to the 'New History of the Tang Dynasty', there were 300 students in the School for the Sons of the State, 500 students in the National University, 1300 students in the School of Four Gates, 50 students in the Law School, 30 students in the Calligraphy School and 30 students in the Mathematics School. At one time, throughout the whole empire, including the provincial colleges, there were 8000 students pursuing higher education, with foreign students coming from nearby countries as well. The whole edifice of state higher education was very well-established in the Tang Dynasty.

The culminating apex of this edifice, the annual state examination, was a grueling experience for many. Some authors in the Tang Dynasty wrote about how candidates stood in a long queue, carrying their own stationery, supply of food and water, candles and charcoal (for preparing meals and for getting warmth), waiting to be admitted to their cells, only to be searched and shouted at by guards who were stationed by the thorny hedge (an ancient analogue of barbed-wire fence) which encompassed the examination venue. Candidates were clad in flimsy clothes and shivered in the freezing weather, for they were not allowed thick clothing to prevent concealment of manuscripts. Throughout the long hours they worked on their examination scripts, the candidates were confined to their cells, in which they would prepare their own meals and take care of their own personal hygiene. In the case of failure in the examination, which was not uncommon, this grueling experience would have to be repeated in another year, and perhaps in yet another year, ... WEI Chengyi (韦承贻), who was awarded the degree of accomplished man of letters in 867, once sneaked into the office of the Ministry of Rites called Nangong, which was in charge of examination affairs, and composed a poem on the wall: "Like a thousand white lotus petals, /The candles lit up the hall, /Which was filled with the peaceful rhymes/Of the Ya and the Song./As the flame of the third candle/Flickered towards its end, /One realized it meant failure/To complete the scene of Nangong." (白莲千朵照廊明。一片升平雅颂声。才唱第三条烛尽。南宫风景画难成。) This poem, with its trace of resignation, depicted vividly those assiduous candidates racing against time with their examination scripts by the light of the three candles allowed them to last through the night.

Modern examinations are definitely much less grueling than that. However, it would be unfair to his ancestors in the Tang Dynasty if the author fails to point out that even over a thousand years ago some good modern examination procedures were already in place. In 759 the Chief Examiner LI Kui (李揆) said, "The empire selects its officials for their talent. The requisite classics are displayed here. Candidates are welcome to consult them at will." This was perhaps the earliest open-book examination! In 742 the Chief Examiner WEI Zhi (韦陟) said, "The performance of a candidate in one single examination may not reflect his true potential, hence his previous essays should also be consulted." This was perhaps the earliest instance of assessment by project work and portfolio! A famous example is the work presented by BAI Juyi (白居易) to the Chief Examiner GU Kuang (顾况). BAI Juyi was awarded the degree of the accomplished man of letters in 800 at a rare early age of 27, and is remembered today as a renowned poet of the 9th century. The "project work" he presented is handed down as one of his very well-known and oft-quoted poems which begins (translated text taken from Y. Xu & Yuan, 2000): "Grass on the plain spreads higher and higher; /Year after year it fades and grows./ It can't be burned up by wild fire, / But revives when the spring wind blows./ ..." (离离原上草。一岁一枯荣。野火烧不尽。春风吹又生。)

5 State Examination in Mathematics in the Tang Dynasty

In the state examination for either Program A or B, in mathematics, the candidate was examined on two types of question. The first type was described in the 'New History of the Tang Dynasty' as: "[The candidates should] write [a composition on] the general meanings, taking as the basic/original task a 'problem and answer'. [They should] elucidate the numbers/ computations, [and] construct an algorithm. [They should] elucidate the structure/principle of the algorithm in detail." (録大义本条为问答。明数造术。详明术理。) For Program B there was added the remark, "If there is no commentary, [the candidates should] make the numbers/computations correspond [to the right ones?] in constructing the algorithm." (无注者合数造术。不失义理。) (For an attempt to explain the latter remark, see Siu and Volkov, 1999.) We will say more about this type of question in Section 6. The second type of question was testing on quotations known as *tie du* (帖读, strip reading). Candidates were shown a line taken from either *shu shu ji yi* or *san deng shu*, with three characters covered up. Candidates had to answer what those three characters were. In to-day's terminology, this type of questions is called "fill in the blank". It is interesting to note that the 'Memoir on Some Traditions of the Mathematical Art' is a short text with only 934 characters, which could be committed to memory with reasonable ease (not to mention that a candidate had seven years to do it!). There may well be other reasons for singling out this book for the purpose of testing on quotations, but that would be the subject of another paper. (See Volkov [1994] for an interesting discussion on the content of 'Memoir on Some Traditions of the Mathematical Art') The book 'Three Hierarchies of Numbers' was lost by the Song Dynasty (960 – 1279). We can only surmise that it might be a text similar to the 'Memoir on Some Traditions of the Mathematical Art' in this respect.

By the way, there was a reason for instituting the practice of testing on quotations. The practice was proposed by the Chief Examiner LIU Sili (刘思立) in 681 (in all subjects) to rectify the deficiency of a prevalent habit of candidates who only studied "model answers" to past questions instead of studying the original classics. Testing on quotations forced candidates to read (at least some) original classics. However, examination being what it is, it is prone to abuse. The setting of questions on quotations got more and more difficult and unreasonable, testing candidates on obscure phrases, sometimes even setting up traps to confound the candidate intentionally. In response, candidates collected such obscurities and memorized them for the sole purpose of passing those unreasonable tests! The laudable purpose of encouraging candidates to read the original classics was totally defeated. In 728 it was decreed that quotations should be set within reasonable bounds. There is a good lesson to be learnt here about making use of examination to direct the curriculum.

6 A "Re-constructed" Examination Question

Since no trace of any examination question is extant, but there is a reference to tasks on elucidation and construction in the state examination in mathematics, we will attempt to "re-construct" some examination questions to lend evidence in support of the thesis that the curriculum in mathematics in the Tang Dynasty was not so elementary nor was it learnt by rote. It is hard to imagine that a group of selected young men spent seven of their golden years in simply memorizing the mathematical classics one by one without understanding just to regurgitate the answers in the state examination at the end! If readers are of the opinion that imagination should have no place in historical study, the author will insert an (apologetic?) self-defense at this point by referring to a wider (but somewhat controversial) view of studying history as propounded by the British philosopher-historian Collingwood (Collingwood, 1946, p. 202), "History is thus the self-knowledge of the living mind. ... For history is not contained in books or documents; it lives only, as a present interest and pursuit, in the mind of the historian when he criticizes and interprets those documents, and by so doing relives for himself the states of mind into which he inquires." Collingwood echoed the view held by the Italian philosopher Croce who said in (Croce, 1919/1920, p. 19), "History is living chronicle, chronicle is dead history; history is contemporary history, chronicle is past history; history is principally an act of thought, chronicle an act of will. Every history becomes chronicle when it is no longer thought, but only recorded in abstract words, which were once upon a time concrete and expressive."

Before giving examples, it is helpful to look at a typical textbook and see how the author did mathematics. Which better choice can one pick than the prime textbook 'Nine Chapters on the Mathematical Art' (with English translation in Shen, Crossley, and Lun, 1999)? With the commentaries by the 3rd centu ry mathematician LIU Hui added, this provides more "circumstantial evidence" for our thesis.

In Chapter 5 of the 'Nine Chapters on the Mathematical Art' some formulae for the volume of various solids are given. In particular, Problem 17 is about that of a tunnel at the entrance of a tomb (*xian chu* 羡除). Mathematically speaking, a *xian chu* is a solid bounded by three trapeziums and two triangles on the two sides. The three trapeziums have opposite parallel sides of length a, b; a, c and b, c, the depth is h and the trapezium on top has length l (see Figure 1).

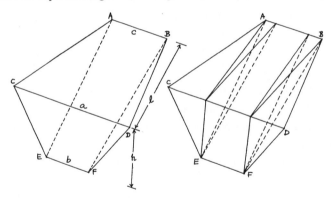

Figure 1.

The formula for the volume of the *xian chu* is given in the text as $V = \frac{1}{6}(a+b+c)hl$. (In the text, numerical data are given in place of a, b, c, but the numerical data are actually generic rather than special.) LIU Hui explains in his commentaries how the volume is calculated. He dissects the *xian chu* into smaller pieces, each of some standard shape such as a triangular prism (*qian du*, 堑堵), a tetrahedron of a particular type (*bie nao*, 鳖臑), or a pyramid with a square base (*yang ma*, 阳马). If you try to do that by yourself, you will find out that the way of dissection is different for different relations between a, b, c. For instance, if $a > c > b$, then you obtain two tetrahedron of a particular type each of volume $\frac{1}{12}(a - b)hl$, two tetrahedron of a particular type each of volume $\frac{1}{12}(c - b)hl$ and one triangle prism of volume $\frac{1}{2}bhl$ (see Figure 1). They add up to $\frac{1}{6}(a + b + c)hl$. But if $a > b > c$, then you obtain two tetrahedron of a particular type each of volume $\frac{1}{12}(a - b)hl$, two pyramid with a square base each of volume $\frac{1}{6}(b - c)hl$ and one triangular prism of volume $\frac{1}{2}chl$. They also add up to $\frac{1}{6}(a + b + c)hl$. In fact, LIU Hui in his commentaries treats all eight different cases except the one case $b > a = c$. The calculation is different for different ways of dissection, but the basic underlying idea is the same. Probably candidates in the examination would be asked to carry out a similar explanation for other formulae on area and volume, possibly with given numerical data. Once the basic idea is understood, such a demand for elucidation is reasonable.

In the same chapter, Problem 10 is about the volume of a pavilion (*fang ting*, 方亭) with square base (see Figure 2).

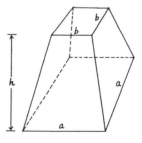

Figure 2.

Mathematically speaking, a *fang ting* is a truncated pyramid with square base. If a, b are the sides of the bottom and top squares respectively and h is the height, then the volume is given in the text as $V = \frac{1}{3}(a^2 + b^2 + ab)h$. Again, LIU Hui in his commentaries explains how to obtain the formula by an ingenious method of assembling blocks of standard shape (called by him *qi*, 棋). There are three kinds of *qi*: cube of side a with volume a^3 (*li fang*, 立方, LF); pyramid of square base of side a and one vertical side of length a perpendicular to the base, with volume $\frac{1}{3}a^3$ (*yang ma*, YM); triangular prism with isosceles right triangle of side a as base and height a, with volume $\frac{1}{2}a^3$ (*qian du*, QD).

He observes that the truncated pyramid is made up of one LF, four YM and four QD. (Careful readers will notice that here we require $h = b$, so that we are talking about blocks of a standard shape.) He then observes that one LF makes up a cube of volume b^2h; one LF and four QD make up a rectangular block of volume abh; one LF, eight QD and twelve YM make up a rectangular block of volume a^2h. (Careful readers will notice that here we require $h = b$ and $a = 3b$ so that each corner piece is a cube formed from three YM.) In problem 15, LIU Hui further explains how to obtain the more general formula of the volume of a pyramid of rectangular base with an arbitrary height by an infinitesimal argument (Wagner, 1979). Altogether, three LF, twelve QD and twelve YM make up a volume $b^2h + abh + a^2h$. Hence the volume of the truncated pyramid is $\frac{1}{3}(a^2 + b^2 + ab)h$ (see Figure 3).

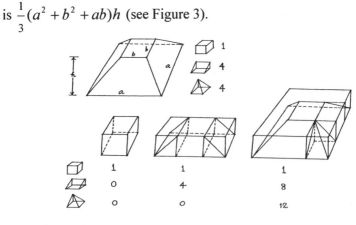

Figure 3.

LIU Hui gives an alternative formula $V = \frac{1}{3}(a-b)^2 h + abh$ by another way of dissection (see Figure 4).

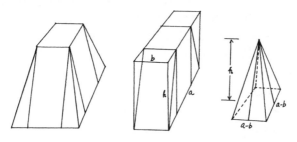

Figure 4.

In the second explanation, there is no need to assume $h = b$, $a = 3b$. But it works only when the bottom and top pieces are squares.

Here is a fictitious examination question: Compute the volume of an "oblong pavilion" of height h with bottom and top being rectangles of sides a_1, a_2 and b_1, b_2 respectively ($a_1 \neq a_2$, $b_1 \neq b_2$). If one understands the argument by LIU Hui, one can easily modify either method to arrive at the answer, which is left as an exercise for the readers. (Readers may also wish to solve the problem in a way commonly known to school pupils of today, *viz* by making use of similar triangles.) The answer turns out to be $V = \frac{1}{3}[a_1 a_2 + b_1 b_2 + \frac{1}{2}(a_1 b_2 + a_2 b_1)]h$. If one merely memorizes the formula given in the textbook by heart, it is not easy to hit upon the correct formula. This is probably what is meant by "constructing a (new) algorithm". Again, such a demand is reasonable, especially when these candidates might well be facing in their subsequent career problems which are variations (e.g., with parameters changed) of the problems they learnt in the textbooks.

7 Is the State Examination Really so Damaging to Learning?

The *ke ju* enjoys the strange ambivalence of being described as a rich cultural heritage as well as a scandalous historical burden of the Chinese, with its strength and shortcoming the subject of controversy to this date (Jin 1990; H.-F. Liu, 1996). We will not enter into another long debate here. To counteract the traditional view that the ancient Chinese studied mathematics only by rote memorization and industrious drilling, we will, however, "magnify" the more positive part of the system, which unfortunately was outweighed by its negative part, especially in later evolution in the Ming and Qing dynasties.

It is strange that a popular view is to equate Confucian learning with rote learning and with submissive learning despite what the Masters themselves had said. (The following translated texts are taken from Legge [1893/1960].) In the 'Confucian Analects' (论语, 5th century B.C.) we find, "Learning without thought is labor lost; thought without learning is perilous." In the 'Doctrine of the Mean' (中庸, 6th-5th century B.C.) we find, "He who attains to sincerity, is he who chooses what is good, and firmly holds it fast. To this attainment there are requisite the extensive study of what is good, accurate inquiry about it, careful reflection on it, the clear discrimination of it, and the earnest practice of it." In the books by the leading neo-Confucian scholar ZHU Xi (朱熹) (1130 – 1200) we find (all translated texts from the books of ZHU Xi quoted below are taken from [Gardner, 1990]), "In reading, if you have no doubts, encourage them. And if you do have doubts, get rid of them. Only when you've reached this point have you made progress." (Book 11, p. 151). Would one call this rote-learning? submissive learning? By reading more extensively in the books by ZHU Xi, we can perhaps understand better what appears to Western observers as rote-learning actually consists of. ZHU Xi said, "Generally speaking, in reading, we must first become intimately familiar with the text so that its words seem to come from our own mouths. We should then continue to reflect on it so that its ideas seem to come from our own minds. Only then can there be real understanding. Still, once our intimate reading of it and careful reflection on it have led to a clear understanding of it, we must continue to question. Then there might be additional progress. If we cease questioning, in the end there'll be no additional progress." (Book 10, p. 135). He also elaborated further, "Learning is reciting. If we recite it then think it over, think it over then recite it, naturally it'll become meaningful to us. If we recite it but don't think it over, we still won't appreciate its meaning. If we think it over but don't recite it, even though we might understand it, our understanding will be precarious. ... Should we recite it to the point of intimate familiarity, and moreover think about it in detail, naturally our mind and principle will become one and never shall we forget what we have read." (Book 10, p. 138). This is an unmistakable differentiation between repetitive learning and rote learning. Contemporary researchers explain the Asian Learner Paradox based on this differentiation (Biggs, 1996; Marton, Dall'Alba, & Tse, 1996).

On the other hand, modern day education in the Western world which arose in the 19th century along with the Industrial Revolution started by emphasizing the 3Rs — reading, writing and arithmetic. In a code issued by Robert Lowe of the Education Department of England in 1862, specific standards for each R were explicitly stated (e.g. Standard I in Reading: Narrative monosyllables; Standard II in Writing: Copy in manuscript character a line of print; Standard IV in Arithmetic: A sum in compound rules [money]) (Curtis, 1967, Chapter VII). The emphasis on mechanical rote learning is captured vividly in the opening sentences (which were intended as a satirical exaggeration) of the 1854 novel *Hard Times* by Charles Dickens (as words uttered by Mr. Gradgrind of Coketown)

"Now, what I want is, Facts. Teach these boys and girls nothing but Facts. Facts alone are wanted in life. ... This is the principle on which I bring up my own children, and this is the principle on which I bring up these children. Stick to Facts, sir!" (Dickens, 1854/1995, p. 9)

About the preparation for state examinations, ZHU Xi has also left us with the following passages (all translated texts from the books of ZHU Xi quoted below are taken from Gardner [1990]):

"Scholars must first distinguish between the examinations and studying, which is less important, which is more important. If 70 percent of their determination is given to study and 30 percent to the examinations, that'll be fine. But if 70 percent is given to the examinations and 30 percent to study, they're sure to be overcome by the 70 percent." (Book 13, p. 191)

"Preparing for the examinations doesn't harm one's studying. Previous generations, when did they ever refrain from taking the examinations? It's simply because people today don't settle their minds that harm is done. As soon as their minds become fixed on success or failure in the examinations, their understanding of the words they read is all wrong." (Book 13, p. 194)

"He was once discussing the examinations and said: It isn't that the examinations are a trouble to men, it's that men become troubled by the examinations. A scholar of superior understanding reads the texts of the sages and worthies and on the basis of his understanding of them writes the essays required in the examinations. He places aside considerations of success and failure, gain and loss, so even if he were to compete in the examination every day he wouldn't be troubled by them. If Confucius were born again in today's world, he wouldn't avoid competing in the examinations, and yet they wouldn't trouble him in the least." (Book 13, p. 194).

Over 800 years ago the Chinese sages already knew that the main shortcoming of examination does not come from the examination itself but from the high stakes it brings with it!

Granted that an examination is not to be passed through rote learning, what good will an examination bring? Let us first compare the ancient Chinese examination format with a modern theory on assessment by Bloom (Bloom, 1956). The modern viewpoint includes both the formative and the summative aspects of assessment, while the ancient Chinese examination focused only on the latter function for selection purposes. The six major classes of taxonomy of Bloom can be matched up with the four different types of question in the ancient Chinese examination, *viz* (i) testing on quotations is about knowledge, (ii) short questions are about comprehension and application, (iii) long questions (on contemporary affairs) are about analysis and synthesis, (iv) composition and poems are about evaluation (H.-F. Liu, 1996, p. 240).

With these varied objectives, an examination can have a beneficial influence on both the student and the teacher, even as a summative process. For the student it is good for consolidation of knowledge, enhancement of comprehension, planning of schedule of study, judgment on what is important to learn, development of learning strategies and motivation and self-perception of competence. For the teacher, besides what has been said above, it is good for monitoring the progress of the class, as a gauge of the receptivity and assimilation of the class and evaluation of the teaching. In this sense, "examination-oriented education" and "quality education" need not be a dichotomy. Crooks says, "As educators we must ensure that we give appropriate emphasis in our evaluations to the skills, knowledge, and attitudes that we perceive to be most important." (Crooks, 1988, p. 470). Viewed in the summative aspect, an examination is a necessary evil. But viewed in the formative aspect, an examination can be a useful part of the learning process. Moreover, it is a false dichotomy to differentiate strictly summative assessment and formative assessment. The important thing to keep in mind is not to let the assessment tail wag the educational dog! (C. Tang & Biggs, 1996, p. 159) The demise of the examination system in Imperial China, even with its initial good intention and with its long life span of 1287 years, is a lesson to be learnt from.

References

Biggs, J. B. (1996). Western misperceptions of the Confucian-heritage learning culture. In D. A. Watkins & J. B. Biggs (Eds.), *The Chinese Learner: Cultural, psychological and contextual influences* (pp. 45-67). Hong Kong: Comparative Education Research Centre, The University of Hong Kong; Melbourne, Australia: Australian Council for Education Research.

Biot, E. (1969). *Essai sur l'histoire de l'instruction publique en Chine, et de la corporation des lettrés, depuis les anciens temps jusqu'à nos jours: Ouvrage entièrement rédigé d'après les documents chinois* [Essay on the history of state education and the literati in China from ancient time to the present: Work written entirely depending on Chinese documents]. Paris: Benjamin Duprat. (Reprinted, 1847, Taipei: Chéng Wen Publ. Co.)

Bloom, B. S. (Ed.) (1956). *Taxonomy of educational objectives, The classification of educational goals, handbook I: Cognitive domain.* London: Longman.

Cai, J. (1995). *A cognitive analysis of U.S. and Chinese students' mathematical performance on tasks involving computation, simple problem solving and complex problem solving.* Reston: National Council of Teachers of Mathematics.

Chen, F. (2002). *Investigation on the part of exposé in state examinations in the Tang Dynasty* [In Chinese 唐代试策考述]. Beijing: Zhonghua Book Company.

Chen, G., & Deng, H. (1997). *Investigation on the system of Shuyuan in China* [In Chinese 中国书院制度研究]. Hangzhou: Zhejiang Educational Press.

Collingwood, R. G. (1946). *The idea of history.* Oxford: Clarendon Press.

Croce, B. (1919/1920). *History: Its theory and practice* (translated from the 2nd edition in Italian). New York: Russell & Russell.

Crooks, T. J. (1988). The impact of classroom evaluation practice on students. *Review of Educational Research, 58*, 438-481.

Curtis, S. J. (1967). *History of education in Great Britain* (7th ed.). London: University Tutorial Press.

des Rotours, R. (1932). *Le traité des examens, traduits de la Nouvelle histoire des T'ang* [Treatise on examinations, translated from 'New History of the Tang Dynasty']. Paris: Librairie Ernest Leroux.

Dickens, C. (1995). *Hard times.* London: Penguin Books. (Original work published 1854)

Ding, G., & Liu, Q. (1992). *The Shuyuan and Chinese culture* [In Chinese 书院与中国文化]. Shanghai: Shanghai Educational Press.

Ding, S., & Zhang, Z.-G. (1989). *Mathematics and education* [In Chinese 数学与教育]. Changsha: Hunan Educational Press.

Franke, W. (1968). *The reform and abolition of the traditional Chinese examination system,* Cambridge: Harvard University Press.

Gardner, D. K. (1990). *Learning to be a sage: Selections from the conversations of Master Chu, Arranged topically.* Berkeley: University of California Press.

Guo, S. C. (Ed.) (1993). *Collection of Chinese classics in science and technology (mathematics)* [In Chinese 中国科学技术典籍通汇(数学卷)] (Vol. 1-5). Zhengzhou: Henan Educational Press.

Guo, S. R. (1991). On the mathematics and astronomy education at state institutions in ancient China [In Chinese 论中国古代的国家天算教育]. In D. Li (Ed.), *Collected papers on research in the history of mathematics* [In Chinese 数学史研究文集] (Vol. 2, pp. 27-30). Huhehaote: Neimenggu University Press.

Jin, Z. (1990). *The Keju examination system and Chinese culture* [In Chinese 科举制度与中国文化]. Shanghai: Shanghai Peoples' Press.

Kracke, E. A., Jr. (1947). Family vs merit in Chinese civil service examinations under the empire. *Harvard Journal of Asiatic Studies, 10*, 103-123.

Lam, L. (1977). *A critical study of the Yang Hui Suan Fa.* Singapore: University of Singapore Press.

Legge, J. (1960). *The Chinese classics, Volume I: Confucian analects, the great learning, the doctrine of the mean* (3rd ed.). Oxford: Clarendon Press. (Reprinted, 1893, Hong Kong: Hong Kong University Press.)

Leung, F. K. S. (2001). In search of an East Asian identity in mathematics education. *Educational Studies in Mathematics, 47*, 35-51.

Li, H. (1994). *Education and examination in the state system of the Song Dynasty* [In Chinese 宋代官学教育与科举]. Taipei: Lian Jing Publishers.

Li, Y. (1954-55). *Collection of essays on history of ancient Chinese mathematics* [In Chinese 中算史论丛] (Rev. ed.). Beijing: Science Press.

Lin, Y. (1997). Evolution of the mathematics curriculum in China [In Chinese 中国数学课程的演变]. *Mathmedia* [In Chinese 数学传播], *21*(3), 31-44.

Liu, D. (1993). *Great indeed is the art of numbering* [In Chinese 大哉言数]. Shengyang: Liaoning Educational Press.

Liu, H.-F. (1996). *The Keju examination from an educational perspective* [In Chinese 科举考试的教育视角]. Hankou: Hubei Educational Press.

Ma, L. (1999). *Knowing and teaching elementary mathematics: Teachers' understanding of fundamental mathematics in China and the United States.* Mahwah, NJ: Lawrence Erlbaum Associates.

Ma, Z., Wang, H., Sun, H., & Wang, Y. (1991). *A concise history of mathematics education* [In Chinese 数学教育史简编]. Nanning: Guangxi Educational Press.

Marton, F., Dall'Alba, G., & Tse, L. K. (1996). Memorizing and understanding: The keys to the paradox. In D. A. Watkins & J. B. Biggs (Eds.), *The Chinese learner: cultural, psychological and contextual influences* (pp. 69-83). Hong Kong: Comparative Education Research Centre, The University of Hong Kong; Melbourne, Australia: Australian Council for Education Research.

Mei, R., & Li, S. (1992). *History of science and technology education in China* [In Chinese 中国科技教育史]. Changsha: Hunan Educational Press.

Needham, J. (with the collaboration of L. Wang). (1959). *Science and civilization in China, Volume 3: Mathematics and the sciences of the heavens and the earth.* Cambridge: Cambridge University Press.

Peng, H. (2001). *Commentary on the Suanshu Shu, a book of Han bamboo strips found at Zhang Jiashan* [In Chinese 张家山汉简《算数书》注释]. Beijing: Science Press.

Ricci, M. (1953). *China in the sixteenth century: The journals of Matthew Ricci, 1583-1610* (L. J. Gallagher, Trans.). New York: Random House. (Original work complied by N. Trigault, 1615)

Shen, K., Crossley, J. N., & Lun, A. W. C. (1999). *The Nine Chapters on the mathematical art: Companion and commentary.* Oxford: Oxford University Press.

Siu, M. K. (1993). Proof and pedagogy in ancient China: Examples from Liu Hui's Commentary on Jiu Zhang Suan Shu. *Educational Studies in Mathematics, 24*, 345-357.

Siu, M. K. (1995). Mathematics education in ancient China: What lesson do we learn from it? *Historia Scientiarum, 4*(3), 223-232.

Siu, M. K. (2001). How did candidates pass the examination in mathematics in the Tang Dynasty (618-917)? — Myth of the "Confucian-Heritage-Culture" classroom. In P. Radelet-de Grave (Ed.), *Actes de la troisième d'été européenne sur l'histoire et l'épistémologie dans l'éducation mathématique* [Proceedings of the third European Summer University on the history and epistemology of mathematics educations] (pp. 320-334). Louvain-la-Neuve/Leuven: Université Catholique de Louvain/Katholieke Universiteit Leuven.

Siu, M. K., & Volkov, A. (1999). Official curriculum in traditional Chinese mathematics: How did candidates pass the examinations? *Historia Scientiarum, 9*(1), 85-99.

Stevenson, H. W., & Stigler, J. W. (1992). *The learning gap: Why our schools are failing and what we can learn from Japanese and Chinese education.* New York: Simon & Schuster.

Stigler, J. W., & Hiebert, J. (1999). *The teaching gap.* New York: Free Press.

Tang, C., & Biggs, J. B. (1996). How Hong Kong students cope with assessment. In D. A. Watkins & J. B. Biggs (Eds.), *The Chinese learner: Cultural, psychological and contextual influences* (pp. 159-182). Hong Kong: Comparative Education Research Centre, The University of Hong Kong; Melbourne, Australia: Australian Council for Education Research.

Teng, S. (1942-43). Chinese influence on the Western examination system. *Harvard Journal of Asiatic Studies, 7*, 267-312.

Volkov, A. (1994). Large numbers and counting rods. *Extrême-Orient, Extrême-Occident, 16*, 71-92.

Volkov, A. (1996). Science and Daoism: An introduction. *Taiwanese Journal for Philosophy and History of Science, 5*(1), 1-58.

Voltaire (F. M. Arouet). (1878). *Oeuvres complètes de Voltaire, t.13* [Complete works of Voltaire, Vol. 13]. Paris: Garnier Frères. (Original work published 1756)

Wagner, D. B. (1979). An early Chinese derivation of the volume of a pyramid: Liu Hui, third century A.D. *Historia Mathematica, 6*, 164-188.

Watkins, D. A., & Biggs, J. B. (Eds.) (1996). *The Chinese learner: Cultural, psychological and contextual influence.* Hong Kong: Comparative Education Research Centre, The University of Hong Kong; Melbourne, Australia: Australian Council for Education Research.

Watkins, D. A., & Biggs, J. B. (Eds.) (2001). *Teaching the Chinese learner: Psychological and pedagogical perspectives.* Hong Kong: Comparative Education Research Centre, The University of Hong Kong; Melbourne, Australia: Australian Council for Education Research.

Wong, N. Y. (1998). In search of the "CHC" learner: Smarter, works harder or something more? In *ICMI-EARCOME Proceedings* (Vol. 1, pp. 85-98). Cheongju: Korean National University of Education.

Wu, Z. (1997). *The state examination system in the Tang Dynasty* [In Chinese 唐代科举制度]. Shenyang: Liaoning University Press.

Xie, Q., & Tang, D. (Eds.) (1995). *History of the state examination system in China* [In Chinese 中国考试制度史]. Hefei: Huangshan Book Company.

Xu, S. (1984). *Journal on the examinations in the Tang Dynasty* [In Chinese 登科记考]. Beijing: Zhonghua Book Company. (Original work published 1838)

Xu, Y., & Yuan, X. (2000). *Gems of classical Chinese poetry.* Beijing: Zhonghua Book Company.

Yan, D. (1965). A brief history of mathematics education in China [In Chinese 中国数学教育简史]. *Mathematics Bulletin* [In Chinese 数学通报], *8*, 44-48; *9*, 46-50.

Yang, X., Zhu, Q., & Zhang, H. (1992). *Compilation of selected historical documents on the state examination system in China* [In Chinese 中国考试制度史资料选编]. Hefei: Huangshan Book Company.

Zhang, Z.-F. (1985). *A sketch of the history of the system of Shuyuan in China* [In Chinese 中国书院制度史略]. Nanjing: Jiangsu Educational Press.

Zhao, L. (1991). *A comparative study of the history of mathematics in the Oriental and Western worlds* [In Chinese 中西数学史的比较], Taipei: Commercial Press.

Zhao, S., & Xue, Z. (1995). *Journals and documents on Shuyuan in China throughout different dynasties* [In Chinese 中国历代书院志] (Vol. 16). Nanjing: Jiangsu Educational Press.

Zhou, D. (1990). A general outline of mathematical studies and Yang Hui's methodology of teaching mathematics [In Chinese 《习算纲目》与杨辉的数学教育思想]. *Journal of Central Normal University (Natural Sciences)* [In Chinese 华中师范大学学报 (自然科学版)], *24*(3), 396-399.

Section 2

CONTEXT AND
TEACHING MATERIALS

Chapter 7

The "Two Basics": Mathematics Teaching and Learning in Mainland China

ZHANG Dianzhou   LI Shiqi   TANG Ruifen

Mathematics education in eastern Asian countries emphasizes the importance of foundations, and in Mainland China the principle of "basic knowledge and basic skills" was explicitly put forward for the teaching of mathematics. This chapter analyzes in a detailed way the benefits and inadequacies of this principle and the practice arising from it from four aspects, namely, its historical roots and social environment, the goals of classroom teaching, teaching characteristics and underlying psychological principles, and education reforms and development in China. The different characteristics of Eastern and Western mathematics education can be complementary to each other, helping strike a balance between foundation and development concerning classroom teaching.

Key words: the "Two Basics" principle, basic knowledge, basic skills, mathematics teaching, mathematics learning, individual development

1   Introduction

Any theory of mathematics education would likely concern two aspects: first, help students gain the basic mathematics knowledge and skills; secondly, let students realize full individual development and foster their creative mathematical thinking. Success is ensured if both of them can be equally emphasized and appropriately interwoven. In fact, commenting on the well-known US NCTM *Standards* (National Council of Teachers of Mathematics, 1989), Bamberger (1998) once pointed out:

"Mathematics educators around the country felt that finally a balance had been struck between understanding concepts and learning skills, between meaningful problem solving and memorization of facts, and between real-life mathematics and experimenting with the patterns and relationships that exist in mathematics."

Due to historical and cultural reasons, eastern Asian countries, including Japan, Korea, Singapore, and China (Mainland China, Taiwan, Hong Kong and Macao), even Russia, emphasize more on the importance of laying foundation. Moreover, the principle of "basic knowledge and basic skills" ("Two Basics") is most typically observed in Mainland China.

A direct consequence of the implementation of the "Two Basics" principle in Mainland China is: acquiring the leading position in numerous international mathematics assessment and contests, for example, topping the accuracy rate in the International Assessment of Education Progress [IAEP] 1989 (Lapointe, Mead, & Askew, 1992), and achieving outstanding results in the past International Mathematics Olympiads (e.g., see Fan & Zhu, this volume).

This chapter will discuss the benefits and inadequacies of mathematics teaching and learning under the "Two Basics" principle in Mainland China.

2   Historical Roots and Social Environment for the "Two Basics" Principle in Mathematics Teaching

A good foundation is essential for the construction of a building. Hence, no one would deny the importance of a solid foundation. But the question is to what level or degree we should emphasize it. In this concern, people have different views and practice. Most Chinese mathematicians and mathematics educators believe that primary and secondary education are foundational education, and establishing a good foundation is the main task of mathematics education. This foundation can only be laid properly when one is young, or else it would be too late. Therefore it is of foremost importance that a good foundation should be laid during primary and secondary school years. Without a solid foundation, it is impossible to realize children's creativity, and ultimately let alone students' differentiated individual development. These beliefs were gradually formed under the influences of culture accumulated through thousands years of Chinese history.

Let us trace back to the factors of forming these beliefs about the foundation in China's traditional education.

First, China is in a sense one of few countries where human's ancient civilization has had a continuous existence. Thousand years of agricultural culture, especially culture developed from plantation of paddy-field crops, required detailed and crafty artifice. Given a small land area, farmers had to rely on well-practiced and efficient techniques to obtain maximum outputs. It was very different from a nomadic society's culture where people can make a living through the extension of rearing areas. Thus, in the Chinese society, to be equipped with effective and efficient "skills" is of vital importance for survival.

Secondly, Confucianism is the orthodox tradition of Chinese culture. In a very long time, Confucianism endorses a clan system, where obedience to the unified emperor is universally required. Individuals have less room for their self-creativity, compared to the West. This is also reflected in the learning process, with more emphasis being put on the uniformity of teaching contents as well as the requirements. The result is the existence of a unified foundation but a lack of individual development among students (Brand, 1987; Murphy, 1987; Wong, 1998).

Thirdly, the strict and unified examination systems have driven students to only learn the contents that will be tested in exams. The system of civil examinations in China can be traced back to as early as the year of 597. Through this system, even a peasant can become government official if he could pass the national examination. This was a highly fair and civilized policy at that time. It is hence rooted in the minds of Chinese that examination can determine one's life. After the Ming Dynasty, the test items used in the unified examinations by the government became "Bagu-oriented" (八股), which refers to a set of extremely condensed and procedure-fixed basic knowledge, and very stereotyped and sophisticated writing skills. Referring to the current mathematics examinations, most of the questions tested are also mathematics procedures and well-practiced skills. As examinations focus on the "basics", for the purpose of scoring well on the examinations students would also learn the basics only (Bishop, 1998; Zhang & Lee, 1990).

Fourthly, in terms of scientific tradition, after the 18th century, the School of Evidential Investigation (考据) became dominant in China, which equated academic research with "bibliographical investigation" and "exegesis of written work". These two approaches of study mainly relied on the basic knowledge of ancient texts and mature skills on written words. In the eyes of many Chinese intellectuals, scientific research is equal to Evidential Investigation (Zhang, 2002).

Fifthly, as an educational wisdom in the Chinese society says, practice makes perfect. It was believed that the primary aim of learning is to achieve familiarization and proficiency. Through practicing and familiarizing, one can naturally become "skillful" (perfect).

Finally, in the 1950s, the mathematics education in Mainland China was heavily influenced by former Soviet Union's mathematics education, which further increased the emphasis on "mathematics foundation" and "basic mathematics skills". As well known, the mathematical education in former Soviet Union emphasized the rules and regulations of basic knowledge, and the rigor of proof, including the basic training of logic reasoning.

Under the above factors, in 1963, the Ministry of Education of China stated in the national mathematics curriculum and teaching standard: "mathematics education should strengthen students' learning of basic knowledge and basic skills", and moreover mathematics instruction should foster students' "basic computation ability, spatial visualization ability and logical reasoning ability". The idea of emphasizing on the basics is still practiced now.

3　Goals of Mathematics Teaching under the "Two Basics" Principle

In Mainland China, the "Two Basics" principle in mathematics teaching is a broad and loose idea without a strict definition. Its general meaning is that in the two aspects of "solid foundation" and "application and creativity", although both are important, more important is the knowing well of basic knowledge and grasp of basic skills. Specifically, the primary goals of mathematics education are:

(1) Fast and accurate calculation with the four arithmetic operations involving integers, decimals and fractions etc., and memorization of the algorithms. Primary students can correctly finish ten questions of addition and subtraction within 100 per minute (For example, see Changshou and Fenghua surveys in Appendices 1 & 2).

(2) Fast and accurate manipulation on polynomial expressions, algebraic fractions, exponential and radical expressions, and memorization of the rules. Finishing twenty questions of factorization and completing the square in ten minutes is the requirement for a pass (see Appendix 3). Students at year 12 are required to correctly solve at least twenty eight manipulative polynomial questions in ten minutes, and thirty one correct averagely in a class.

(3) Accurate memorization of definitions and formulas, the formula for finding the roots of quadratic equation, the definitions and properties of curves of the second order, trigonometric formulas and the formulas for changing the base in logarithm, etc. Take trigonometric formulas as an example. In actual teaching, students are required to recite angle-sum formulas, doub le-angle formulas and half-angle formulas and the formulas for changing sum to product and vice versa, concerning Sine, Cosine and Tangent (Formulas on triple-angles have not been required for students to memorize in recent years). Otherwise it is impossible for them to fulfill the speed requirements for taking the high school or college entrance examination.

(4) Logical and formal expressions of mathematical concepts and an awareness of logical accuracy of categorization and mathematics propositions (For example, see 1991 National College Entrance Examination, Question 15).

(5) The conformity of reasoning in solution process to rigorous logical rules with sufficient reason and being expressed in a clear and formal way.

(6) Familiarity with solution patterns. Memorizing certain basic solution patterns, and using them on similar problems through fast imitating and transferring. For example, in the 2003 College Entrance Examination, there were twenty three questions and time allowed was one hundred and twenty minutes. Candidates had an average of five

minutes and twenty seconds for each question. Speed plays the key role there.

These six goals above are the bottom line for mathematics teaching. All teachers must remind themselves all the time that their students are required to meet these targets. Of course, teachers must first meet these targets themselves.

In his PhD dissertation, Bao (2002) elaborately compared the basic knowledge and skills in the curriculum and exercise papers of China and those of the United Kingdom in five dimensions: "computation", "reasoning", "topic coverage", "context" and "investigation". He found that the requirement of China's curriculum was better than UK's in the first three dimensions, but not in the other two dimensions.

4   Characteristics of Mathematics Teaching under the "Two Basics" Principle

To fulfill the above goals of mathematics learning, teaching students to acquire basic knowledge and skill to solve mathematics problems, especially examination questions, accurately and speedily become the primary task of mathematics education. It is also necessary to maximize students' problem solving ability, to raise the objective of "effective learning" and to closely monitor the progress of mathematics classroom teaching. Therefore, under the principle of "Two Basics", the following ideas and teaching methods are put into practice:

(1) Teachers play a central role in classroom. Since the class size can reach as many as 40–50 students, it is impossible for teachers to practice individualized teaching. Therefore, individualized teaching is not a primary goal. What topic to teach in every period and how long to let students stay at every stage in a class are decided by teachers. The pace of classroom teaching is led by teacher's judgment based on most students' learning ability in the class. Students are required to follow the pace of progress. The central role demands teachers to have profound understanding on the topic and to find the best way to organize own teaching.

(2) Effective teaching is emphasized. It requires teachers to present

the main mathematics contents as quickly as possible so that students won't spend too much time in a winding path. One of the criterions to evaluate classroom teaching is to examine whether teacher completes the objectives that are set in advance. In this aspect, investigation, group discussion and real-life application would be considered a waste of time if such activities are relatively far away from the main topic. "Discovery", "constructivist teaching", "group discussion" and "real-life mathematics" could only be practiced in a very limited amount of time in classroom, certainly not on a daily basis. However, it does not mean that whole class lecture is a spoon-fed teaching. Oral questioning is a very popular interaction in practical teaching. Classroom observations show that in teaching process, teacher usually asks a series of relatively easy questions about the topic and students answer them individually, in a group or teacher provides answer. On average, a teacher would raise fifty questions in each period of lesson and the number can amount to as many as one hundred twenty. Questioning process guides students to reach the learning objectives step by step instead of their own discovery. This is so called "small step" teaching.

(3) The pattern of "teach only the essential and ensure plenty of practice" is used in teaching. It does not support the idea of "understanding first", but insists that both understanding and manipulation are of equal importance. This means that what teacher explain and demonstrate should be essential in order to save time for students to do more exercises and problem solving. It is not necessary for them to spend much time to make students understand, as it is believed that this is unlikely to be accomplished through first explanation. It is better that students do exercises after they have understood. However without thorough understanding, students could practice first and then develop their understanding through their plenty of exercises. This is probably the way most people learn mathematics. For example, when teaching the idea of "a negative number times a negative equals a positive one", teachers do not need to explain much but just demonstrate how multiplying a number with (−1) equals to its opposite number. Students will understand gradually when they practice more.

Teachers in China believe that students should have sufficient exercises in order to consolidate the knowledge learned. Generally, students are given a large number of exercises to practice. Students' ability to used mathematics procedures proficiently is often an indicator of their "Two Basics" level. However it is not complete if we only think that this way means emphasizing meaningless memorization, imitation, and manipulation (Watkins & Biggs, 1996). "Practice makes perfect" is a traditional proverb in Chinese education. Based on Sfard's (1991) theory of dual nature of mathematics concept, research on "practice makes perfect" has revealed that having proficiency and flexibility in mathematics manipulation can facilitate the formation of mathematics concept (Li, 1999). Adequate practice can lead to thorough understanding and enable students to preserve, search and apply the contents efficiently. The ability to apply formulas and patterns can transfer mechanical manipulation skill to mathematical calculation ability. Skillful calculation and memorization of formulas can make mathematical thinking more condensed and faster, lead to a higher level of mathematics thinking.

(4) There is a distinctive way of mathematics teaching called "teaching with variation" in China. Research on "variation" pointed out that the "Two Basics" in China can develop into meaningful learning since students' practices are not meaningless symbol games. Ma (1999) described a typical example in her research. Chen, an experienced teacher, could propose five different "non-conventional" strategies to help students solve the problem of 123×645. Those five strategies create a framework for students to understand the "standard" procedure from different angles. All these serve to make students understand the essential theory – the place value system – underlying multi-digit number multiplication procedure. This kind of sophisticated way of teaching is much more effective than the simple repetition of tasks. With teachers' profound understanding, subject matters presented in classroom are carefully chosen and well organized so that it has meaningful variation in different aspects.

Theoretically, there are many kinds of variations, including concept variation and process variation, as well as explicit variations and implicit variations (Huang, 2002; Gu, Huang, & Marton, this volume). The focal point of variation is the procedure or form in which problems are proposed. It is carefully designed such that only the non-fundamental elements of knowledge and skills are changed in a variety of ways. By comparing and differentiating, students struggle to identify invariant properties: the essence of mathematics ideas and procedures. An example is "The line $y = ax^2 + bx + a$ intersects the x-axis at two points. Draw the locations of 'a' and 'b' on the ab-plane." This is a typical question to promote understanding of variation with "Two Basics" principle. Since it only involves a reasonable variant of the original quadratic equation formula and the trivial concept of analytic geometry.

Psychologically, under the teaching with variation, the knowledge and skill mastered by students is not enforced by merely doing extensive amount of boring exercises but can be understood in a meaningful and appropriate context.

(5) Mathematics teachers in China usually believe in the maxim that "mathematics is gymnastics of thinking". The "Two Basics" principle emphasizes the importance of fostering mathematics thinking. Since the 1990s, with the effort of numerous mathematics teachers, the "Two Basics" principle has been used to teach higher level of thinking in mathematics teaching. Curriculum standards set a higher level of teaching objectives in this aspect. Students need to master many "basic ways of thinking" flexibly, such as classification without overlapping, four types of prepositions and the conversions among them, necessary and sufficient conditions, induction and deduction, analysis and synthesis and mathematical method of reversion-mapping-inversion, etc. In particular, during review stage for examination, teachers especially emphasize on summarization and exploration of new thinking methods through reviewing the old knowledge and skills. This kind of training is a typical case of applying the "Two Basics" principle at a higher level.

(6) Under the "Two Basics" principle, logical deductive reasoning is thought as the core of thinking ability. Emphasis is put on logical analysis of mathematics content and the logical reasoning in the solution of problems. The minimum requirement is logical correctness. For instance, although the teaching of definitions also emphasizes on "practical context of the concept" and on the appropriateness of introducing new knowledge, heavier emphasis is however put on the logical analysis of "genus + the differences of species". In some cases, students are even required to memorize definitions, recite together in

class (eighth graders and below), and be quizzed repeatedly on them. Especially, Euclidean geometry is always an important content in mathematics curriculum at school since it is useful in teaching rigorous deductive reasoning and formal proof. Compared to "verification", "proof" is more valued. For example, to prove Pythagoras Theorem, one needs to use rigorous algebraic or geometric methods, while demonstrating a cut-and-paste method is not acceptable.

5   Basic Skills: Diminishing Differences between the East and the West

The eastern and western mathematics education is looking for a balance between fundamentals and development (Leung, 1998; Lim, 1998). In the International Conference on Mathematics Education held in Chongqing in 2002, the description of basic mathematics skills is a concern of various countries in their secondary school mathematics curriculum (Zhang, Cheung, & Song, 2003).

According to the findings of the Third International Mathematics and Science Study (TIMSS), students in the eastern countries do better than their counterparts in the western countries in mathematics. However, there are signs that the gap is narrowing down to some extent. Specifically, it is observed that in the eastern countries, students' basic mathematical skills are not as good as before whereas the students in the western countries are more skilled. Such improvement might be due to that they are required to acquire stronger basic skills in mathematics.

In the United States, NCTM *Standards* has paid more attention to computational fluency, which should develop in tandem with understanding, at the first stage of schooling:

- Knowing basic number combinations (the single-digit addition pairs and their counterparts for subtraction) that build on their thinking about, and understanding of, numbers.
- Fluency with basic addition and subtraction number combinations is a goal for the pre-K-2 years.

(NCTM, 2000, p. 84)

An interesting remark is that if the students by the end of the year four are still not able to use the combination of multiplication and division fluently, they must either develop strategies so that they are fluent with these combinations or memorize other harder combinations.

In eastern Asian countries, the situation seems different. Sawada used a set of seventeen questions to examine whether calculation abilities of Japanese pupils in decimals and fractions have declined. He found that when the test items were first administered in 1982, the average correct rate was 69 percent. By 1994, it dipped slightly to 65 percent. However, in the last test the result sunk to 58 percent (Sawada, 2002).

In Mainland China, the "Two Basics" principle has gradually combined with "education reform" beliefs. The teaching under the principle of "Two Basics" in China is pursuing a balance between students' foundation and development. The meaning of the "Two Basics" has been expanded. Mathematics modeling and application will be treated as a part of basic mathematics knowledge and skill. Especially, the "investigation study course" is put into practice. Investigative topics are added to the original program with a clear regulation on the number of teaching hours. Questions of mathematics application and modeling also appear in the College Entrance Examinations.

Many Chinese teachers are reducing routine problem solving and emphasizing the variation of problems in teaching. Meanwhile, mathematics teachers are paying more attention to students' thinking process in the study of basic knowledge and skill. In particular, open-ended problem has been introduced to the Curriculum Standards, textbooks and College Entrance Examination as well. Through research and teaching of open-ended problems in these years, many traditional problems (close-ended questions) are effectively designed to turn into open-ended ones so that students can develop the ability of divergent thinking. For example, the question "what is a common factor in the two expressions: $8a^2b^2c^3$ and $12x^2y^3a^2$?" has many answers, but it is closely related to the "Two Basics". Another example is the "clock-face problem" (There are two numbers on the clock-face, please add positive or negative sign before somes numbers so that the algebraic sum of them becomes zero). It is also closely related to the foundation of addition and subtraction of numbers (Dai, 2002).

Reference

Bamberger, H. J. (1998). Using a "standards-based" approach to teaching mathematics. *The Business Monthly*. (Also retrieved from http://www.bizmonthly.com/1_1998_com/1_1998_focus/Bamberger.html)

Bao, J. (2002). *Comparative study on composite difficulty of Chinese and British school mathematics curricula* [In Chinese 中英两国初中数学课程综合难度的比较研究]. Unpublished doctoral dissertation, East China Normal University, Shanghai, China.

Bishop, A. J. (1998). Culture, value and assessment in mathematics. In Korea Sub-Commission of ICMI etc (Ed.), *Proceedings of ICMI-EARCOME 1* (Vol. 1, pp. 27-38). Korea National University of Education.

Brand , D. (1987, August 31). The new whiz kids: Why Asian Americans are doing well and what it costs them (cover story). *Time*, 42-50.

Dai, Z. (2002). *A new mathematics teaching approach: Open-ended problem solving* [In Chinese 开放题—数学教学的新模式]. Shanghai: Shanghai Education Press.

Huang, R. (2002). *Mathematics teaching in Hong Kong and Shanghai: Analysis from prospective of variation*. Unpublished doctoral dissertation, Hong Kong University, Hong Kong.

Lapointe, A. E., Mead, N. A., & Askew, J. M. (1992). *Learning mathematics*, New Jersey: Educational Testing Service.

Leung, F. K. S. (1998). The traditional Chinese views on mathematics and education - Implications for mathematics education in the new millennium. In H. S. Park, Y. H. Choe, H. Shin, & S. H. Kim (Eds.), *Proceedings of the ICMI East Asia Regional Conference on Mathematics Education 1* (Vol. 1, pp. 61-76). Seoul, South Korea: Korea Society of Mathematics Education.

Li, S. (1999). Does practice make perfect? *For the Learning of Mathematics, 19*(3), 33-35.

Lim-Teo, S. K. (1998). Seeking a balance in mathematics education - The Singapore story. In H. S. Park, Y. H. Choe, H. Shin, & S. H. Kim (Eds.), *Proceedings of the ICMI East Asia Regional Conference on Mathematics Education 1* (Vol. 1, pp. 315-329). Seoul, South Korea: Korea Society of Mathematics Education.

Ma, L. (1999). *Knowing and Teaching Elementary Mathematics*. Mahwah, NJ: Lawrence Erlbaum Associates.

Murphy, D. (1987). Offshore education: A Hong Kong perspective. *Australian Universities Review, 30*(2), 43-44.

National Council of Teachers of Mathematics. (1989). *Curriculum and evaluation standards for school mathematics*. Reston, VA: Author.

National Council of Teachers of Mathematics. (2000). *Principles and standards for school mathematics*. Reston, VA: Author.

Sawada, T. (2002, August). *The reform of mathematics curriculum and its issues in Japan.* Paper presented at ICM2002-ICRMCE, Chongqing, China.

Sfard, A. (1991). On the dual nature of mathematical conception: Reflections on processes and objects as different sides of the same coin. *Educational Studies in Mathematics, 22*(1), 1-36.

Watkins, D. A., & Biggs, J. B. (Eds). (1996). *The Chinese learner: Culture psychological and contextual influences*. Hong Kong: Comparative Education Research Centre, The University of Hong Kong; Melbourne, Australia: The Australian Council of Educational Research.

Wong, N. Y. (1998). In search of the "CHC" learner: Smarter, works harder or something more? Plenary Lecture. In H. S. Park, Y. H. Choe, H. Shin, & S. H. Kim (Eds.), *Proceedings of the ICMI East Asia Regional Conference on Mathematics Education 1* (Vol. 1, pp. 85-98). Seoul, South Korea: Korea Society of Mathematics Education.

Zhang, D. (2002). Textual research in Qing Dynasty and mathematics education. [In Chinese. 清末考据学派与中国数学教育] *Science* [In Chinese 科学], *54*(2), 43-48.

Zhang, D., Cheung, K. C, & Song, N. (2003). Curriculum reform in the 21st Century. *Acta of Southwest Normal University, 2003*(1), 1-21.

Zhang, D., & Lee, P. Y. (1990). Examination culture and mathematics teaching. In Beijing Normal University etc (Ed.), *Proceedings of ICMI-China Regional Conference* (pp. 141-145). Beijing: Beijing Normal University.

Appendix 1

A Survey on Farmers' Mathematics Literacy in Changshou County, Chongqing, Western China

The survey was conducted under the charge of Tan Caixing, the chair of the Changshou Representative Committee. Sixty-four farmers were randomly sampled, using in-depth interviews and face-to-face conversations to measure their realistic calculation ability. They are physical laborers who require least mathematics skills among different professions.

Years of Education the 64 Farmers Received

6 Years	9 Years	12 Years
12	38	11

Age Distribution of the 64 Farmers

Below 30	30-39	40-49	50 or above
12	18	14	20

Question 1: Solve 34 + 48 =? and 5 × 23 =? (Oral Calculation)

Correct	Only able to add	Unable to solve
57	5	2
89%	8%	3%

Question 2: Solve 1/2 + 1/3 = ?

Correct	Answered 2/5	Unable to solve
28	13	23
44%	15%	41%

Question 3: How much water is needed to add if a farmer wants to dilute 100 catties of 60% concentrated insecticide to 12% concentrated insecticide?

Correct	Used rate	Unable to solve
3	27	34
4 %	42 %	53 %

In Changshou County, another 103 people were interviewed individually. The rate of correct answers to the first two questions is similar to the finding from the survey of the 64 farmers, only 3 to 4 percent higher than the former. The result for Question 3 is different. 10 of 103 people answered correctly. Among them one was tertiary educated, eight were high school graduates and one graduated from junior high school.

Appendix 2

A Survey on Primary Students' Arithmetic Ability in Jinpeng, Fenghua County of Zhejiang Province[1]

Zhejiang Province is a relatively developed area compared to others. However, the economy of Fenghua County is only moderately developed, so is its education quality. The aim of this test is to find out primary students' calculation speed and accuracy under normal circumstances. This test was carried out without prior notice to both teachers and students. Two primary schools, one in town and the other at rural area, participated the investigation. First graders and third graders from a total of 4 classes took part in this test.

(1) Test contents:
  i. First graders: 50 questions on addition and subtraction of numbers within 100, and the other 10 questions each with 4 blanks. A total of 90 questions are to be completed within 15 minutes.
  ii. Third graders: 20 questions on one-step multiplication and division, 10 questions on addition, subtraction, multiplication and division of whole numbers, which should be completed in 25 minutes.

(2) Test results and analysis:
  i. Results and analysis of mathematics ability of the first graders

---

[1] This survey is conducted by Zhou Leiming and Hu Yixiang.

School	No. of test samples	Quickest	Slowest	Average time used	Highest points	Lowest points	Average points	Excellence rate	Passing rate
Jinpeng town centre school	48	6'	15'	9'38"	100	66	90.1	46.65%	100%
Xi'qi School	23	6'3"	14'	9'52"	100	57	87.4	36.7%	96%

Results show that first graders are faster at oral calculation. On average, they can complete about 10 questions on addition and subtraction within 100 in a minute. The accuracy of oral calculation meets the requirements of the standards and students often lost points when the calculation involved renaming during subtraction, and mixed addition and subtraction.

ii. Re sults and analysis of mathematics ability of the third graders

According to the test results, third graders could finish about two questions on addition, subtraction, multiplication and division of whole numbers in a minute. Students in the town-centre primary school had higher percentages in excellence rate, passing rate and average points. For calculation techniques, students had firmly mastered ordered calculation, but not many students could solve the question flexibly in simple and convenient ways. It indicates that teachers need to strengthen students' flexibility in problem solving.

School	No. of test samples	Quickest	Slowest	Average time used	Highest points	Lowest points	Average points	Excellence rate	Passing rate
Jinpeng town centre school	54	8'10"	23'	14'17"	100	44	87.4	61.1%	98.1%
Xi'qi School	29	10'	21'	15'12"	95	36	78.6	21.5%	85%

Appendix 3

A Survey on Rural and Urban Secondary Students' Ability in Calculation Involving Algebraic Expressions in Jiangsu Province

(1) Test subject and method

In 1998, a test was done on 2049 students from 8 schools, a total of 43 classes in Jiangsu Province, China. The content is algebra expressions (included grouping, completing the square and factorization). There are 38 questions of various levels of difficulties and students are required to complete them within 10 minutes. It was a test of students' basic mathematics skills, especially the speed of calculation.

(2) Test data

Results are shown in the following table, X is the average number of correct answers, σ_n is the standard differentiation of the number of correct answers, Y (%) is the accuracy rate. The accuracy is defined as: (the total number of correct answers in the respective grade level) ÷ (the number of students in that level × the number of questions) × 100%.

Average Number of Correct Questions, Standard Differentiation and Accuracy

Grade Variable	8 th	9 th	10 th	11 th	12 th	Total
X	17.82	20.73	28.11	29.43	31.00	25.78
σ_n	6.08	7.05	4.22	4.34	4.20	7.29
Y (%)	46.89	54.55	73.97	77.45	81.58	67.84

(3) The testing criteria of secondary students' ability in calculation involving algebraic expressions

In mathematics education the main goal is to teach students' basic knowledge and to train them to have high standards of mathematics ability.

Based on the statistical analysis of the above samples and the experiences of Mathematics teachers, three indices can be proposed and they are namely average points, pass points and excellent points. According to statistical results, the following reference standard is compiled:

Standard Reference Chart of the Equation Solving Test Results

Standard Grade	Average Correct answers	Pass Correct answers	Excellent Correct answers
8 th	17.90	$\geqslant 13$	$\geqslant 27$
9 th	21.84	$\geqslant 16$	$\geqslant 32$
10 th	27.67	$\geqslant 24$	$\geqslant 34$
11 th	30.06	$\geqslant 26$	$\geqslant 36$
12 th	31.29	$\geqslant 28$	$\geqslant 36$

Note. The maximum number of correct answers is 38.

Chapter 8

A Comparative Study on Composite Difficulty between New and Old Chinese Mathematics Textbooks

BAO Jiansheng

If one compares the old middle school mathematics syllabus to the newly published National Mathematics Standards one can notice numerous changes both to curriculum framework and to mathematics contents. In fact, these new standard-based mathematics textbooks are being used in experimental districts in Mainland China. However, these changes may lead us to ask the following questions: What precisely are the differences between the new and old mathematics textbooks? How do these differences affect the styles of both mathematics teaching and learning?

In order to answer these questions, this paper uses a model developed by the author (Bao, 2002a, 2002b) to evaluate the composite difficulties of new and old eighth grade mathematics textbooks using five factors of difficulty. From the initial findings, we can see some typical characters in the two samples. For example, the new textbooks have advantages in areas such as "Investigation" and "Context" levels. However, the level of difficulty for "Symbolic computation", "Complex reasoning" and "Topic coverage" has been reduced.

Key words: composite difficulty, curriculum standards, Chinese mathematics textbook, comparative study

1 Introduction

Since the *National Mathematics Curriculum Standards* for Compulsory Education (Ministry of Education, 2001) was issued, several series of new standard-based mathematics textbooks have received government approval. The first two new textbooks (Ma, 2002; Wang, 2002) are now being used in all schools in the experimental districts, and the first round of tests should be completed by the summer of 2005.

In non-experimental districts, however, the old mathematics textbooks based on the *National Mathematics Teaching Syllabus* for Compulsory Education (People's Educational Press [PEP], 2000) are still being used. Of these, the most widely used textbooks are the PEP textbooks published by the People's Education Press.

In comparison to the old Syllabus, the new Standards Course has made numerous changes not only with regard to curriculum framework but also with regard to mathematical content. Obviously, this leads us to ask: What are the differences between the new and old mathematics textbooks? How do these differences affect styles of mathematics teaching and learning?

Many approaches are possible in performing a comparative study of the two textbooks. However, this study will use a composite difficulty model developed by the author (Bao, 2002a, 2000b), which compared Chinese and British mathematics curricula. The initial findings of the early study show that there are significant differences between the two mathematics curricula. For example, the old Chinese mathematics curriculum attaches more importance to understanding mathematical knowledge and methods than to activities which investigate the use of mathematics. That is, in old Chinese textbooks there are few mathematical problems related to the daily life of students. In addition, the level of "two basics" in the Chinese mathematics curriculum is much more advanced than that found in the British mathematics curriculum; and so on. In this paper, however, we want to know whether or not the case is similar with the new Chinese mathematics textbooks.

2 Methods

2.1 *The modification of composite difficulty model*

The original model (Bao, 2002a, 2002b) was developed from the model of Overall difficulty (Nohara, 2001). It has five factors (see Figure 1).

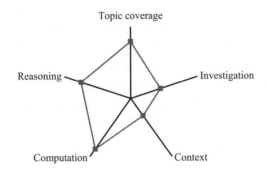

Figure 1. Composite difficulty model (Bao, 2002a, 2002b)

Each factor in the model is further divided into several levels (see Table 1).

Table 1
Difficult Levels of Composite Difficulty Factors (Bao, 2002a, 2002b)

Factor	Level			
Investigation	Knowing	Understanding	Investigating	
Context	None	Personal	Public	Scientific
Computation	None	Number computation	Simple symbolic computation	Complex symbolic computation
Reasoning	None	Simple reasoning	Complex reasoning	
Topic coverage	Single topic	Two topics	Above three topics	

In this study, the original model has been modified in the following way:

Firstly, the third level of "Topic coverage" is divided into two levels, because there are many mathematical problems in Chinese textbooks which contain more than three topics. Thus, Table 1 is changed into Table 2.

Table 2
Difficult Levels of Composite Difficulty Factors

Factor	Level			
Investigation	Knowing	Understanding	Investigating	
Context	None	Personal	Public	Scientific
Computation	None	Number computation	Simple symbolic computation	Complex symbolic computation
Reasoning	None	Simple reasoning	Complex reasoning	
Topic coverage	Single topic	Two topics	Three topics	Above four topics

Secondly, the method used to compute the difficulty index of the last three factors is simplified according to the levels defined by Table 2, but the general formula remains the following:

$$d_i = \frac{\sum_j n_{ij} d_{ij}}{n} \quad (\sum_j n_{ij} = n; i = 1, 2, 3, 4, 5; j = 1, 2, \cdots) \qquad (*)$$

Where d_i ($i = 1, 2, 3, 4, 5$) corresponds to five factors; d_{ij} represents the i'th power index of the j'th level; n_{ij} is the total number of items which belong to the j'th level of the i'th factor, the sum of n_{ij} is n.

2.2 Samples

In Bao's research (Bao, 2002a, 2002b), the Chinese sample was two chapters of grade eight PEP textbooks (PEP, 2001a, 2001b). That is "Chapter Nine" in "Algebra Book Two" and "Chapter Five" in "Geometry Book Two". As in Bao's earlier studies, the two textbooks are still used as the samples for the "old textbooks" in this study although all the chapters in these books will be considered and evaluated.

The sample for the "New textbooks" will include "Mathematics Book I" and "Mathematics Book II" (grade eight) published by East China Normal University Press (ECNUP) (Wang, 2002). As with the old sample textbooks, all the items in the two ECNUP textbooks will be examined.

Table 3 shows the numbers of items in each chapter for the two sample textbooks.

Table 3
Numbers of Items in Two Sample Textbooks (Grade Eight)

PEP textbooks			ECNUP textbooks	
Content		Number of items	Content	Number of items
Algebra book two	Ch 8. Factorization	352	Ch 11. Translations and Rotations	58
	Ch 9. Rational Expressions	292	Ch 12. Parallelograms	58
	Ch 10. Evolution of Numbers	229	Ch 13. Linear Inequalities	121
	Ch 11. Square Root Expressions	461	Ch 14. Multiplication of Polynomials	198
Geometry book two	Ch 3. Triangles	372	Ch 15. Frequency and Chance	42
	Ch 4. Quadrilaterals	244	Ch 16. Evolution of Numbers	111
	Ch 5. Similarities	167	Ch 17. Functions and Graphs	196
			Ch 18. Similarities	89
			Ch 19. Solving Right Triangles	77
			Ch 20. Handling and Interpreting Data	54
Total		2117		1004

The numbers of items in each chapter is calculated using the following rules (Bao, 2002a):

- The term of "items" in the above table includes all "Samples", "Practices", "Exercises", "Review Exercises",

"Self-test problems", and mathematics problems described as "Think a moment", "Hands on" and "Just try" in the textbooks. The items in a textbook will indicate what the curriculum wants students to do, so we may use the composite difficulty of the item system of a textbook to represent the composite difficulty of the textbook.

• In the two sample textbooks, the first numbering of items is all by 1, 2, 3, ..., which are called "big items". The second numbering of items is by (1), (2), (3), ..., which are called "small items". The total number of items in a textbook is calculated on the second level. That is to say, if a big item includes three small items, it will be counted as three items.

From Table 3 we can see that the number of chapters in the PEP textbooks is noticeably less than that found in the ECNUP textbooks. Although, the number of items in the former textbooks is double of that found in the later ones. Therefore, the old textbooks allocate more time for each single topic. For example, the same chapter "Evolution of numbers" appears in the different sample textbooks. Yet, in the old textbook the number of items in the chapter totals 229, whereas in the new textbook it totals only 111. A comparison of the quantities of items in the two samples shows that the old one demands that, with this topic, students do more practice.

The comparison of item numbers of the two sample textbooks has a research limitation, however, since it can only indicate the quantity of the item system of the textbooks. Therefore, we intend to use the composite difficulty model to analyze the quality of the item systems of the textbooks. Table 4 shows the numbers and percentages of items on each level for each factor in the two sample textbooks.

Table 4
Numbers and Percentages of Sample Items on Each Difficulty Level

Factors	Levels	Number of Items		Percentage		Weighted Mean	
		Old Book	New Book	Old Book	New Book	Old Book	New Book
Investigation	Knowing	690	274	33.59	27.29	1.68	1.83
	Understanding	1404	631	66.32	62.85		
	Investigating	23	99	1.09	9.86		
Context	None	2032	747	95.98	74.40	1.07	1.38
	Personal	20	145	0.94	14.44		
	Public	64	104	3.02	10.36		
	Scientific	1	8	0.05	0.80		
Computation	None	544	290	25.70	28.88	2.42	2.13
	Number	466	349	22.01	34.76		
	Simple Symbolic	788	307	37.22	30.58		
	Complex Symbolic	319	58	15.07	5.78		
Reasoning	None	1063	477	50.21	47.51	1.66	1.54
	Simple	712	515	33.63	51.29		
	Complex	342	12	16.15	1.20		
Topic Coverage	Single	437	275	20.64	27.39	2.24	2.07
	Two	842	410	39.77	40.84		
	Three	767	287	36.23	28.59		
	Above Four	81	31	3.83	3.09		

Note. 1. The weighted mean is calculated by formula (*); 2. Percentage and weighted mean are rounded to 0.01.

3 Findings

The following part of this paper will first compare difficulty levels on each factor of the PEP Eighth Grade Textbooks (Old Books) with the

ECNUP Eighth Grade Textbooks (New Books). Then, the composite difficulties of the two samples will be analyzed.

3.1 *Investigation levels*

As shown in Table 4, 33.59 per cent of items in the old eighth grade books belong to the "Knowing" level, whereas with the new sample the percentage is 27.29 per cent. The percentages for items belonging to the "Understanding" level in each sample are respectively 66.32% and 62.85%; The percentages for items belonging to the "Investigating" level are 1.09% and 9.86% (see Figure 2).

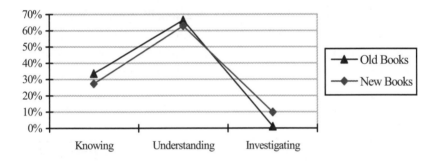

Figure 2. Comparison on investigation levels between new and old textbooks

Figure 2 shows, that the percentages in the new textbooks, compared to the old textbooks, are lower on the "Knowing" and "Understanding" levels, but higher on the "Investigating" level.

In the old textbooks, the items on the "Investigating" level mainly appear as "Think a moment" in two special sections. One is section "9.6 Investigating Activity: $a = bc$ Type Relationship of Variables". The other is section "4.8 Practice activity". There are few investigating activities in the standard "samples" or "exercises". This situation has been changed in the new textbooks. In fact, many kinds of "Investigating" items can be found in every part of the new textbooks. These new types include open-ended problems, hands-on activities, fieldwork, and real world projects.

Compared to the related data of the British mathematics curriculum, we find that the percentage of items on the "Investigating" level in the

British intended curriculum is 22% (Bao, 2002a, 2002b). This is still higher than that found in the new Chinese textbooks.

3.2 *Context levels*

The contexts of mathematics problems can be divided into four levels by the "distance" of the material to the students (Bao, 2002a; Organization of Economic Cooperation and Development, 2000). The closest is (personal) daily life, next is public/occupational life, and the most distant contexts for students are scientific ones. As shown in Table 4, 95.98% of items in the PEP eighth grade books do not provide any real-life contexts, whereas in the ECNUP sample the percentage is 74.40 per cent. The percentages of items belonging to "Personal" context level in each sample are respectively 0.94% and 14.44%; The percentages of items on "Public" context level are 3.02% and 10.36%. There are few items related to "Scientific" contexts in both samples (see Figure 3).

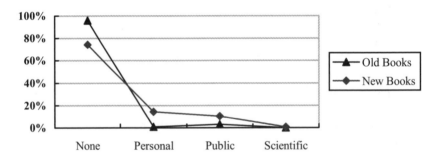

Figure 3. Comparison on context level between new and old textbooks

Figure 3 shows that there are more items in the new textbooks connected to real-life situations. In the old textbooks, almost all the items are "pure mathematics" problems. The few items which are related to real-life contexts are usually associated with a traditional workplace. In the new textbooks, the situation has improved. The percentage of items that offer different contexts in the new textbooks is significantly higher. This is highlighted by the fact that the percentage of items relating to students' personal life has increased from 0.94% in the old textbooks to 14.44% in the new textbooks.

The great improvement on "Context" level in the new textbooks is not only due to changes in curriculum ideas in the new Standards, but is also due to the arrangement of the teaching content in the new textbooks. The old grade eight mathematics curriculum is split into an algebra book and a geometry book, both of which focus on symbolic computation and formal mathematical deductive reasoning. In the new mathematics textbooks, algebraic topics and geometric topics are joined together with other new mathematics topics such as "Frequency and Chance" and "Handling and Interpreting Data", which are more closely connected to the real world.

It is interesting to note, however, that the percentage of items related to "real" contexts in the Chinese new textbooks is still much lower than that found in British textbooks. For example, more than 41 per cent of items in Mathematics Enhancement Programme (MEP) year 8 textbooks are connected to real life, with more than 30 per cent of items connected to students' personal life (Bao, 2002a). It is more than double the percentage found in the new Chinese textbooks. The big gap between the Chinese mathematics curriculum and the British mathematics curriculum may due to the choice of teaching contents. For example, there are up to 20 chapters in MEP year 8 textbooks (Table 5).

Table 5
Contents of MEP Textbooks (Year 8)

Y8A		Y8B	
1	Mathematical Diagrams	12	Formulae
2	Factors	13	Money and Time
3	Pythagoras' Theorem	14	Straight Line Graphs
4	Rounding and Estimating	15	Polygons
5	Data Analysis	16	Circles and Cylinders
6	Nets and Surface Area	17	Units of Measure
7	Ratio and Proportion	18	Speed, Distance and Time
8	Algebra: Brackets	19	Similarity
9	Arithmetic: Fractions and Percentages	20	Questionnaires and Analysis
10	Probability – Two Events		
11	Angles, Bearings and Maps		

Table 5 shows that most topics in MEP textbooks are connected closely to the real world, such as "Rounding and Estimating", "Nets and Surface Area", "Angles, Bearings and Maps", "Money and Time", "Speed, Distance and Time", and so on. Therefore, the "real world" mathematics problems in the textbooks are far greater in number than the number found in Chinese textbooks.

It is necessary to note, however, that the percentage of items that have "scientific" contexts is still very low in sample textbooks both in Mainland China and in the UK. The new teaching and learning styles, such as "Project Learning", "Cross Subjects activity", "Scientific Investigation", are increasingly popular in many countries, although this leads us to question whether scientific situations can be better integrated into the mathematics curriculum. Obviously, this issue requires further research.

3.3 *Computation level*

Figure 4 shows the percentages of items for different difficulty levels of computation in the new and old Chinese textbooks.

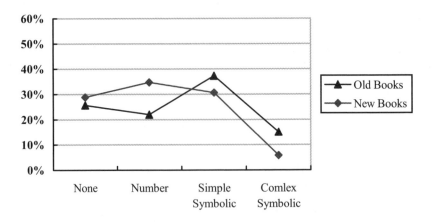

Figure 4. Comparison on computation level between new and old textbooks

According the above figure, the percentages of items that do not require any computation in the two samples are almost same. These items usually appear in geometric topics. The percentage of items that need numeral computation in the new textbooks is significantly higher than that found in the old textbooks. But with the "Complex symbolic computation" level, the percentage of items in the new books is about 10 per cent lower than that found in the old textbooks.

The above differences between the new and old textbooks are mainly due to the following factors:

Firstly, the complexity and difficulty of computation in the new mathematics curriculum are strictly limited by the new *National Standards*. For example, as explained in the Standards, "Multiplication of Polynomials" only means "A linear expression times a linear expression"; Steps of factoring by applying formulae shouldn't occur "more than twice"; the number of fractional expressions in a equation should be "less than two"; and so on (Ministry of Education, 2001). Because there are no such regulations in old mathematics syllabus, the difficulty level of computation found in the old textbooks is certainly much higher than that found in the new textbooks.

Secondly, in the old textbooks, the topics are more consistent than in the new textbooks. The adjacent chapters in the old textbooks are usually closely related. So, solving a problem often demands the use of some former knowledge. For example, in the PEP textbook "Algebra Book Two" there is a computation exercise (PEP, 2001a, p. 221):

Simplify: $\dfrac{n+2+\sqrt{n^2-4}}{n+2-\sqrt{n^2-4}} + \dfrac{n+2-\sqrt{n^2-4}}{n+2+\sqrt{n^2-4}}$ $(n > 2)$.

Solution: $\dfrac{n+2+\sqrt{n^2-4}}{n+2-\sqrt{n^2-4}} + \dfrac{n+2-\sqrt{n^2-4}}{n+2+\sqrt{n^2-4}}$

$$= \frac{\sqrt{(n+2)^2}+\sqrt{(n-2)(n+2)}}{\sqrt{(n+2)^2}-\sqrt{(n-2)(n+2)}} + \frac{\sqrt{(n+2)^2}-\sqrt{(n-2)(n+2)}}{\sqrt{(n+2)^2}+\sqrt{(n-2)(n+2)}}$$

$$= \frac{\sqrt{n+2}+\sqrt{n-2}}{\sqrt{n+2}-\sqrt{n-2}} + \frac{\sqrt{n+2}-\sqrt{n-2}}{\sqrt{n+2}+\sqrt{n-2}}$$

$$= \frac{(\sqrt{n+2}+\sqrt{n-2})^2}{4} + \frac{(\sqrt{n+2}-\sqrt{n-2})^2}{4}$$

$$= n$$

As shown above, the solution of the given item that belongs to Chapter 11 is related to topics in Chapters 8 and 9. These kinds of situations do not occur as often in the new textbooks.

Thirdly, there are more "real world" items in the new textbooks. These items are often only related to number computations. So, the chance for complex symbolic computation is lower in new textbooks than in the old ones.

In the MEP year 8 textbooks, however, only 20 per cent of items need "Simple symbolic computation" and no items need "Complex symbolic computation" (Bao, 2002a, 2002b). So, compared to its British counterpart, the computational difficulty level in the new Chinese textbook is still very high.

3.4 *Reasoning levels*

Mathematical reasoning is a strong point in traditional Chinese mathematics curriculum, especially in the geometry curriculum. Compared to the old mathematics syllabus, however, the greatest change which has taken place in the new mathematics standards can be found with geometry. So, the question is: Are there any differences in mathematical reasoning between the new and old textbooks? Let's consider Figure 5.

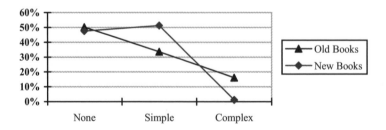

Figure 5. Comparison on reasoning level between new and old textbooks

Figure 5 shows, about half the items in both the new and old samples don't need any mathematical reasoning. But with the items that need "Complex reasoning", the percentage has dropped from 16.15% in the old textbooks down to 1.20% in the new textbooks. That is to say, of the 1004 items in the new textbooks, only about 12 items need "Complex reasoning" whereas the corresponding number in the old textbooks totals about 300.

The decline in the level of reasoning required in the new textbooks is mainly due to the changes caused by the new Standards. In the new national Standards, there are only four theorems that can be used as arguments for geometric proofs. These are:

- When two parallel lines are cut by a single straight line, the corresponding angles are equal.
- Straight line falling on two straight lines makes the corresponding angles equal to one another, then the straight lines are parallel to one another.
- If two sides and the angle between them (two angles and the side between them, or three sides) in one triangle have the same measures in another triangle, then the triangles are congruent.
- In congruent triangles, the corresponding sides and angles have the same measures.

Compared to the new Standards, however, propositions highlighted in boldface in the old textbooks can be counted as arguments for mathematics proofs. These propositions (which total 84 in Geometry Book Two) form a new level based on mathematics conceptions in the knowledge structure. We call this curriculum a "Theorem-based curriculum" because the geometric proofs in the curriculum are mainly "theorem-based" deduction (Chin & Tall, 2000, 2001). Of course, the reasoning level in a "Theorem-based curriculum" will be higher than that found in a "Definition-based curriculum".

Although the new Chinese mathematics curriculum appears to lean towards a "Definition-based curriculum" from a "Theorem-based curriculum", the reasoning level of the Chinese new textbooks is still significantly higher than that of its British counterpart. For example, there are no items that need "Complex reasoning" in MEP year eight textbooks.

3.5 *Topic coverage levels*

In this paper, the concept "Topic coverage" indicates the number of topics in a single item, and the term "topics" is defined by the Standards or Syllabus (Bao, 2002a). The following figure is based on Table 4.

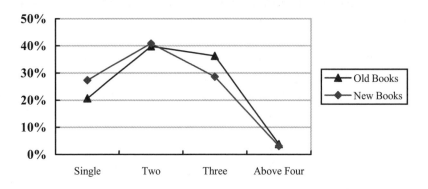

Figure 6. Comparison on topic coverage level between new and old textbooks

Figure 6 shows that the percentages on the four levels of the two sample textbooks are close, especially on the second and fourth levels. On the other two levels, there are a few differences between the two textbooks. For example, the percentage of "Single topic" items in the new textbook is a little higher than that found in the old textbooks, whereas the percentage of items containing "Three topics" in the new textbooks is a little lower.

In the MEP textbooks in the UK, however, more than 64% of items in year 8 only have a "single topic" and less than 1% of items have more than "Three topics" (Bao, 2002a). That is to say, there is little connection between the different topics. In fact, the two countries' mathematics curricula have different emphases. The MEP textbooks focus on the connection between mathematics and the real world whereas the Chinese textbooks attach more importance to relationships between different mathematical concepts.

3.6 *Composite difficulties*

In the above five sections, we have compared the difficulty levels on different factors with the new and old Chinese textbooks.

In this section, we will use the composite difficulty model to compare these two samples as a whole. By Table 4 and formula (*), we could get the weighted mean for each factor (Table 6) and the composite difficulties of the textbooks (Figure 7).

Table 6
Weighted Means of Five Difficult Factors

Textbook	Investigation	Context	Computation	Reasoning	Topic Coverage
Old	1.68	1.07	2.42	1.66	2.24
New	1.83	1.38	2.13	1.54	2.07

Note. The weighted means are corrected to 0.01.

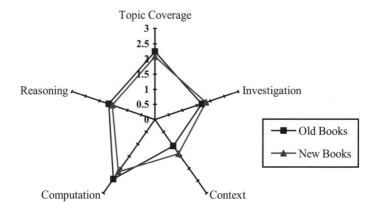

Figure 7. Comparison on composite difficulty between new and old textbooks

From Figure 7, we can see some typical characters in the two samples. For example, the new textbooks have advantages in areas such as "Investigation" and "Context" levels. However, the level of difficulty for "Symbolic computation", "Complex reasoning" and "Topic coverage" has been reduced.

4 New Question

The initial findings of this study show that in the new Chinese textbooks there are more investigating activities (e.g., open-ended problems, hands-on activities, cross subjects projects), more items connected to real life (especially to students' personal life), and fewer complex computations and reasoning.

However, will these changes in mathematics textbooks lead to innovations in teaching and learning styles?

The traditional Chinese mathematics textbooks have the following characteristics (Figure 8):

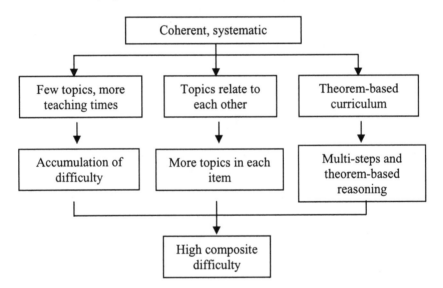

Figure 8. Characteristics of traditional Chinese textbooks

As shown in Figure 8, the traditional Chinese mathematics textbooks have three characteristics. Firstly, there are only a few mathematics topics in each grade and more teaching time is devoted to each topic. Secondly, there are close links between the different topics. This is especially the case because later topics are usually related to preceding topics, as in a logic chain. Thirdly, the geometry textbooks are typical "Theorem-based curriculum", and the geometric reasoning is typical of "Theorem-based deduction".

Based on the above characteristics of Chinese traditional mathematics textbooks, there are three typical Chinese mathematical teaching styles:

The first is "Teaching with variation" (Gu & Marton, this volume). In Chinese mathematics textbooks, most items usually have multi-steps and cover several topics. There are often different variations from the original item in three ways: (1) Change the given conditions or conclusions of the proposition; (2) Using different methods to solve the problem; (3) Applying the solutions of the item to other situations (called a problem-solving trilogy by Chinese mathematics teachers). So, "Teaching with variation" is the most popular teaching style in Mainland China.

The second is "Grouped-items training". Because the traditional Chinese mathematics curriculum is a "Theorem-based curriculum", the basic principle of problem-solving is to transfer unsolved problems to solved ones, and complicated problems to simple ones. The success of transferring not only depends on the mastery of the "Two basics", but it also depends on the accumulation of "Typical sample problems" and "transferring strategies". In Chinese mathematics classes, experienced teachers usually integrate several "transferring strategies" into a series of "Typical sample problems", which is called "Grouped-items training".

The third involves overlapping review and knowledge re-construction. In the traditional Chinese mathematics curriculum, there are rich relationships between different topics and items, and the learning of a topic or the solving of a problem often depends on the mastery of former topics or problems. Thus, in traditional Chinese mathematics classes, a large amount of teaching time is spent reviewing what was learned before so as to systemise the knowledge gained.

Similar to the notion in nature of "survival of the fittest", the Chinese traditional teaching and learning style, after decades of "evolution" has proved itself the most fit for the traditional mathematics curriculum. But now, the mathematics curriculum has changed in many ways. So, the question is: What styles of teaching and learning will best fit the new curriculum?

To find answers to the above question, it is important to note that reform of teaching and learning styles is more difficult to attain than reform of curriculum. Additionally, traditional teaching and learning styles do not always fit the new curriculum.

Finally, it would be pertinent to highlight TIMSS findings in concluding this paper. Recent reports of the TIMSS curriculum study state that "Textbooks, not standards, drive U.S. mathematics and science achievement" and that "Textbooks affect which topics teachers teach and how much time they spend on them. They also affect gains in student achievement" (Schmidt et al., 2001). In fact, the relatively poor comparative performance of U.S. eighth graders is viewed "Nationally, (as)… related to a middle-school curriculum that is not coherent, and is not as demanding as that found in other countries we studied. U.S. eighth-grade students study arithmetic, for example, but the children in the top-achieving countries study algebra and geometry" (Schmidt, McKnight, Cogan, Vakwerth, & Houang, 1999).

Yes, indeed, a textbook does matter.

References

Bao, J. (2002a). *Comparative study on composite difficulty of Chinese and British school mathematics curricula*[In Chinese 中英两国初中数学课程综合难度的比较研究]. Unpublished doctoral dissertation, East China Normal University, Shanghai.

Bao, J. (2002b). Comparative study on composite difficulty of Chinese and British intended mathematics curricula [In Chinese 中英两国初中数学期望课程综合难度的比较研究]. *Global Education* [In Chinese 全球教育展望], *31*(9).

Chin, E.-T. & Tall, D. O. (2000). Making, having and compressing formal mathematical concepts. In T. Nakahara & M. Koyama (Eds.), *Proceedings of the 24th Conference of the International Group for the Psychology of Mathematics Education* (Vol. 2, pp. 177-184). Hiroshima, Japan: Hiroshima University.

Chin, E-T. & Tall, D. O. (2001). Developing formal mathematical concepts over time. In M. van den Heuvel-Pabhuizen (Ed.), *Proceedings of the 25th Conference of the International Group for the Psychology of Mathematics Education* (Vol. 2, pp. 241-248). Utrecht, The Netherlands: Freudenthal Institute, Utrecht University.

Ma, F. (Ed.) (2002). *Experimental mathematics textbooks (Year eight)* [In Chinese 数学实验教科书(八年级)]. Beijing: Beijing Normal University Press.

Ministry of Education. (2001). *National mathematics standards* (experimental edition) [In Chinese 国家数学课程标准(实验版)]. Beijing: Beijing Normal University Press.

Nohara, D. (2001). A comparison of the National Assessment of Educational Progress (NAEP), the Third International Mathematics and Science Study Repeat (TIMSS-R), and the Programme for International Student Assessment (PISA). *NECS Working Paper*, No. 2001-07.

Organization of Economic Cooperation and Development. (2000). *Measuring student knowledge and skills: The PISA 2000 assessment of reading, mathematical and scientific literacy.* Retrieved from http://www.pisa.oecd.org

People's Educational Press. (2000). *National mathematics teaching syllabus for compulsory education* [In Chinese 义务教育数学教学大纲]. Beijing: Author.

People's Educational Press. (2001a). *Algebra book two* [In Chinese 代数第二册]. Beijing: Author.

People's Educational Press. (2001b). *Geometry book two* [In Chinese 几何第二册]. Beijing: Author.

Schmidt, W. H., McKnight, C. C., Cogan, L. S., Jakwerth, P. M., & Houang, R. T. (1999). *Facing the consequences: Using TIMSS for a closer look at US mathematics and science education.* Dordrecht, The Netherlands: Kluwer Academic Press.

Schmidt, W. H., McKnight, C. C., Houang, R. T., Wang, H., Wiley, D. E., Cogan, L. S., et al. (2001). *Why schools matter: A cross-national comparison of curriculum and learning.* San Fancisco, CA: Jossey-Bass Press.

Wang, J. (2002). *Standard-based experimental textbook: MATHEMATICS I & II* (year eight) [In Chinese 课程标准实验教科书: 数学 (八年级(上), (下))]. Shanghai: East China Normal University Press.

Chapter 9

Textbook Use within and beyond Mathematics Classrooms: A Study of 12 Secondary Schools in Kunming and Fuzhou of China

FAN Lianghuo   CHEN Jingan

ZHU Yan   QIU Xiaolan   HU Jiuzhong

This chapter presents a study which investigated how teachers and students used textbooks within and beyond Chinese mathematics classrooms. Data were collected from 36 mathematics teachers and 272 students in 12 secondary schools in Fuzhou and Kunming, two major cities in Mainland China, through questionnaires, classroom observations, and interviews. The study provided a general picture of the textbook use by Chinese teachers and students of mathematics. The results showed that textbooks were the main but not the only source for teachers to make decisions about what to teach and how to teach. For students, textbooks were their main learning resource for both in-class exercise and homework. No significant differences were found between teachers with different genders, experiences, from different regions and schools in their use of textbooks, though some significant differences were found between students in the two cities in their use of textbooks. Explanations for the results are offered in the chapter.

Key words: Chinese mathematics classrooms, learning materials, problem solving, teaching materials, textbook use

1 Introduction

Over the last two decades, the role of textbooks in both teachers' teaching and students' learning of mathematics has received increasing attention from researchers (e.g., see Ball & Cohen, 1996). Many studies have revealed that the availability of textbooks (i.e., the presence of textbooks in class) was positively associated with student achievement, especially in the developing countries (e.g., Fuller & Clarke, 1994; Heyneman, Farrell, & Sepulveda-Stuardo, 1978; Schiefelbein & Simmons, 1981). Moreover, researchers around the world have consistently reported the extensive use of textbooks in classrooms. For example, in Germany and Switzerland, teachers used one main textbook for mathematics teaching for each year and overall followed the book fairly closely (Bierhoff, 1996). In England, the majority of teaching approaches in classroom practice were found to essentially reflect those embodied in the textbooks (ibid.). In the US, researchers found that 75 to 90 percent of instructional time was structured around textbooks (Tyson & Woodward, 1989; Woodward & Elliott, 1990). In Japan, Fujii (2001) indicated that the majority of teachers taught the contents in textbooks in a straightforward way; they usually neither went beyond the materials nor offered less than what was included in the books, which he called "a very honest manner".

Studies on how teachers use textbooks in their teaching practice have so far generated different conclusions. Relatively speaking, earlier studies (i.e., before the mid-1980s) showed more evidence that school teachers adhered closely to textbooks in terms of content selection and sequencing. The teaching approaches adopted by the teachers were also highly similar to those presented in the books (e.g., McCutcheon, 1982; National Advisory Committee of Mathematics Education, as cited in Kuhs & Freeman, 1979; Woodward & Elliott, 1990). However, more recent studies revealed that there existed significant differences on the ways in which teachers used textbooks in class. For instance, Schmidt, Porter, Floden, Freeman, and Schwille (1987) found that there were four patterns of textbook use by eighteen primary mathematics teachers in Michigan, US: (1) classic textbook-follower (six teachers), (2) textbook follower/strong student influence (six teachers), (3) follower of district objectives (three teachers), and (4) follower of conception and past experiences (three teachers). Similarly, Freeman and Porter (1989) also found that there are three styles of textbook use by four primary mathematics teachers: (1) textbook-bound (one teacher), (2) focus on the basics (two teachers), and (3) focus on district objectives (one teacher).

The inconsistency in the findings of different researches about how teachers used textbooks in their teaching suggests that teachers' use of textbooks is a complex activity. Many factors could affect teachers' behavior and decision about how textbooks are used. Textbooks themselves could be such a factor that has direct impacts on the ways in which teachers used them. In other words, teachers might use different textbooks in different ways (e.g., Barr, 1988; Fan & Kaeley, 2000; Krammer, 1985).

Another reason for the inconsistency might be related to the fact that many of the studies on how teachers used textbooks were, as Fan and Kaeley (2000) indicated, of small scale. As Love and Pimm (1996) pointed out, collecting research data in this area is rather difficult. Understandably, there could be problems concerning the external validity of findings from such small-scale studies. In this sense, more studies, especially those with a larger scale, are still needed.

Naturally, large-scale studies would involve more subjects. However, the data in currently available large-scale studies were often just collected by questionnaire surveys, as we can see from the Second International Mathematics Study (SIMS) and the Third International Mathematics and Science Study (TIMSS). Some researchers have questioned about the (internal) validity of findings obtained merely from this research method, that is, teachers' self-reports on textbook use. In fact, some researchers have reported a conflict between how teachers reported their use of textbooks and how they really used textbooks in practice (e.g., Sepulveda-Stuardo & Farrell, 1983). Sosniak and Stodolsky (1993) pointed out that many teachers were not concerned or self-conscious about how they used textbooks in their own teaching.

Overall, among the limited number of studies on textbook use in teaching and learning, most were conducted in Western educational contexts. As Zhu and Fan (2002) noted, there were few such studies conducted in Asian countries, particularly in Chinese school settings. In addition, most studies were from a perspective of teaching, that is, on how teachers use mathematics textbooks in their teaching, and few were from a perspective of learning, namely, on how students use textbooks in their learning.

The main purpose of this study was to investigate how mathematics teachers in secondary schools in two major cities, Kuming and Fuzhou, of China used mathematics textbooks in their teaching. The study was also partially designed to look into how students there used mathematics textbooks in their learning of mathematics. Through investigating the ways in which teacher and students in those two cities used mathematics textbooks both within and beyond classrooms, we hope to provide useful empirical evidence and shed light on what role textbooks play in the teaching and learning of mathematics in Chinese educational environment and how they shape the way Chinese students learn mathematics. In addition, the study also examined some factors that might affect the ways in which the teachers and students used the textbooks.

2 Research Design and Procedures

2.1 *Population and sample*

There are several series of mathematics textbook currently being used in Mainland China, all being approved by the Ministry of Education. In each year, the ministry issues an approved textbook list for schools to select. In the past, there were totally eight series of mathematics textbooks being used at junior high school level. The majority of Chinese students (around 70%) used the books published by People's Education Press (PEP) (Zeng, 1997; also see Li Jianhua this volume). Mainly because of its popularity, the PEP series was chosen for this study[1].

However, in the latest major curriculum reform, new textbooks were nation-widely introduced progressively from 2000 (Lian, 2000) and that the PEP series will be finally completely phased out. As a matter of fact, students in both Fuzhou and Kunming have stopped using the PEP series from Junior High 1 (JH1) since 2002, though students at Junior High 2 (JH2) were still using the series. Therefore, only JH2 students in both

---

[1] Another reason for us to select this series is that we have undertaken a study on the textbooks and hence obtained reasonable knowledge about the textbooks, particularly on their content, structure, and ways of representing mathematics problem solving (see Zhu, 2003).

cities were involved in this study, the target population of the study. Correspondingly, *Algebra II* and *Geometry II* of the PEP series are the two textbooks being then used by the teachers and students.

The research subjects of this study consisted of 36 mathematics teachers and 272 students from 12 secondary schools (6 in Fuzhou and 6 in Kunming), a stratified sample from the population. More specifically, in each city, two schools were selected from high-performing schools (School Cohort I), two schools were selected from average-performing schools (School Cohort II), and the other two were selected from low-performing schools (School Cohort III).

Table 1 presents the background information of the 36 participating teachers, including their gender, highest education level, length of mathematics teaching experience, and the experience of teaching with the textbooks. All the information was gathered from the first four questions in the teacher questionnaire used in this study (see below).

Table 1
A Profile of the 36 Participating Teachers

	Fuzhou						Kunming						Total
	I		II		III		I		II		III		
	A	B	C	D	E	F	G	H	I	J	K	L	
Gender of teachers													
Male	0	1	1	1	1	0	0	3	0	2	0	1	10
Female	2	1	1	1	1	2	5	4	2	4	2	1	26
Highest level of education													
Teacher College	0	0	1	1	1	0	1	0	0	1	1	0	6
Normal University	2	2	1	1	1	2	3	6	2	5	1	2	28
Other University	0	0	0	0	0	0	1	1	0	0	0	0	2
Experience of teaching mathematics[1]													
< 10 years	1	1	1	1	1	1	3	2	1	2	1	1	16
≥ 10 years	1	1	1	1	1	1	2	4	1	4	1	1	19
Experience of teaching with the PEP series													
< 10 years	1	1	1	2	1	1	4	3	2	3	1	1	21
≥ 10 years	1	1	1	0	1	1	1	3	0	3	1	1	14

[1] One teacher in School H did not report the year of teaching mathematics and that of teaching with the PEP series.

As for the students, 121 were from Fuzhou and the other 151 were from Kunming. In each city, the numbers of participating male students and female students were nearly equal.

2.2 *Instruments and data collection*

Three instruments were designed for this study: questionnaires, classroom observation, and interviews.

2.2.1 *Questionnaire*

The questionnaire survey used two questionnaires, one for teachers and the other for students. Both questionnaires are in multiple-choice format. The construction of the questionnaires was mainly based on the structure of the PEP books.

There are 27 questions in the teacher questionnaire. Questions 1 to 4 are set to collect teachers' background information, as shown in Table 1, which is helpful to understand and analyze teachers' responses to the questionnaire. Questions 5 to 14 are about teachers' general use of the textbooks. For example, Question 7 asks teachers how often they used textbooks (student edition) in class. Questions 15 to 24 focus on how teachers used different groups of problems in the textbooks, such as example problems. Questions 25 and 26 are on teachers' understandings of the importance of various teaching materials, including textbooks, in teachers' teaching and students' learning. The last question asks teachers whether there had been changes in their textbook use since they became mathematics teachers.

The student questionnaire consisted of 14 questions; its design is similar to that of the teacher one. Questions 1 to 5 are about students' general use of the textbooks. Questions 6 to 12 focus on how students used different parts of texts, including various groups of problems, in the textbooks. Question 13 is about students' understandings of the importance of various learning materials, including textbooks, in their mathematics learning. The last question asks students whether there had been changes in their textbook use from year JH1 to year JH2.

A pilot test of the teacher questionnaire with 2 teachers in Fuzhou and 3 teachers in Kunming selected from the population but not in the sample showed that the questionnaire could be completed within 30 minutes. Moreover, none of the five teachers had difficulty in answering the questionnaire.

2.2.2 *Classroom observation*

Having noticed the validity issue concerning the questionnaire survey method as raised by researchers mentioned earlier, we also employed two other instruments: classroom observation and interview, for data collection.

Two teachers in each sample school with different teaching experience, that is, one teacher with less than 10-year teaching experience and the other with no less than 10-year teaching experience, were observed for their actual classroom teaching. All the teachers in Fuzhou were observed for once (one class period), whereas those in Kunming were observed twice.

The classroom observation was used to investigate what really happened in class, with the focus being on textbook use by both teachers and students. Instruction for classroom observation was pre-designed. All classroom observations were documented with field notes. Those in Kunming were also tape recorded.

2.2.3 *Interview*

The interviews were conducted with all the teachers who received classroom observation. Interviews were used to ask teachers open-ended questions which were not covered or difficult to be asked in questionnaires; in particular, they were used to explore the underlying reasons why teachers were using the textbooks in the ways which they have reported in questionnaires or been observed in classroom teaching.

General instruction for interviews was also pre-designed in order to keep the interviews focused and consistent. Understandably, in the actual interviews, questions were posed based on what the teachers had demonstrated in the classroom observation and other actual situations. Each interview was scheduled to take about 30 minutes.

2.2.4 *Data collection*

Data collection from schools took place in the second quarter of 2003[2]. In Fuzhou, the questionnaires were distributed to about 20 JH2 students and 2 mathematics teachers in each of the 6 sample schools with a response rate being 100% from both the students and teachers. In Kunming, the questionnaires were distributed to all the JH2 students and their mathematics teachers in the 6 sample schools with a response rate being, around 88% from the students and 80% from the teachers.

As mentioned before, in each sample school, 2 teachers with different lengths of teaching experience were observed for their classroom teaching. In total, 36 lessons consisting of 14 algebra lessons and 22 geometry lessons were observed. In Fuzhou each teacher was observed for one lesson (class period) and in Kunming each teacher was observed for two lessons, Among the 36 lessons observed, 25 lessons were normal lessons and 11 were review lessons.

Before the classroom observation, the information relevant to the observed classes was gathered by the researchers, including student background, teaching content, and the structures and characteristics of the corresponding texts in the textbooks.

All the 12 teachers were interviewed after the classroom observation. The interviews focused mainly on the reasons why the teachers used textbooks in the ways that displayed in the classroom observations. Correspondingly, the questions asked in the interviews varied from teacher to teacher. All the interviews were documented with field notes. Those conducted in Kunming were further tape recorded.

2.2.5 *Data processing and analysis*

The data in tape-recorded form obtained from classroom observations and interviews were first transcribed verbatim. Together with the transcriptions, all the collected data were translated from Chinese into

---

[2] In Mainland China, a school academic year usually starts from the beginning of September and ends around the end of next June, and when the data were collected in the study, the two textbooks had been used by the teachers and students for close to two semesters.

English before analysis. The data from the questionnaires were then stored, processed, and analyzed using SPSS mainly by quantitative methods. The analysis is intended to get a general picture about how students and teachers use textbooks in mathematics class.

The data from the other two instruments were analyzed mainly by qualitative methods. It is used to examine how textbooks were actually used by students and teachers in mathematics class and also the reasons why textbooks were used in this way or that way.

In addition, to detect the factors that might affect the ways in which textbooks were used, three criteria were respectively employed to classify both students and teachers into different groups for comparison:

1. *Region*: Fuzhou *vs.* Kunming
2. *School quality*: high-performing schools, average-performing schools, and low-performing schools (i.e., School Cohort I, School Cohort II, and School Cohort III)
3. *Gender*: Male *vs.* Female

For teachers, two more dichotomies were created according to their responses to the first four questions in the teacher questionnaire:

4. *Teaching experience*: Novice teachers *vs.* Experienced teachers;
5. *Teaching experience with the PEP series*: Novice users *vs.* Experienced users.

In this study, "Novice teachers" refer to the teachers who had taught mathematics for less than 10 years and the remaining teachers are defined as "Experienced teachers". Similarly, the time period of 10 years was also used to distinguish "Novice users" from "Experienced users".

We were initially also interested to know if teachers' educational background would affect the way in which they use the textbooks. However, as showed in Table 1, it is quite homogenous among the 36 participating teachers in this aspect. In particular, more than four fifths of the teachers were university graduates and all but two of them were from normal universities. Therefore, it is difficult for this study to detect whether teachers with different education background would use textbooks differently, and "education background" was not used as a variable for classification and hence no comparison was made against it.

3 Results and Discussions

The results of this study are reported in the following sequence: general use of the textbooks, use of various parts of texts in the books, and some other issues (including teachers' understanding of the role of textbooks in mathematics teaching and learning and their changes in textbook use over the years), which is parallel to the sequence of the questions arranged in the questionnaires.

3.1 *General use of the textbooks*

Ten questions in the teacher questionnaire and 5 questions in the student questionnaire were specifically focused on the general use of the textbooks.

According to teachers' response to the questionnaire survey, about 22% teachers "always" followed the order presented in the textbooks, the others "often" or "sometimes" did so, and no one "seldom" or "never" followed the order. Moreover, it was found that there was significant difference among the teachers from different school cohorts, χ^2 (2, $N = 36$) = 8.25, $p < .05$. In particular, significantly more teachers from low performing schools "always" followed the sequence in the textbooks than those from high performing schools, χ^2 (1, $N = 25$) = 7.68, $p < .05$. The result seems understandable. As some teachers commented in the interview, it was convenient for students to understand better and review well what had been taught in class if teachers followed the textbooks closely in their teaching. It appears that students from low performing schools who were relatively slow learners could benefit more from such a textbook use strategy.

In the questionnaire survey, the percentages of the teachers who reported that they "always", "often", and "sometimes" used the textbooks in their classroom teaching were 22%, 59%, and 19% respectively, while no teacher claimed that he/she "seldom" or "never" used the textbooks. No significant difference was found across different comparison groups in this aspect of textbook use.

The classroom observation confirmed the above result. In particular, except for 5 lessons in Kunming and 1 in Fuzhou, in all the lessons observed teachers used textbooks in their classroom teaching. The five lessons in Kunming were review lessons taught by five teachers. Nevertheless, all these teachers used textbooks in the other lesson observed. Moreover, four out of the five teachers were found using textbooks over 60% of the instructional time, with an average being 71.6%. The lesson in Fuzhou observed was a typical lesson. When being asked why he did not use textbooks in the lesson, the teacher explained that "it was the second lesson on Section 12.4 and the content was more difficult so that the examples and exercises were all not from textbooks." In fact, in the lesson, the examples and exercises used were either taken from past examination papers or designed by the teacher himself. Examining the teacher's questionnaire, we found that the teacher actually reported that he conducted his lesson "always" following the order suggested by the textbook and he "often" used textbooks in his class.

Different from the finding that more than 80% of the teachers "always" or "often" used textbooks in their lessons, students' responses to the questionnaire showed that they used the books in classes less frequently. According to the responses, 7% of the students "seldom" or "never" used textbooks in mathematics classes, 29% of the students "sometimes" did so, and the percentages of "often" or "always" using the textbooks in classes were 41% and 23%, respectively. The difference between teachers and students in the frequency of using textbooks in classes, to some extent, suggests that textbooks serve more as a teaching resource than as a learning resource in Chinese classrooms. In other words, textbooks are indeed used more as "teaching materials" than as "learning materials"[3]. By the way, no significant differences were found among different comparison groups of students in this aspect.

The data collected from the teacher questionnaire revealed that the percentage of instructional time being structured by textbooks in

---

[3] In fact, "textbooks" in Chinese are usually called *ke ben* (课本, literally "texts for lessons"), or simply *jiao cai* (教材, literally "teaching materials").

mathematics classes varied from 20% to 90%, with an average being 66.7%. No significant difference was detected across comparison groups of teachers. According to the classroom observation conducted in Kunming, which recorded the time structure of all the lessons in detail, we found that excluding the five review lessons without using textbooks, there was 72.4% of the instructional time involving the use of textbooks. The result is largely consistent with available findings from US classrooms, where around 75 to 90 percent of instructional time was found to be centered on textbooks (Tyson & Woodward, 1989; Woodward & Elliott, 1990).

The TIMSS study found that in five out of 34 educational systems, mathematics teachers relied more on the curriculum guides than textbooks when they made decisions on "what to teach". As to teaching approaches, most used textbooks as their main resources (see Beaton et al., 1996). In this study, we set two similar questions. The results showed that the teachers used textbooks (student edition) most frequently among all the teaching materials for both content and approach decisions (see Figure 1).

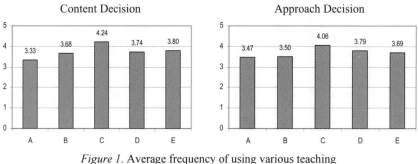

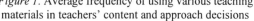

Figure 1. Average frequency of using various teaching materials in teachers' content and approach decisions

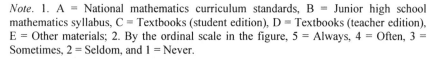

Note. 1. A = National mathematics curriculum standards, B = Junior high school mathematics syllabus, C = Textbooks (student edition), D = Textbooks (teacher edition), E = Other materials; 2. By the ordinal scale in the figure, 5 = Always, 4 = Often, 3 = Sometimes, 2 = Seldom, and 1 = Never.

Consistent with the results from the above analysis based on the average frequency, an ordinal regression (PLUM) using SPSS revealed that in both content and approach decision making procedures, the teachers used textbooks (student edition) with the highest frequency. Table 2 shows that the order of the frequency of using the five teaching materials for content decision is, from highest to lowest, "textbooks (student edition)" (C), "other materials" (E), "textbooks (teacher edition)" (D), "junior high school mathematics syllabus" (B), and "national mathematics curriculum standards" (A). Furthermore, it can be found that the teachers used "textbooks (student edition)" for content decisions significantly more often than "textbooks (teacher edition)" at the 0.01 level, whereas the frequency of using the other three materials was at the same level as that of using "textbooks (teacher edition)". The order for the approach decisions is quite similar to that for the content decisions: "textbooks (student edition)" (C), "textbooks (teacher edition)" (D), "other materials" (E), "junior high school mathematics syllabus" (B), and "national mathematics curriculum standards" (A).

Table 2
Log-Linear Regression Results on the Data about Content Decisions by Teachers

Parameter Estimates

		Estimate	Std. Error	Wald	df	Sig.	95% Confidence Interval	
							Lower Bound	Upper Bound
Threshold	[FREQUENC = 1]	-4.485	1.293	12.021	1	.001	-7.020	-1.949
	[FREQUENC = 2]	-2.694	1.187	5.156	1	.023	-5.020	-.369
	[FREQUENC = 3]	-1.164	1.173	.986	1	.321	-3.463	1.134
	[FREQUENC = 4]	1.294	1.170	1.224	1	.269	-.998	3.586
Location	[STANDARD=0]	.8005	.456	3.079	1	.079	-9.370E-02	1.695
	[STANDARD=1]	0[a]	.	.	0	.	.	.
	[SYLLABUS=0]	4.644E-02	.455	.010	1	.919	-.846	.939
	[SYLLABUS=1]	0[a]	.	.	0	.	.	.
	[SBOOK=0]	-1.2249	.470	6.782	1	.0092	-2.147	-.303
	[SBOOK=1]	0[a]	.	.	0	.	.	.
	[OTHERS=0]	-2.41E-02	.471	.003	1	.959	-.947	.899
	[OTHERS=1]	0[a]	.	.	0	.	.	.
	[TBOOK=0]	0[a]	.	.	0	.	.	.
	[TBOOK=1]	0[a]	.	.	0	.	.	.

Link function: Logit.
a. This parameter is set to zero because it is redundant.

Note. STANDARD = National mathematics curriculum standards, SYLLABUS = Junior high school mathematics syllabus, SBOOK = Textbooks (student edition), TBOOK = Textbooks (teacher edition), and OTHERS= Other materials.

In the interview, many teachers reported that they always used textbooks in their lesson preparations. When being asked for the purposes of using textbooks at this stage, most mentioned that to decide teaching contents and approaches was one of the main concerns. In addition, some teachers also selected example problems, in-class exercises, and homework from the textbooks during their lesson planning.

The frequency of using various teaching materials in the two processes across different teacher groups was more or less the same. Chi-square tests revealed that school quality was the only factor having significant influence on the frequency of using syllabus (χ^2 [8, N = 34] = 16.83, p < .05) and textbooks (teacher edition) (χ^2 [6, N = 34] = 13.94, p < .05), when teachers decided teaching approaches. In particular, significantly more teachers from School Cohort II at least "sometimes" resorted to syllabus for teaching approaches than those from School Cohort III, χ^2 (1, N = 19) = 3.96, p < .05; significantly more teachers from School Cohort II "always" or "often" used textbooks (teacher edition) in preparing for teaching approaches than those from School Cohort III, χ^2 (1, N = 19) = 4.00, p < .05.

The questionnaire also asked teachers how often they referred to various teaching materials to select example problems, in-class exercises, and homework. In terms of the average frequency, the results showed that textbooks (both student and teacher editions) were used most frequently in the three activities (see Table 3), which is largely confirmed from the interviews as mentioned earlier. No significant difference was found across different comparison groups.

Table 3
Average Frequency of Using Various Teaching Materials to Select Tasks for Example, In-class Exercise, and Homework Assignment

	Example	In-class exercise	Homework
A	3.13	3.10	3.07
B	3.27	3.43	3.39
C	4.17	4.37	4.34
D	3.90	3.94	3.81
E	3.60	3.68	3.73

Note. 1. A = National mathematics curriculum standards, B = Junior high school mathematics syllabus, C = Textbooks (student edition), D = Textbooks (teacher edition), E = Other materials; 2. By the ordinal scale in the figure, 5 = always, 4 = often, 3 = sometimes, 2 = seldom, and 1 = never.

Log-linear regression analysis again obtained consistent results. It indicates that the five teaching materials from the most frequently used one to the least one in all the three activities were "textbooks (student edition)" (C), "textbooks (teacher edition)" (D), "other materials" (E), "junior high school mathematics syllabus" (B), and "national mathematics curriculum standards" (A). Moreover, the analysis showed that when selecting both example problems and in-class exercises, the teachers significantly more often referred to "textbooks (student edition)" than "other materials" at the 0.01 level, whereas the frequencies of using the other four teaching materials were at the same significant level. For homework assignment, the frequency of using "textbooks (student edition)" was again significantly higher than that of using "other materials" and the difference reached at the 0.001 level, meanwhile the use of "national mathematics curriculum standards" was less frequently than the use of "other materials" at the 0.05 level.

It should be pointed out that the above finding has been consistently found by many other researchers in different educational settings. For instance, in a survey of 28 Australian secondary mathematics teachers' preferences in textbook characteristics and uses, Shield (1989) found that the most important textbook use was for student exercises in class and for homework (also see National Advisory Committee on Mathematics Education, as cited in Nicely, 1985; Porter, Floden, Freeman, Schmidt, & Schwille, as cited in Flanders, 1987; Zhu & Fan, 2002).

In the student questionnaire, students were asked to estimate how much of their homework was directly from textbooks. Around 60% of the students claimed that "almost all" or "large part" of their homework were assigned from textbooks, while more than 20% of the students reported that only "small part" or "very little" of the homework were from the books. It was further found that students in Kunming received significantly more homework from textbooks than those in Fuzhou, χ^2 (4, $N = 266) = 42.52$, $p < .001$. School quality was another factor that had significant influence on the source of homework; students' homework in high performing schools was assigned from textbooks significantly more than that in both average (χ^2 [4, $N = 186$] = 35.02, $p < .001$) and low (χ^2 [4, $N = 169$] = 15.27, $p < .01$) performing schools. The reason might be that students in lower performing schools were assigned more extra homework for reinforcement; nevertheless more evidences are needed concerning this result.

The classroom observation revealed that a higher percentage of teachers in Kunming (41.7%) assigned homework entirely from textbooks than those in Fuzhou (25.0%). However, we did not find teachers from different school cohorts had significant difference on homework assigning, in terms of the source of homework. The fact that only a limited number of lessons were observed might be one reason for the inconsistency between the result obtained from the classroom observation and that from the student questionnaire.

The importance of textbooks in lesson preparations was highly evaluated by the teachers. In particular, all the teachers gave positive evaluation and 62.9% of them rated "textbooks (student edition)" "very important" and 54.5% gave the same evaluation to "textbooks (teacher edition)". Moreover, an ordinal regression (PLUM) revealed that the importance of "other materials" was significantly lower than that of textbooks in both student and teacher versions at the 0.01 level. It was found that teachers from different comparison groups had no significant differences on the evaluations of the importance of various teaching materials in their lesson preparations.

In the teacher questionnaire, teachers were also asked how often they required students to read textbooks before, during, and after classes. Correspondingly, students were asked in the student questionnaire how often they read the textbooks at the three time periods. The results were displayed in Table 4.

Table 4
Teachers' Requirements (TR) on Reading Textbooks and Students' Actual Reading (S) Before, During, and After Classes

	Before the class		During the class		After the class	
	TR	S	TR	S	TR	S
Always	9 (26.5%)	22 (8.1%)	8 (22.9%)	36 (13.4%)	6 (17.6%)	14 (5.3%)
Often	15 (44.1%)	66 (24.4%)	14 (40.0%)	110 (40.9%)	18 (52.9%)	72 (27.2%)
Sometimes	7 (20.6%)	115 (42.4%)	9 (25.7%)	90 (33.5%)	7 (20.6%)	112 (42.3%)
Seldom	3 (8.8%)	52 (19.2%)	4 (11.4%)	26 (9.7%)	3 (8.8%)	60 (22.6%)
Never	0 (0%)	16 (5.9%)	0 (0%)	7 (2.6%)	0 (0%)	7 (2.6%)

Table 4 suggests that students read textbooks most often during the class and least before the class. An ordinal regression (PLUM) further revealed that students read textbooks significantly more frequently during the class than after the class at the 0.001 level. Teachers' direct instruction on reading textbooks during the class might be one motivation for students to do the in-class reading. It can be seen from the table that more than 88% of the teachers at least "sometimes" required their students to read textbooks in class.

The classroom observation found that the majority of teachers (62.5%) asked students to read textbooks in class, including reading main texts and example problems. Most lessons with reading instruction were normal lessons (16 out of 18). The results from the follow-up interview consistently revealed that the majority of teachers at least "sometimes" asked their students to read textbooks in class. However, in students' views, the main reason for them to read textbooks in class is not teachers' requirement on reading but their own desires (teachers' instruction: 21.1%, self motivations: 70.5%, other reasons: 8.4%).

Table 4 also shows that teachers less frequently required students to read the textbooks during the class than to do so during the other two time periods. No statistically significant differences were found among teachers from different comparison groups about this requirement. In the interviews, many teachers also expressed their preference for students to read textbooks before classes. In doing so, teachers expected students to have some ideas about what they were going to learn in the next lesson so as to achieve better learning effects. However, some teachers also doubted whether their students would really read textbooks before and after classes. One teacher from School Cohort II pointed out that she required students' parents to check students' reading outside the classroom. Students' self-reports showed that nearly 25% of the students "seldom" or "never" read textbooks before or after classes, and most of them (68.2%) claimed that they did not read textbooks because they did not have such a habit.

A further analysis with respect to different comparison groups of students revealed that the students in Fuzhou read textbooks both before classes and during classes significantly more frequently than their peers in Kunming (Before: χ^2 [4, $N = 271$] $= 20.79$, $p < .001$; During: χ^2 [4, $N =$

269] $= 12.73$, $p < .05$]. Further study is needed to explore why there is such a difference. Nevertheless, no significant difference was found on teachers' requirement on reading during the two time periods between the two cities.

3.2 *Use of various parts of texts*

In the PEP textbooks, a regular chapter usually consisted of several parts: introduction, main text (including example problems and their solutions), various exercise problems[4] (i.e., Drill, Practice, Revision, Self-Test, Think-it-Over), summary and revision, and enrichment materials[5] (i.e., Read-it, and Do-it[6]) (see more details in Zhu, 2003). To investigate how these components of the texts are used by both students and teachers, specific questions were designed in the questionnaires.

Mathematics textbooks, particularly Asian ones, normally devoted much space to example problems and their solutions, including explanations. For instance, earlier studies found that 63% of text space in Japanese textbooks and 67% in Chinese textbooks was used for worked-out examples and related explanations (Carter, Li, & Ferrucci, 1997; Mayer, Sims, & Tajika, 1995). As Love and Pimm (1996) noted, examples were intended to offer students a model to be emulated in the exercises which followed. In this sense, examples with their explanations played a very important role in the process of teaching and learning.

In the present study, we found that in all but two normal lessons (92%), teachers presented examples to students in the classes observed.

Where the examples used by the teachers in class came from was one of our concerns. Questions 15 to 17 in the teacher questionnaire were

---

[4] According to the textbook authors, "Drill" problems (练习) are mainly for in-class use for consolidation; "Practice" problems (习题) are mainly for in-class or after-class assignment; "Revision" problems (复习题) are designed for chapter revision; "Self-Test" problems (自我测验题) are for self checking after completing learning of one chapter; "Think-it-Over" problems (想一想) are mainly for students to do high order thinking (PEP, 1993a, 1993b).
[5] Not all chapters have enrichment materials.
[6] Only geometry books have problems entitled "Do-it", which provide students with "hands-on" activities.

targeted on this issue. The results showed that the percentages of examples illustrated in class which were from textbook examples varied from 10% to 100%, with an average being 74.4%. Nevertheless, the teachers also reported that around 65% of in-class examples were taken from various types of non-example problems provided in the books. It seems to us that some teachers were not clearly aware how they selected in-class examples.

The results from classroom observations showed that only around 35.2% of the in-class examples were textbook examples. The main texts also contained some worked-out problems which were not designed as examples. In the classroom observations, quite a number of teachers used these problems as in-class examples. Including these problems, we found that the corresponding percentage of in-class examples being worked-out problems in the textbooks was 52.7%. In addition, no exercise problems in the textbooks were used by the teachers as in-class examples in the classes observed.

The questionnaire survey revealed that about 81.7% of the textbook examples were used by teachers in their classroom teaching practices. We also compared the examples actually used in the classes observed and the example problems presented in the corresponding texts, and the result showed that 80% of the textbook examples were used in class by those teachers who were observed. When including all the non-example problems in the main text, we found that the percentage reached 88.2%.

The classroom observations found that 75% of the teachers who conducted normal lessons used examples which were not from textbooks or simply designed by themselves. In the 17 normal lessons observed in Kunming, teachers presented a total of 52 in-class examples, while there were only 20 example problems available in the corresponding texts. Although the teachers used nearly all of these textbook examples as in-class examples and some of them further used the non-example worked-out problems in the main text, 22 in-class examples were either taken from other teaching materials or designed by the teachers themselves.

In the interview, all the teachers reported that in general they would use textbook examples as in-class examples, meanwhile they also often selected in-class examples from other types of problems in the textbooks and other reference books. Although no teacher claimed that the shortage of textbook examples was one reason for he/she used examples from outside materials, most teachers indicated that the purpose for them to resort to other resources was to deepen students' understanding, widen students' views, and promote the development of students' ability in problem solving. It appears that the examples provided in the textbooks were not sufficient in both quantity and quality for teachers to use in their classrooms.

With respect to the way in which the textbooks presented the solutions to the example problems, we found that the majority of teachers (75.8%) "always" or "often" used the ways presented in the textbooks but with some modifications. No one reported that he/she strictly followed the textbooks all the time, and a minority (18.5%) of the teachers said that they often used the ways different from the textbooks. By the way, further analysis revealed that female teachers used the ways presented by the textbooks without modifications significantly more frequently than their male colleagues, χ^2 (2, $N = 30$) = 6.47, $p < .05$. Moreover, male teachers tended to use different ways from the textbooks more often than female teachers and the difference was statistically significant at the 0.05 level (χ^2 [2, $N = 27$] = 8.00).

The classroom observations also showed that many teachers illustrated the examples in the ways which were presented in the textbooks. Moreover, the teachers in many cases added some alterative solutions to those example problems, either demonstrated by themselves or asked students to provide alterative solutions. In the observed classes, we did not find any teacher who used the ways significantly different from the textbooks.

During the interviews, teachers were asked why they in the observed lessons used some different ways from the textbooks for presenting the examples. Almost all the teachers told us that they would basically follow the ways presented in the textbooks, since those ways were usually fundamental, simple, and easy for students to understand. Using the ways in textbooks was also convenient for students to do revision after class. However, the ways in the textbooks might not be best ones so that they often provided students with alterative ways to broaden students' minds and encourage them to think.

Various exercise problems designed for students to work through are another important component of mathematics textbooks. As reported earlier, teachers often selected in-class exercises and homework tasks from this component of the books. Teachers' self-reports in the questionnaire showed that the problems under the rubrics of "Drill" and "Practice" had the highest rates of utilization, whereas the problems entitled "Think-it-Over" were used least (see Figure 2).

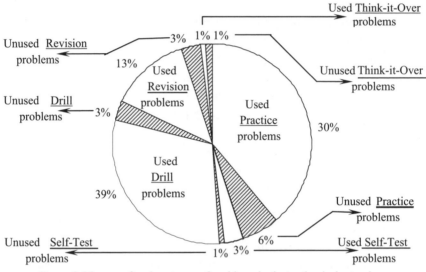

Figure 2. The use of various types of problems in the textbooks by teachers

The t-tests revealed that the teachers used the various types of exercise problems significantly differently across the problem categories. The results are displayed in Table 5.

It can be seen that the teachers used significantly fewer problems under the rubric "Think-it-Over" than all the other types of problems in class. The difficulty of these problems could be one possible reason. An analysis on the features of the various types of problems in the textbooks revealed that more non-routine problems were in these exercise problems (Drill: 0.3%, Practice: 0.1%, Revision: 0%, Self-Test: 0%, Think-it-Over: 9.5%; see more details in Zhu, 2003). According to the textbook authors, the purpose of providing "Think-it-Over" problems was to enrich students' knowledge and inspire their interest. The contents involved in these problems can go beyond the normal curriculum requirement (PEP, 1993a, 1993b). Therefore, it is reasonable that the teachers used those problems less frequently than other problems.

Table 5
T-test Results on Teachers' Use of Various Exercise Problems Offered in the Textbooks.

	Drill	Practice	Revision	Self-Test	Think-it-Over
Drill	–	1.153	3.01^{**}	2.47^{*}	4.29^{***}
Practice		–	3.06^{**}	1.981	4.02^{***}
Revision			–	0.87	3.04^{*}
Self-Test				–	2.53^{*}
Think-it-Over					–

Note. $^{*}p < .05$, $^{**}p < .001$, $^{***}p < .001$. "Drill" problems were not used significantly more than "Self-Test" problems, but the difference approached significance, $p = .056$.

From the table, we can also find that the teachers used significantly more "Drill" and "Practice" problems than "Revision" and "Self-Test" problems. The main reason appears to be the fact that "Drill" and "Practice" problems were provided for each lesson to reinforce what students have learned, and hence were fundamental in students' learning, whereas "Revision" problems were provided at the end of a chapter for chapter review purpose.

Although "Self-Test" problems were also offered at the end of a chapter, they were not as challenging as those in "Revision" and "Practice" (Group B[7]), in terms of the number of steps involved in problem solutions. As described on the book preface, "Self-Test" problems were intentionally designed for students' self-checking whether they have achieved basic learning objectives (PEP, 1993a, 1993b). Since these problems were particularly set for students' self-learning, it was reasonable that teachers did not use them much but left them to students themselves.

In general, there was no much difference on the use of various types of problems offered in the textbooks by the teachers across different comparison groups. The only significant difference was detected on the

---

[7] The textbooks divided problems in both "Practice" and "Review" into two groups: A and B. Problems in Group A were basic ones and meant for all the students, whereas those in Group B were relatively challenging and meant for students of higher ability.

use of "Self-Test" problems. Experienced teachers and users used significantly more of these problems than novices at the 0.05 level. Being more familiar with teaching contents and the problem features could be one possible reason for the difference. Moreover, the concern that some students might not do these problems without teachers' requirement so that they would possibly miss something important (e.g., specific problem solving skills) could also be possible motivation for the experienced teachers/users to more often use the "Self-Test" problems.

The teacher questionnaire revealed that while teachers in Kunming did not use significantly more "Self-Test" problems than those in Fuzhou, the difference approached significance, $t (13) = -2.14$, $p = .051$. However, in the classroom observations, we did not see any teacher from both cities used these problems in actual classroom teaching. It might be because the fact that only a limited number of lessons were observed.

Besides the frequency of using the different types of problems, teachers were asked about the functions that these problems were used to serve in their instruction. Five particular usages were defined in the questionnaire. They were "in-class exercises", "homework", "in-class examples", "tests", and "discussions". Figure 3 displays the number of teachers who used the various types of exercise problems for the different purposes.

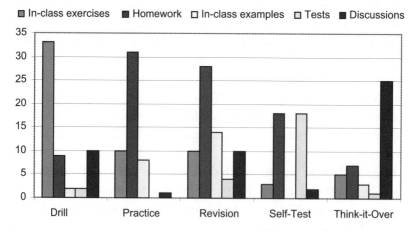

Figure 3. The usage of various types of exercise problems provided in the textbooks
Note. Three teachers did not give answers to the corresponding questions in the questionnaire.

It can be seen that all the teachers used "Drill" problems for in-class exercises, while around 30% of the teachers also used these problems for students' homework or in-class discussions. It was quite consistent with the book authors' intentions, as described on the book preface (PEP, 1993a, 1993b). In the classroom observations, we also found that in the majority of lessons (55.6%), teachers asked students to do the "Drill" problems in class.

The figure shows that both "Practice" and "Revision" problems were more used for students' homework. Consistently, in the observed lessons, the majority of teachers (81.8%) assigned homework from "Exercise" sections, although many teachers also often used other materials (45.8%) or self-designed problems (20.8%) for homework assignment. Moreover, only one teacher from each city selected homework from "Revision" in our observations and both lessons were understandably review lessons. In the interview, the teachers reported that around 65.4% of students' homework was assigned from the textbooks.

Compared to the other types of problems, "Self-Test" problems were more often used for in-class tests by the teachers. It was consistent with the textbook authors' intentions, as mentioned before. In addition, many teachers (54.5%) reported in the questionnaire that they also assigned these problems as students' homework. Nevertheless, this practice was not found in the classroom observation.

The teacher questionnaire data showed that the majority of teachers (75.8%) used "Think-it-Over" problems for in-class discussions. As said earlier, those problems were designed to enrich students' knowledge and inspire their interest, moreover a higher percentage of problems in this section were non-routine problems (Zhu, 2003). Therefore, the result seems understandable.

Figure 2 revealed that around 14% of all types of the problems in the textbooks were not used by the teachers in their teaching. In the student questionnaire, five questions were particularly designed on these unassigned problems. Table 6 lists the number (percentage) of students who worked on these unassigned problems under each type. The results showed that many students did the unassigned problems.

In general, there was no significant difference among the students from different comparison groups about the unassigned problems, except students from low performing schools did significantly more unassigned "Self-Test" problems than those from both high (χ^2 [4, N = 180] = 9.67, p< .05) and average (χ^2 [4, N = 180] = 16.92, p < .01) performing schools. It was found that all the "Self-Test" problems were routine problems and the majority of them (58.6%) were single-step problems (Zhu, 2003). It appears reasonable that student in School Cohort III were relatively slow learners so that they might need to do more elementary problems. When answering the reason for students to do these unassigned problems, many students indicated that it was their own choice. Only about 12.8% of the students claimed that the reason was that their teachers required them to do so and 7.8% of the students reported that the reason is that their parents asked them to do so.

Table 6
Students' Usage of Unassigned Exercise Problems Offered in the Textbooks

	Drill	Practice	Revision	Self-Test	Think-it-Over
Almost all	27 (10.0%)	21 (7.8%)	22 (8.2%)	31 (11.5%)	16 (6.0%)
Most	58 (21.6%)	51 (19.0%)	60 (22.4%)	51 (18.9%)	38 (14.3%)
About half	75 (27.9%)	84 (31.2%)	69 (25.7%)	66 (24.4%)	47 (17.7%)
Some	72 (26.8%)	73 (27.1%)	83 (31.0%)	74 (27.4%)	85 (32.1%)
Very few	37 (13.8%)	40 (14.9%)	34 (12.7%)	48 (17.8%)	79 (29.8%)

On the unassigned "Revision" problems, the study found that students in Fuzhou did significantly more than their peers in Kunming at the 0.05 level (χ^2 [4, N = 268] = 11.79). Again, the motivation of doing these problems was mainly from students themselves (69.3%).

Like many other textbooks, all but two textbooks (i.e., *Geometry II* and *Geometry III*) in the PEP series provided answers to some non-maintext problems at the back of the books. These answers were prepared for students' self-checking (PEP, 1993a). Figure 4 depicts the usage of the answer sections by the students according to the questionnaire data.

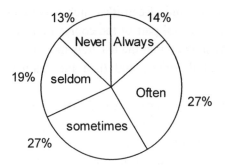

Figure 4. Use of answer sections by students

The results showed that only about 40% students often or always used the answer sections for self-checking. One reason for the low usage of the answer sections provided in the textbooks might be that the exercise problems were relatively easy for students, and hence they did not feel such a need to check the answers. Another reason might be that some students had not developed such a habit of self-checking. By the way, it is interesting to note that students in Fuzhou used the answer sections significantly more frequently than those in Kunming at the 0.05 level (χ^2 [4, N = 266] = 13.21).

"Do-it" problems were only included in the PEP geometry textbooks. In *Geometry II* there were only four problems under this category. These problems were intended to provide students extracurricular hands-on activities (PEP, 1993b). According to the teacher questionnaire, there were actually more than 54% of the teachers who "always" or "often" used these problems for in-class activities and no one claimed that he/she "never" used such problems. Nevertheless, in the classroom observation, there were three lessons (1 in Fuzhou and 2 in Kunming) whose corresponding texts had "Do-it" problems, but no one used the problems in classes observed.

As reported earlier, the majority of teachers required their students to read texts before, during, or after class. We further asked in the questionnaire how frequently the teachers required students to read the various parts of texts. They included the main text, "Summary and Revision" provided at the end of each chapter, which summarized all the key points in that chapter so as to provide a convenient source for students to do revision, and "Read-it" which was mainly for enrichment purpose and not an essential part of the course requirement (PEP, 1993a, 1993b). The results showed that the teachers most often asked students to read "Summary and Review", and then the main text, but least for "Read-it".

The classroom observations revealed that teachers seldom discussed the "Summary and Review" section with students in class. We believe that teachers would more likely leave it for students' self-learning. In addition, as pointed out in the preface of the textbooks, the requirement explained in "Summary and Review" was slight higher than that being reflected in the main texts within the chapter. More reading requirements on this part of texts from teachers were therefore understandable.

Concerning the main texts, a few teachers in the interview pointed out that if students had understood what had been taught in class, it was not necessary to ask them to read the corresponding texts again. In contrast, some teachers believed that it was good for students to read main texts before they started to do their homework. Therefore, more diversity was found among the teachers in their requirement for students' reading of this part compared to the part of "Summary and Review". The classroom observations also found that some teachers asked their students to read the main texts in class. Moreover, the results from the questionnaire showed that the longer the teachers used the books, the more frequently they would asked their students to read the main texts, χ^2 $(3, N = 33) = 7.54, p < .05$.

Similar questions were also included in the student questionnaire. Consistently, the students reported that they read "Read-it" least frequently and the difference between this part and the other two parts reached statistically significant level. In particular, only 4.6% of the students "seldom" or "never" read the main texts, and the percentage for "Summary and Review" was 20%. In addition, it was found that students in Fuzhou significantly more frequently read both text parts than their peers in Kunming (Main text: χ^2 [4, $N = 259$] = 13.14, $p < .01$; Summary and Review: χ^2 [4, $N = 255$] = 9.99, $p < .05$). In contrast, teachers' self-reports in the questionnaire showed that teachers in Kunming required their students to read "Summary and Review" with a significantly higher frequency than those in Fuzhou, χ^2 (3, $N = 33$) = 8.47, $p < .05$. Given the complexity of the teaching and learning process, the discrepancy between teachers' teaching and students' leaning seems plausible. Nevertheless, a further discussion of this discrepancy is beyond the scope of this chapter.

Table 7 presents a summary of descriptive statistics based on the data collected from the questionnaires. The gap between teachers' requirement and students' practice can be also found from the table.

Table 7
Teachers' Requirements (TR) on Reading and Students' Corresponding Practice (S)

	Main Text		Read-it		Summary and Review	
	TR	S	TR	S	TR	S
Always	5 (15.2%)	115 (44.4%)	4 (12.1%)	32 (12.5%)	11 (33.3%)	36 (14.1%)
Often	22 (66.7%)	82 (31.7%)	19 (57.6%)	60 (23.5%)	16 (48.5%)	91 (35.7%)
Sometimes	5 (15.2%)	50 (19.3%)	8 (24.2%)	110 (43.1%)	5 (15.2%)	77 (30.2%)
Seldom	1 (3.0%)	10 (3.9%)	2 (6.1%)	43 (16.9%)	1 (3.0%)	42 (16.5%)
Never	0 (0%)	2 (0.8%)	0 (0%)	10 (3.9%)	0 (0%)	9 (3.5%)

3.3 *Some other issues*

In the questionnaires, teachers and students were respectively requested to evaluate the importance of various instructional materials in their mathematics teaching and learning, with a 5-point Likert scale from the highest "very important" to the lowest "no importance". The majority of teachers (90.9%) and students (91.5%) chose the highest two evaluations (i.e., "very important" or "important") for the textbooks (student edition). None of the teacher and only 3 out of 259 students rated the textbooks as "little important" or "no importance", respectively. In addition, teachers in Kunming rated the importance of textbooks significantly higher than those in Fuzhou, χ^2 (2, $N = 33$) = 6.42, $p < .05$.

Overall, the questionnaire surveys showed that textbooks (student edition) were the most important materials in both teachers' teaching and students' learning. To students, the importance of the textbooks was significantly higher than that of any other learning materials at the 0.001 level. Consistently, the data revealed that the majority of teachers (84.8%) believed that the textbooks were also "very important" or "important" in students' learning of mathematics.

According to teachers' responses, the next two important teaching materials to their teaching were school mathematics syllabus and national mathematics standards. It is somehow surprising to us that the teachers from both cities gave a relatively low evaluation to the importance of the textbooks of teacher edition. We think it suggests that only the textbooks of student edition, but not teacher edition, is essential to teachers, especially experienced teachers.

The last question in both teacher and student questionnaires asked whether there had been changes in their textbook use since they became mathematics teachers (for teachers) or from year JH1 to year JH2 (for students). The results were displayed in Figure 5.

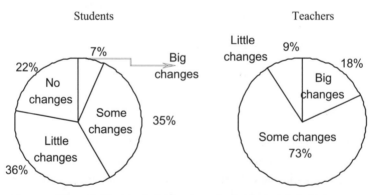

Figure 5. Changes in textbook use by teachers and students

It can be seen that teachers made more changes than their students in textbook use. In particular, only 42% of the students, but 91% of the teachers had some or big changes in their textbook use.

An open-ended sub-question was included in the last question to invite students and teachers to describe what kinds of changes they had made in textbook use. The most frequently cited change by the students was that they started to read the texts more (main text [1][8], Example [11], Summary [4], Read-it [6]). Many students reported that they did more preview (18) and review (7) this year than the last year. Moreover, quite a number of students also mentioned that they did more unassigned problems in the textbooks now than before, and six students particularly cited the problems under the rubric "Think-it-Over".

The last question in the student questionnaire further asked the reasons for the changes in their textbook use. Several reasons were identified by the students. One main reason was that the mathematics at JH2 becomes more challenging than that at JH1, in terms of both the amount of content (10) and its difficulty level (30). The second reason was that many students (41) realized that mathematics was increasingly important to them, although five of them just related the importance of mathematics to school examinations. It is interesting to note that there were four students attributed their changes in textbook use to the textbook developers. In particular, two of them noted that since the textbooks made changes, they made changes correspondingly. A few students also reported that they changed the ways in which they used textbooks in mathematics learning because of their teachers (4) or parents (1).

The teacher questionnaire data showed that the changes made by the teachers were more related to the ways in which they presented the topics and structured their classroom instruction. The most obvious change was that teachers encouraged more participation from students, including more discussions and less repetition of what has been said in the textbooks. Many teachers believed that learning through self-discovery can help students to get a better and deeper understanding about what they have learned. Four teachers claimed that their teaching was less dependent on textbooks now and the ways in which they used textbooks

---

[8] The number in the brackets refers to the number of students who gave the corresponding answers.

became more flexible, such as reorganizing the order of topics presented in the textbooks.

In the interview, many teachers attributed their changes in textbook use to the growth of their teaching experience and familiarity with the textbooks that they had used for teaching. One teacher explained, "When I just began to be a teacher, I was not familiar with the textbooks I used and my teaching thus followed the textbooks very closely. Along with the increase in teaching experience, I gained a deeper understanding of the textbooks and hence the ways in which I dealt with the textbooks became more flexible." Getting to know more learning theories, such constructivism, was another important factor that motivated teachers to make changes in their textbook use. In addition, some teachers pointed out that some changes they made were based on their own reflections on the effectiveness of their teaching and correspondingly students' performance. The change in the characteristics of students in class was also one factor for teachers to make changes in using textbooks. Many teachers also related their changes in textbook use to the development in mathematics education, especially the on-going development of "Quality Education", a change from education for test to education for students' overall quality.

4 Summary and Conclusions

The results presented and discussed above provided us with useful empirical evidence and insight on what role textbooks play in the teaching and learning of mathematics in Chinese educational settings and how they shape the way in which Chinese students learn mathematics.

Overall, the study revealed that textbooks were the main resource for mathematics teachers in their classroom teaching. In particular, textbooks were the most important source for teachers to make decisions on what to teach and how to teach, and the majority of instructional time was structured around the textbooks. In addition, teachers largely followed the textbooks closely in their use of various parts of the textbooks, though noteworthily about half of the in-class examples were from other resources due to the insufficiency in both the amount and quality of the examples offered in the textbooks, and moreover many teachers also often introduced alternative solutions to the example problems.

Textbooks were also the main resource for students' learning of mathematics. In particular, most problems for students' in-class exercises and homework were taken from textbooks, and many students also read the textbooks and actively worked on the unassigned exercise problems in the textbooks.

On the other hand, the study also found that many teachers have changed the ways in which they used the textbooks for classroom teaching over the years, and particularly they used textbooks in a more flexible way, with the main reason being the growth of their teaching experience and knowledge of the textbooks.

In general, the study revealed more similarities rather than differences in the textbook use by the teachers and students within and beyond the Chinese classroom. In particular, the study found there were overall no significant differences between teachers with different genders, experiences, from different regions and schools in their use of textbooks, though there were some significant differences between students in the two cities in their use of textbooks. Due to the design of this study, we were not able to address this issue in a more detailed way. It would be interesting and helpful to further study what it signals in mathematics instruction and why there exist such differences.

References

Ball, D. L., & Cohen, D. K. (1996). Reform by the book: What is – or might be – the role of curriculum materials in teacher learning and instructional reform? *Educational Researcher, 25*(9), 6-8, 14.

Barr, R. (1988). Conditions influencing content taught in nine fourth-grade mathematics classrooms. *The Elementary School Journal, 88*(4), 378-410.

260   *How Chinese Learn Mathematics: Perspectives from Insiders*

Beaton, A. E., Mullis, I. V. S., Martin, M. O., Gonzalez, E. J., Kelly, D. L., & Smith, T. A. (1996). *Mathematics achievement in the middle school years: IEA's Third International Mathematics and Science Study*. Chestnut Hill, MA: TIMSS International Study Center, Boston College.

Bierhoff, H. (1996). Laying the foundations of numeracy: A comparison of primary school textbooks in Britain, Germany and Switzerland. *Teaching Mathematics and its Applications, 15*(4), 1-157.

Carter, J., Li, Y., & Ferrucci, B. J. (1997). A comparison of how textbooks present integer addition and subtraction in PRC and USA. *The Mathematics Educator, 2*(2), 197-209.

Fan, L., & Kaeley, G. S. (2000). The influence of textbook on teaching strategies: An empirical study. *Mid-Western Educational Researcher, 13*(4), 2-9.

Flanders, J. R. (1987). How much of the content in mathematics textbooks is new? *Arithmetic Teacher, 35*(1), 18-23.

Freeman, D. J., & Porter, A. C. (1989). Do textbooks dictate the content of mathematics instruction in elementary schools? *American Educational Research Journal, 26*(3), 403-421.

Fujii, T. (2001). The changing winds in Japanese mathematics education. *Mathematics Education Dialogue, 2001*(November). Retrieved June 19, 2002, from http://www.nctm.org/dialogues/2001-11/20011105.htm.

Fuller, B., & Clarke, P. (1994). Raising school effects while ignoring culture? Local conditions and the influence of classroom tools, rules, and pedagogy. *Review of Educational Research, 64*(1), 119-157.

Heyneman, S. P., Farrell, J. P., & Sepulveda-Stuardo, M. A. (1978). *Textbooks and achievement: What we know*. Washington, DC: World Bank.

Krammer, H. P. M. (1985). The textbook as classroom content variable. *Teaching & Teacher Education, 1*(4), 273-278.

Kuhs, T. M., & Freeman, D. J. (1979, April). *The potential influence of textbooks on teachers' selection of content for elementary school mathematics*. Paper presented at the annual meeting of the American Educational Research Association, San Francisco.

Lian, Y. (2000, January 27). Some grades will change to use new textbooks [In Chinese 中小学部分年级换用新教材]. *Guangming Daily* [In Chinese 光明日报], A2. China.

Love, E., & Pimm, D. (1996). 'This is so': A text on texts. In A. J. Bishop, K. Clements, C. Keitel, J. Kilpatrick, & C. Laborde (Eds.), *International handbook of mathematics education* (pp. 371-410). Dordrecht, The Netherlands: Kluwer.

Mayer, R. E., Sims, V., & Tajika, H. (1995). A comparison of how textbooks teach mathematical problem solving in Japan and the United States. *American Educational Research Journal, 32*(2), 443-460.

McCutcheon, G. (1982, March). *Textbook use in a central Ohio elementary school*. Paper presented at the annual meeting of the American Educational Research Association, New York. (ERIC Document Reproduction Service No. ED 216968)

Nicely, R. F., Jr. (1985). Higher-order thinking skills in mathematics textbooks. *Educational Leadership, 42*(7), 26-30.

People's Education Press. (1993a). *The compulsory education three-year junior secondary school textbooks: Algebra II* [In Chinese 九年义务教育三年制初级中学教科书: 代数,第二册]. Beijing: Author.

People's Education Press. (1993b). *The compulsory education three-year junior secondary school textbooks: Geometry II* [In Chinese 九年义务教育三年制初级中学教科书: 几何,第二册]. Beijing: Author.

Schiefelbein, E., & Simmons, J. (1981). *The determinants of school achievement: A review of the research for developing countries*. Ottawa: International Development Research Center.

Schmidt, W. H., Porter, A. C., Floden, R. E., Freeman, D. J., & Schwille, J. R. (1987). Four patterns of teacher content decision-making. *Journal of Curriculum Studies, 19*(5), 439-455.

Sepulveda-Stuardo, M. A., & Farrell, J. P. (1983). The use of textbooks by teachers and students in learning and teaching. In E. Schiefelbein, J. P. Farrell, & M. A. Sepulveda-Stuardo (Eds.), *The influence of school resources in Chile: Their effect on educational achievement and occupational attainment* (pp. 72-109). Washington, DC: International Bank Reconstruction and Development Staff Working Paper No.530.

Shield, M. (1989). Mathematics teachers' preferences in textbook characteristics. *Mathematics Education Research Journal, 1*(1), 11-15.

Sosniak, L. A., & Stodolsky, S. S. (1993). Teachers and textbooks: materials use in four fourth-grade classrooms. *The Elementary School Journal, 93*(3), 249-275.

Tyson, H., & Woodward, A. (1989). Why students aren't learning very much from textbooks. *Educational Leadership, 47*(3), 14-17.

Woodward, A., & Elliott, D. L. (1990). Textbook use and teacher professionalism. In D. L. Elliott & A. Woodward (Eds.), *Textbooks and schooling in the United States: Eighty-ninth yearbook of the National Society for the Study of Education* (Part I, pp. 178-193). Chicago, IL: University of Chicago Press.

Zeng, T. (1997). *On curriculum* [In Chinese 教材论]. Jiangxi, China: Jiangxi Education Press.

Zhu, Y. (2003). *Representations of problem solving in China, Singapore and US mathematics textbooks: A comparative study*. Unpublished doctoral dissertation, National Institute of Education, Nanyang Technological University, Singapore.

Zhu, Y., & Fan, L. (2002). Textbook use by mathematics teachers at lower secondary school level in Singapore. In D. Edge & B. H. Yeap (Eds.), *Proceedings of EARCOME-2 & SEACME-9 Conference* (Vol. 2, pp. 194-201). Singapore.

Chapter 10

Thorough Understanding of the Textbook – A Significant Feature of Chinese Teacher Manuals

LI Jianhua

Through an analysis of a popular Chinese elementary school mathematics teacher manual, this chapter discusses a significant feature of teacher manual, namely, the manual is designed to help teachers achieve a thorough understanding of student text mathematically and pedagogically. Using multi-digit number multiplication, this chapter discusses the in-depth analyses and detailed suggestions for the core part of a lesson with concrete examples. In particular, it argues that an in-depth analysis of student text is the main focus of the guide. It also argues that concerted efforts are made to help create an environment that helps teachers professionally and teachers need to study the student text carefully in order to conduct classroom instruction effectively.

Key words: textbook, teacher manual, multiplication, algorithm, pedagogical knowledge

1 The Role of Teacher Manuals

Pedagogy is culturally bound. While the general school curriculum of a country reflects the government's priority and basic philosophy in education, the design of student textbooks and teacher manuals speaks of the characteristics and preferences of the people, that is, students, teachers, and parents. In countries where the use of textbook is the norm and textbook publishing is competitive, the attractiveness of a textbook often consists in how good the assistance it offers to teachers. "Good" here usually means the supply of sufficient examples in problem solving, accessible page-layout for skimming or any other time saving tools in class preparation. These criteria are important especially when a teacher has a heavy teaching load. But the shortcomings of this practice are obvious. The teacher's preoccupation with his or her convenience may cause oversights in detecting drawbacks in the textbook from pedagogical effectiveness point of view as well as from the student's perspective. Moreover, minimal class preparation time could easily lead to less adaptive and effective teaching in the face of unpredictable classroom situations.

In contrast, teachers in Mainland China do not look into the teacher manual for quick ideas and user-friendly guidelines. For them, the teacher manual, instead of being a collection of instant ideas for quick classroom consumption, is but a reference that requires careful studying. The student texts and teacher manuals in China are authoritative texts that many teachers feel they have to diligently consult in order to perfect their teaching skills and to achieve successful teaching. This is particularly the case for elementary school teachers because of their lacking of resources. Teachers acquire this mentality in part through their training offered in the normal schools or colleges. In the official textbook for prospective math teachers, the *Elementary School Mathematics Textbooks and Teaching* (Elementary Mathematics Department [EMD], 1995), for example, stressed that teachers should study student textbooks carefully and observe the "standard" set by the Ministry of Education. Moreover, schools in China have regular class preparation sessions during school years. The main purpose of these sessions is to have a thorough understanding of the student text. Thus, in China, understanding thoroughly the student text and the topics taught is considered the key to successful teaching. The teacher manual is designed to help teachers acquire this key.

Through analyzing the pedagogical materials for multi-digit number multiplication in one of China's most widely used mathematics teacher manuals, this chapter illumines a central characteristic of mathematics teacher manual, that is, the thoroughness of teachers' understanding of student text.

The teacher manuals[1] described in this chapter are from the most commonly used series published by the People's Education Press (PEP hereafter). The PEP, which was established in 1950, a year after the founding of the People's Republic of China, is directly affiliated with the Ministry of Education. It served as the only official developer of national curriculum and teaching materials until the late 1980s when a reform on school curriculum introduced a competition mechanism in the development of teaching and learning materials. Since then, a textbook committee in the Ministry of Education has acted as the final decision maker in admitting the teaching and learning materials to the official textbook list. Only until a few years ago the PEP series had dominated the textbook market, constituting more than 70 percent or more of the market's supply. However, other publishers have been providing more and more textbooks for schools, especially since 2002, textbooks published by other publishers have been widely used. Nevertheless, the PEP is generally considered a powerhouse in China's development of curriculum and pedagogical materials, with in-house editors as designers and authors of textbooks. Although a new series by the PEP has been for testing since 2001 in some schools in a number of provinces, the series I am to discuss was first published in 1995, and changes between the two series are small.

Since the Ministry of Education introduced the competition mechanism in providing school textbooks, provincial publishing houses and major normal universities have been very active in developing new learning materials and taken more market shares. We are still not clear about how this competition plays it out. We still need more time to see how the new system works best concerning questions of the status of the PEP and local protection, just name a few. But one thing is for sure, that is, the PEP as the only textbook publisher has become a history.

With the above in mind, the readers are reminded that there are many teacher manuals available now in the Mainland China because many publishers have provided textbooks and teacher manuals to schools, so

---

[1] The use of teacher manuals is for the convenience of chapter. The actual books used by Chinese teachers are called teachers' reference books (教学参考书).

what are true in the teacher manual examined in this chapter might not be true in the new teacher manuals published in recent years.

On a whole, textbook development and publishing in China have been treated as a powerful tool of promoting deep understanding of curriculum materials. In developing and designing teacher manuals, in particular, the Chinese publishers tend to focus less on the issues of formatting and user-friendliness at the surface level, but more on in-depth analysis of the technical side of the topics taught.

The way in which the teacher manual is used in China helps explain the manual's overall design and inherent complexity. As an example, Table 1 shows the "Table of Contents" of the fifth volume (Grade 3, first semester) of the PEP teacher manual[2] (EMD, 1997a).

Table 1
Table of Contents of Volume 5 of the Teacher Manual (Partial)

An Introduction to the Nine-Year Compulsory Education Five-Year Elementary School Mathematics Volume 5
    1   Instructional content and goals
    2   Characteristics of text
    3   Teaching Aids and Munipulatives for students to be prepared for instruction
    4   Pacing chart
Notes on each chapter and instructional suggestions for each unit
    1   Multiplication of 2-digit multipliers
        A   Instructional goals
        B   Notes on the text
        C   Notes and suggestions on each subsection
            a.   Mental multiplication
            b.   Paper-and-pencil multiplication
                 Multiplication of 2-digit multipliers (A)
                 Multiplication of 2-digit multipliers (B)
                 Multiplication of 2-digit multipliers (C)
            ...

---

[2] Following the semester system in China, the mathematics series published by the PEP comprises 10 volumes of textbooks for Grades 1–5, one per every semester. Each of the volumes has a teacher manual. At the beginning of an academic year, schools will provide each teacher with a new copy of the textbook and teacher manual for each course he or she is going to teach. The Grades 1-5 is based on the 5-4-3 system, meaning 5 years of elementary schooling, 4 years of junior high schooling, and 3 years of senior high schooling. Roughly half of China's schools follow this system. The alternative system is 6-3-3 (i.e., 6 years of elementary schooling, 3 years of junior high schooling, and 3 years of senior high schools). The curricula for the 5-year and 6 year elementary schooling are very similar with the 5-year curriculum stretched into the 6-year curriculum.

Like all the other 9 volumes, Volume 5 bears a 2-part structure. The first part is a comprehensive introduction to the textbook. This includes issues such as the special features of the text, the rationale behind the design, pedagogical approaches to main topic, etc. The second part is a lesson-to-lesson teaching guide based on the textbook. In addition to an in-depth discussion of the topic taught in each lesson, it offers considerable examples and alternative approaches for creative teaching.

2 Teaching and Learning of Whole Number Multiplication

Table 2 provides the scope and sequence of the PEP Mathematics on whole number multiplication[3].

Table 2
Scope and Sequence of Multiplication of the PEP Mathematics*

	Grade 1		Grade 2		Grade 3	
	First half	Second half	First half	Second half	First half	Second half
Meaning**		X				
Basic facts		X	X			
Of 1-digit numbers				X		
Of 2-digit numbers					X	
Of 3-digit numbers						X

* Compiled from the Table of Contents of the PEP Mathematics.
** Other topics, such as "relation to addition/division" and "choosing a computation tool", are listed in the scope and sequence of the PEP mathematics teacher manuals. Only four major topics are listed in this table.

Multiplication is first introduced in the second semester of Grade 1. Then multiplication facts and multiplication of 1-digit multipliers are taught in Grade 2. In Grade 3, students learn multiplication of 2-digit and 3-digit numbers. Since multiplication of 2-digit numbers is the step bridging between multiplication of 1-digit numbers and multiplication of 3-digit numbers, the way in which the "bridge" is structured can be used

---

[3] In addition to the topics in multiplication, which are covered in Chapter 1, the following topics are also covered in other chapters in Volume 5: Chapter 2: Kilometer and ton, Chapter 3: Division of 2-digit divisors, Chapter 4: Mixed operation and word problems, Chapter 5: Introducing fractions, Chapter 6: Areas of rectangles and squares, and Chapter 7: Review (EMD, 1997b).

as a yardstick to gauge how well-developed the curriculum is in terms of connecting topics of progressive difficulty and pacing the progress for students. In the following, we use Volume 5 to illustrate what are included in the two parts of the volume.

We have learned from cross-cultural mathematics curriculum studies (e.g., Schmidt, Valerde, Houang, Wiley, & McKnight, 1997) that the Chinese mathematics curriculum usually covers a topic within a short time of the curriculum and other countries usually cover a topic over a longer period of time. This is evident by looking at Table 2. Once a topic has been taught, it will not be recapitulated. Yet, when a topic is taught, it is taught with considerable thoroughness.

3 Thoroughness for Teacher's Understanding of the Student Text

The thoroughness of the manual in promoting a deep understanding of the student text is reflected in the comprehensive introduction, the detailed analysis in each chapter, and teaching suggestions for the core part of a lesson. The comprehensive introduction to the book gives an introduction to the main themes of the student text, major topics in the chapters, and key concepts of each topic. This part briefly discusses the rationale and the structure of the student text, as well as the key components and concepts. It also provides the instructional goals of the student text. Additionally, this part is aligned with the National Syllabus of the Elementary School Mathematics. Although many areas of the student text are covered, the emphasis of the introduction is placed on the characteristics of the student text. It provides rich mathematical and pedagogical knowledge to the teacher. A case in point is the discussion in this part of the manual of multiplication of 2-digit multipliers.

In the Characteristics of the Text the manual first discusses the major changes of the current volume compared to the same volume of its earlier edition:

"... Compared to the last series, we reduced instruction on naming large numbers and their computations and some abstract theories according to the Elementary School Mathematics

Syllabus. Based on the multiplication of 1-digit multipliers and division of 1-digit divisors, which is developed in Grade 2, the text presents multiplication of 2-digit multipliers and division of 2-digit divisors. Because the numbers are not very large, it will be easier for students to grasp the computing methods and transfer these methods in computing large numbers." (EMD, 1997a, p. 4)

Teachers know how to do multiplication. However, without knowing the above analysis, teachers might spend more time on letting students solve complicated multiplication problems and pay less attention to having students have a good understanding of the algorithm. Thus, in the subsection on multiplication, the manual gives an analysis of how difficult multiplication of 2-digit multipliers is, despite that students have learned multiplication of 1-digit multipliers, what measures are taken in the textbook to help students connect the new topic with the old ones. For instance, certain mental mathematics of multiplications is introduced in this section to prepare student to get ready for multiplication of 2-digit multipliers.

For the key worked examples in this section, the manual explains how they are arranged such that effective instruction can be made.

"When presenting the examples of multiplication of 2-digit multipliers using a standard paper-and-pencil method, the text tries to stress the algorithm by using typical examples and a pattern of multiplication. For instance, the text first presents a problem of a 2-digit number multiplying a 2-digit number. Then the text provides a problem of a 2-digit number multiplying a 3-digit number. The text leads students to think that regardless how many digits the multiplicand is, the order of multiplication is the same: first use the ones digit to multiply the multiplicand, then use the tens digit to multiply the multiplicand." (EMD, 1997a, p. 4)

In addition to explaining the student text, there is one subsection that is devoted to explaining the elements that foster students' thinking and reasoning abilities. For instance, on fostering students' analytical and syntheses ability, the manual points out that when teaching multiplication of 2-digit multipliers, through a concrete model the text leads students to analyze the computation procedure. Multiplication of 2-digit multipliers can be divided into two steps: the first step is to use the ones digit to multiply the multiplicand; the second step is to use the tens digit to multiply the multiplicand; and the third step is to add the two partial products. Based on these steps, the text leads students to combine the steps into one vertical form. Other abilities are also discussed in the subsection on fostering students' thinking abilities, such as fostering students' judging and reasoning ability (EMD, 1997a, pp. 9-10).

The *Introduction* also specifies the instructional objectives. At the end of above quoted subsection, a table of suggested average error percentage and speed goal is provided. The part on multiplication is shown in Table 3. The most significant feature of this table is that the instructional objectives are quantified. It helps the teacher to keep in mind how much a topic is more difficult than another topic. For example, everyone knows that 2-digit multiplication is more difficult than 1-digit multiplication. But by how much? By giving the teacher a quantified figure, this table helps the teacher to decide how much more time he/she needs to spend on a topic. In addition, this allows the teacher to check how well each individual student perform and whether the instruction has been effective and whether students are ready to move on to next topic.

These discussions in the teacher manual help the teacher to know more about the student text. It also helps the teacher to learn the role the current volume and the topics play in the whole series.

In each chapter, chapter overall analysis follows a pattern similar to that in the Introduction. It covers the teaching objectives, the characteristics of the student text and the main sections in the chapter. Again, emphasis is placed on the characteristics of the student text.

We know that the design of a chapter of student text can be very different from one series to another. For instance, what part the manipulatives should play in a lesson can differ greatly from one design to another. Or how to introduce the paper-and-pencil algorithm can vary significantly from one series to another. However, regardless of what the arrangement of a topic is, letting the teacher know the authors' thinking about the mathematical and pedagogical aspects of the student text is to the advantage of the teacher for effective instruction.

Table 3
Instructional Objectives in the Teacher Manual

Instructional Objectives

	At the end of the chapter		At the end of the semester	
	Average error percentage	Speed	Average error percentage	Speed
Mental computation of one-digit numbers (product within 100), multiplying multiple of tens and hundreds and tens	Within 10%	Most students can do four problems per minute	Within 8%	Most students can do five problems per minute
Multiplication of 2-digit numbers using paper-and-pencil method	Within 18%	Most students can solve 1.5 problems per minute	Within 15%	Most students can do one problem per minute
Two-step story problems	Within 20% (choosing wrong operation types)	-	Within 16%	-

Chapter One of the first semester (Volume 5 in the series) of Grade 3 teacher manual is on multiplication. The *jiao cai shou ming* (教材说明, notes on student text) of Chapter 1 discusses the mathematical and pedagogical aspects of the chapter without discussing individual lessons. It gives the teacher an introduction to the chapter on sections of the chapter and groups of lessons. For instance, the manual first outlines the first section: mental mathematics of multiplication of 1-digit multipliers and multiples of ten serves as the base of learning paper-and-pencil algorithm of multiplication of 2-digit multipliers. The manual uses 24 x 53 as an example to illustrate the connections between the mental mathematics and the paper-and-pencil algorithm: 24 x 53 can be decomposed into 24 x 3, 4 x 50, and 20 x 50. Add all these partial products will give the answer to 24 x 53.

Next, the manual illustrates the second (also the main) part of the chapter – multiplication using paper-and-pencil method. It focuses on how the developers treat this topic in order to emphasize the multiplication algorithm as well as on developing students' ability in reasoning. It first states that once students have mastered multiplication of 2-digit multipliers, it will be easier for them to transfer the method to multiplication of 3-digit multipliers. It further explains that since students have studied multiplication of 1-digit multipliers in the second grade and learned multiplication with different multiplicands, such as zero(s) in the middle or in the end of a multiplicand, the key is to emphasize the order of multiplication, that is, to use ones digit of the multiplier to time the multiplicand and to use tens digit of the multiplier to time the multiplicand. The other important point stated in the manual is about helping students understand that when multiplying a number by the tens digit of the multiplier, the result is how many tens. This explains why the last digit of the partial product should be aligned with the tens digit of the multiplicand.

After explaining the key concepts for the algorithm of multiplication of 2-digit multipliers, the manual outlines the pedagogical approach that the student text takes. Because at the beginning of learning this part students are prone to make mistakes of various kinds, such as to multiply the numbers on the same place, or be confused with the order of multiplication and thus to miss to multiply one digit, the student text does not arrange the lessons by the digits of multiplicand. Rather, it arranges the lessons by the difficulties of different types of multiplications. The student text first introduces a 2-digit multiplier multiplication involving small numbers on each place that needs less carryings. The manual argues that this arrangement has the advantage of highlighting the order of multiplication. Then, students will learn multiplication of large numbers in which many carryings will be needed (EMD, 1997a, pp. 16-17).

The manual further notes that after students have learned the general method of multiplication of 2-digit numbers, the student text presents examples of multiplication with zeros at the end of multiplier or multiplicand using shortcut method and fostering students' ability of choosing appropriate method when computing.

Like what we have seen in the *Introduction*, the above illustrations on Chapter One of the PEP series show the same characteristic of the manual, that is, an in-depth pedagogical analysis of the student text. In particular, we see that the analysis pays close attention to the sequence of the topics and the connections among different parts of the chapter, as well as their relation with division, which is closely related to multiplication topics. The discussion also explains to readers the developers' thinking and argument about why certain topics are included in the chapter. For instance, why mental mathematics is important and what role it plays in the chapter. These illustrations are mathematical and pedagogical knowledge that many mathematics educators value highly.

For each chapter, the PEP teacher manual provides detailed analyses on key lessons. These analyses analyze the worked-out examples and selected exercise problems and clearly explain to readers the purpose of each part of the lesson, the sequence of the worked-out examples, the connections between one part and the other, what to emphasize, and trouble-shooting for students.

The PEP teacher manual usually groups two or three lessons together and discusses them in one section. Unlike many teacher's editions (or teacher's guide), which usually have a format of a duplicated copy of student text in the center of a page and teaching suggestions in the margin (see Li, 2003), the notes on student text and teaching suggestions are provided in regular book format. This gives the authors greater freedom in developing the comments and suggestions for the lesson.

We use the materials in Chapter One to illustrate the above points. There are three lessons in the first section (mental mathematics). The manual covers the three lessons together in one section. The second section covers the paper-and-pencil algorithm of multiplication and there are 11 lessons in this section. The manual covers the lessons in five groups, namely, the Paper-and-Pencil Multiplication (1), (2), (3), Rounding Number and the "Four-down, Five-up" rule, and Estimation of Multiplication. Each group of lessons usually includes one or two new lessons and one or two practice lessons. In fact, these groups can be viewed as subsections. For each group of lessons, the manual has two parts: *Notes on the Text* (教参说明) and *Instructional Suggestions* (教学建议). The first part discusses lesson structure, worked-out examples and some exercise problems in detail, while the second part provides detailed suggestions on the core part of lessons.

We take a look at the Notes on text for the Paper-and-Pencil Multiplication (1) (see Appendix for the actual student text). The manual first states that relatively small numbers are used and very few carryings are needed in giving students an initial grasp of the multiplication order by a 2-digit multiplier. Then it explains the purpose of the two review problems in the student text.

Next, the teacher manual describes Example 1 in great detail. The manual explains how the student text uses concrete model to help students think, that is, how to write a multiplication to represent the word problem and how to change 13 times 24 into some calculations they have learned. The manual states that the key to the new lesson is to know how 10 x 24 and 3 x 24 are connected with 13 x 24. The manual explains that the student text uses three steps to explain the algorithm. The first step is to find out how many crayons are in 3 boxes with 24 crayons in each box. Students should know how to find this out as they learned this before. The second step is to find out the number of crayons in 10 boxes. This is to find 10 times 24. Student learned how to solve this in the mental mathematics lessons before this lesson. The approach to solving 10 times 24 is 24 tens or 240. The third step is to find the number of crayons in 13 boxes. The manual tells us that in the student text, the vertical form of multiplication shown in the dotted box is to help students understand how the above three steps can be combined into one vertical form, namely, the recording of the vertical form of multiplication of a 2-digit multiplier is actually a shortcut of the vertical forms of multiplication of 1-digit multipliers, multiplication of multiples of ten, and the addition of the two partial products (EMD, 1997a, pp. 23-25).

The teacher manual continues to analyze Example 2, a 2-digit number times a 3-digit number, further illustrating that one needs first to use the ones digit to multiply every digit of the multiplicand, and then to use the tens digit to multiply every digit of the multiplicand. Finally, one adds the two partial products to get the final answer. It is clear that the algorithm of multiplication has been emphasized throughout the whole lesson. In the following, the teacher manual explains how the practice problems are designed to help students understand the algorithm through different kinds of problems. For instance, students are asked to complete half completed problems; the vertical form of a multiplication is shown and students are asked to explain the meaning of each step in the computation process; error-checking problems that require students to have a good understanding of the computation process are also presented.

The core part of these illustrations is to explain to the teacher how the algorithm of the paper-and-pencil is designed in a way that promotes both conceptual understanding and mastery by using carefully designed practice problems. These illustrations analyze the worked-out examples and selected exercise problems and clearly explain in detail to the teacher the purpose of each part of the lesson, the sequence of the worked-out examples, the connections between one part and the other, where to give emphasis, and where students may have troubles in learning the topic.

The thoroughness of the teacher manual does not stop at providing thorough analyses of the student text it is also shown by the detailed instructional suggestions. Based on the analysis of student text, teaching suggestions that provided in *Teaching Suggestions* (教学建议) sections of the teacher manual further help the teacher teach. These suggestions are mainly provided for the core part of lessons.

For the beginning of teaching of multiplication of 2-digit multipliers (see Appendix), the suggestion first states that the key to Example 4 is the carrying rule and in order to help students grasp the rule, the teacher should pay attention to using the manipulatives while teaching the example. On how to lead students to use sticks to model the example, the manual suggests that:

First place two bundles (ten sticks in each bundle) in a row, and then 4 sticks next to the two bundles, to represent 24. Next, place another two bundles of sticks below in another row. Then let students observe while you post the following questions: How many sticks are there in the first row? How many rows of sticks are there? If we want to know how many sticks all together are there, what number expression can you use to compute the total number of sticks? After students give an expression 24 × 3, the teacher tells the class while demonstrating using sticks that to find how many sticks there are in three bundles of 24 sticks, first, one needs to find out that three of the 4 sticks are 12 sticks, then tie 10 sticks together to make a bundle and place it under the three groups of sticks and place the other 2 sticks to the right of the bundles of sticks. The second step is to compute the three groups of 2 bundles, which are 6 bundles, and place these 6 bundles of sticks to the left of the bundle tied up before (see the illustration on page 64 of this guide). All together, there are 7 bundles and 2 single sticks. You may also ask students to talk about how $24 \times 3 = 72$ reaches to its answer with these questions: What to do first? What to do next? Based on all of these, write out the vertical form $\begin{array}{r} 24 \\ \times\ 3 \\ \hline \end{array}$ to finish the computation.

Here, you should relate the modeling process using manipulatives and explain to students that 3 times 4 in the multiplicand is 12, write $\begin{array}{r} 2\ 4 \\ \times\ 3 \\ \hline 12 \end{array}$. Then use 3 times 2 in the tens place of the multiplicand, yielding 60. Write $\begin{array}{r} 24 \\ \times\ 3 \\ \hline 12 \\ 60 \end{array}$. At the end, add the two products and write $\begin{array}{r} 24 \\ \times 3 \\ \hline 12 \\ 60 \\ \hline 72 \end{array}$ on the blackboard. In order to record the process in an efficient way, the vertical form can be written as $\begin{array}{r} 24 \\ \times 13 \\ \hline 72 \end{array}$. The emphasis of the teaching of this example should be on the rule of how to do the carrying. If necessary, you can write the following on the blackboard:

$$2\ 4$$
$$\underline{\times 1\ 3}$$

$7\ 2\ \rightarrow$ 3 times 4 on the ones place of the multiplicand is 12. Carry 1 to the next place and write 2 on the ones place of the
$\downarrow$ product.

3 times 2 on the tens place of the multiplicand is 6. Plus the carried 1 is 7. Write 7 on the tens place of the product.

The detailed suggestions cited above illustrates how the PEP teacher manual treats the core part of a lesson. On the other parts of a lesson, the manual only provides sketchy or short suggestions.

One other measure that applied in the PEP teacher manual is to provide some lesson plans at the end of each chapter. One to three lesson plans are provided for the teacher to use them directly or derive his/her own lesson plan based on these lesson plans. These lesson plans seem to be helpful to novices in particular.

4 Summary and Discussion

We have shown that in the teacher manual, the emphases are placed on the rationale of the content, pedagogical aspects of the student text as well as the detailed suggestions for the core part of a lesson. In the Introduction, the PEP teacher manual discusses the basic idea of multiplication and division. In particular, the manual states that the multiplication and division are the two main topics of the first semester of Grade 3 and they also serve as a basis for multiplication and division of decimal numbers. Similar discussions on other topics are presented in the Introduction.

The discussion on the multiplication is further extended to the details at the chapter level. As discussed earlier in this paper, the algorithm of multiplication of 2-digit multipliers is present to readers with an example of 24 x 53. The manual emphasizes the key points of multiplication of 2-

digit multipliers, namely, the multiplication order and an understanding the difference of each partial product, such as when one uses the tens digit of the multiplier to multiply the multiplicand, the result is in tens. So the last digit of the partial product should be aligned with the tens place.

The connections among multiplication and other topics are also discussed. The importance of multiplication as a prerequisite for learning division and the relation between multiplication and division are discussed with an example of $48 \div 16$. The teacher manual states that the mental mathematics of multiplication plays a special role in that chapter because it not only has practical use in daily life but also plays an important role in finding quotient. For instance, if students are familiar with the mental mathematics of 15 or 25 multiplying a number they can speed up the process of division.

We also see that the PEP teacher manual tells the teacher how the examples of the section (e.g., teaching the paper-and-pencil algorithm) are organized in order to reduce the difficulty of each lesson and where the teaching should emphasize and thus foster students' thinking and computation skills. For instance, the first examples of the section on multiplication of 2-digit multipliers are of smaller numbers with no or few carryings needed during the calculation. Thus, students can have more time to concentrate on the rules of multiplication. The subsequent lessons focus on more difficult problems (EMD, 1997a, p.16).

For instructional suggestions, detailed suggestions for the core part of new lessons are given. The suggestions for the worked-out example of multiplication of a 2-digit multiplier are almost step-by-step. It is evident that the teacher plays a dominant role in conducting the core part of the lesson. As a contrast, only sketchy and short suggestions are provided for practice lessons.

All of the above show the thoroughness that the PEP teacher manual provides for the teacher. Everything is centered on a thorough understanding of the student text. As we discussed earlier, a key component of instructional activities is the practice of teacher studying the textbook. It makes sense that the teacher manual is written in this way so that teachers can have a comprehensive understanding of the curriculum and prepare for their lessons with in-depth understanding of topic taught. In fact, the demand of teacher's thorough understanding of textbooks is explicitly expressed in preservice pedagogical courses (EMD, 1995).

Researchers have suggested that what teachers really need is subject matter knowledge for teaching (Ball, 1990; Ball & Bass, 2001). Ma (1999) argues that Chinese elementary mathematics teachers have a profound understanding of elementary mathematics. We have discussed that in China there is the demand for the teachers to have a deep understanding of the textbooks and there exists a favorable environment for teachers to study the curriculum. The PEP teacher manuals provide an example that shows how to help teachers understand the curriculum and student text in one of many areas of teachers' professional development.

This chapter is an attempt to characterize teacher manual by a case study of its material on multiplication. In order to understand the way the teacher manual is written, we need to look at other areas that are closely connected to teacher manual. We see that there is a concerted effort on improving teachers' professional expertise in China. Prospective teachers' pedagogy course is geared towards a better understanding of the curriculum and towards implementing the "standard" mathematics textbook. Both schools and parents expect that mathematics teachers are specialists in mathematics teaching. Group class preparation sessions are held many times during school years. All these demand that a teacher manual is written in such a way that can help teachers understand the mathematics curriculum and the topics in each volume, rather than a quick classroom instruction guide. In a way, the teacher manual must be studied in order to obtain a better learning result for the teachers.

The thoroughness of the teacher manual illuminated here certainly would constitute the strength of mathematics education in China, if the manual is studied carefully, critically and used creatively. I hope that future research on how the teacher manual is used by the Chinese teachers will greatly enrich our understanding on this issue.

References

Ball, D. L. (1990). The mathematical understandings that prospective teachers bring to teacher education. *The Elementary School Journal, 90*(4), 449- 466.

Ball, D. L., & Bass, H. (2001). What mathematical knowledge is entailed in teaching children to reason mathematically? In National Research Council (Ed.), *Knowing and learning mathematics for teaching: Proceedings of a workshop* (pp. 26-34). Washington, DC: National Academic Press.

Ma, L. (1999). *Knowing and teaching elementary mathematics.* Mahwah, NJ: Lawrence Erlbaum Associates.

Li, J. (2003). *A comparative study of U.S. and Chinese elementary mathematics teacher's guides.* Unpublished doctoral dissertation. University of Chicago, Chicago, IL.

Elementary Mathematics Department. (1995). *Elementary school mathematics textbook and teaching (Vol. 2).* [In Chinese 小学数学教材教法第二册]. Beijing, China: People's Education Press.

Elementary Mathematics Department. (1997a). *PEP mathematics teacher manual, Grade Three (Vol. 1)* [In Chinese 义务教育五年制小学数学第五册教学参考书]. Beijing, China: People's Education Press.

Elementary Mathematics Department. (1997b). *Mathematics, Grade Three (Vol. 1)* [In Chinese 义务教育五年制小学数学第五册]. Beijing, China: People's Education Press.

Schmidt, W. H., Valverde, G. A., Houang, R. T., Wiley, D. E., & McKnight, C. C. (Eds.) (1997). *Many visions, many aims: A cross-national investigation of curricular intentions in school mathematics.* Dordrecht, The Netherlands: Kluwer Academic.

Appendix

English Translation of Student Text of Multiplication of 2-digit Numbers, Grade 3, PEP Mathematics

Multiplication Using Paper & Pencil

Multiplication of 2-digit numbers

Review

(1) 14 x 2   31 x 30   214 x 3

(2) One box of crayons has 24 crayons, how many crayons are there in three such boxes?

Example 1

3 boxes of crayons: 10 boxes of crayons: 13 boxes of crayons:
                   tens' digit of "1"   add the two sub
                   multiplies 24 is 24   results.
                   of ten.

```
    2  4              2  4                       7  2
     \ |               \               +  2  4  0
  x   1 3           x  1  0
  ---------         ----------               ----------
    7  2              2  4  0                 3  1  2
```

How to combine the above steps into one formula?

```
      2  4
   ×  1 3
   --------
      7  2   ...... Product of 24×3
    2 4 0    ...... Product of 24×10 ("0" may be ommited)
   --------
    3 1 2
```

Think about this question: Can you write down the top-down format multiplication for this problem? Can you change 13 multiplies 24 into something you have learned?

Try These

Finish the following multiplication.

```
   2 3          1 2           1 3
 x 1 3        x 4 2         x 2 4
   6 9          2 4           5 2
 _____      _____       _____
```

Example 2   212 x 34 = 7208

```
        2 1 2
      x   3 4
        8 4 8
        6 3 6
       7 2 0 8
```

Try These

```
   3 2 1        1 3 2         2 1 4
 x   1 3        x 3 2         x 2 3
   9 6 3        2 6 4
 _____      _____       _____
```

Let's summarize the multiplication procedure for multiplication of 2-digit numbers.

1. Start using the number in the one's place of the multiplier to multiply every digit of the multiplicand, align the last digit of the partial product with one's place;
2. Then use the number in the ten's place of the multiplier to multiply every digit of the multiplicand, align the last digit of the partial product with the ten's place;
3. Last add the two partial products.

Chapter 11

Effects of Cram Schools on Children's Mathematics Learning

HUANG Hsin Mei

This chapter begins with a literature review of the role of cram schools and how parents and children perceive them in Taiwan. Interviews were conducted to understand the view of primary school teachers concerning the impact of cram schools on school mathematics learning and instruction. Despite controversial opinions on the merits of cram schools, their growing popularity can be attributed to the increasing demand from parents and children. On the one hand, primary school teachers perceive a positive impact of cram school attendance on children's mathematics learning, as evidenced by better computation skills, completion of homework, and greater self-confidence in mathematics. However, they disagree with rote-learning emphasized in cram school instruction and criticize its failure to develop concepts among children. Cram schools have a negative influence on children's understanding of mathematical concepts as well as flexible application of knowledge. Suggestions for improving children's mathematics ability and learning in cram schools are made.

Key words: cram schools, mathematics learning, school mathematics instruction, parents' influence, self-confidence

1 Introduction

For the past three decades, cross-national comparisons of mathematics achievement have favored students in Japan, Taiwan, Mainland China, Singapore, and Korea (Grow-Maienza, Hahn, & Joo, 2001; Stevenson et al., 1990). Taiwan's eighth graders participated in the Third International Mathematics and Science Study (TIMSS) and showed outstanding performance in science and mathematics (TIMSS-Forum, 2003).

However, local scholars and researchers have cautioned that we should not be overly-satisfied with the results, because excellence in other areas such as social science, humanities, and creativity as well as scientific exploration, rather than mere rote-learning, is more important (The China Post Staff, 2000). According to the report, the TIMSS survey did not take into account the fact that a huge number of Taiwanese students attended cram schools (*bu shi ban*, 补习班) for extra classes. However, several studies on children's mathematics learning have reported the positive effects of cram school attendance on school-age children's mathematics achievement. The positive effects of cram school attendance on children's mathematics achievement are more significant for children in higher grades (H. P. Huang, 2002; J. S. Hsieh, 2001).

In recent years, western researchers have paid much attention to the following five major factors which influence children's mathematics learning and achievement: the quality of the school curriculum, the quality of instruction (e.g., Mason & Waywood, 1996; Szendrei, 1996), psychological factors, personality variables, and physical variables (Slavin, 1997). In addition to the aforementioned factors, the cram school classes after school hours have been defined as a variable in mathematics learning in primary and middle education. However, relatively little is known about the influence of cram school attendance on children's learning. Therefore, the role of cram schools and their impact on children's mathematics learning have aroused great interest among researchers.

Cram school education is an extra-curricular program that provides supplementary education in service of persons with special needs (Her, 1977). It covers a number of complex issues related to how the Chinese culture values academic success, the educational system, the administration system for selecting capable persons, and the modern social structure in transition (K. M. Huang, 1993). Parents in traditional Chinese society attach great importance to scholastic achievement of their children. The growing popularity of cram schools is due to the parents' belief that children can benefit from joining extra-curricular programs (Y. Y. Huang, 1995; C. S. Sun & Hwang, 1996; Yeh, 1989). Consequently, various types of cram schools have mushroomed all over Taiwan. Thus, it would be of interest to understand why parents send their children to cram schools.

Alexander and Entwisle (1988) pointed out that one of the most important consequences of schooling for elementary school children is how they view their own capabilities. How do children perceive cram schools? What are children's ideas about the relationship between attending cram schools and mathematics learning? The above issues have drawn researchers in mathematics education to further exploration.

In this chapter, previous empirical studies will be used to provide evidence concerning how parents and children perceive the relationship between mathematics learning and cram school attendance. Besides parents, teachers also play a key role in children's academic development (Alexander & Entwisle, 1988; Stevenson et al., 1990). "Teacher-centered lecturing" was a prevalent mode of school mathematics instruction before the introduction of mathematics education reforms in Taiwan. Such an instruction mode was quite consistent with that used in cram schools (K. M. Huang, 1993). However, 1993 saw the initiation of mathematics education reforms on the basis of constructivism and the launching of the national mathematics curriculum of Taiwan (Taiwan Ministry of Education, 1993; N. Y. Wong & K. M. Wong, 1997). Furthermore, this new mode of teaching is compatible with the latest wave of the First– Ninth Grades Curriculum Alignment (九年一贯课程) reform and its mathematics ramifications in mathematics teaching and learning (Taiwan Ministry of Education, 2000). Recent reform efforts in school mathematics have focused primarily on the effectiveness of curriculum content and instructional approach in promoting students' learning through mathematical discourse and problem-solving (Chung, 2000; Chung & Chu, 2001; H. M. E. Huang, 2001, 2002; Taiwan Ministry of Education, 1993, 2000). In fact, there is now a big gap in instructional modes between ordinary schools and cram schools. Few studies have taken note of this. Nor have they taken note of how teachers view the influence of cram schools on school-based mathematics learning and instruction.

This chapter begins with a literature review of the concept of cram school education, its background in Chinese society, its trend of development in Taiwan after the implementation of current educational reforms, and the current multi-entrance admission program to senior high schools and universities. Since there is little literature on teachers' views on cram schools, interviews were conducted to understand how teachers perceive the role played by cram schools and their influence in Chinese education.

This chapter focuses on the following five aspects.

1. The role of cram schools and the trend of their development in Taiwan;
2. Parents' influence on children's attendance of cram schools;
3. Factors affecting children's willingness to attend cram schools;
4. Children's perception of the relationships between cram school attendance and mathematics learning;
5. Primary school teachers' perception of the interaction between cram schools and school-based mathematics learning and instruction.

2 The Role of Cram Schools and the Trend of their Development in Taiwan

2.1 *The role of cram schools in students' education*

Supplementary education is for young people and adults who missed out an opportunity for education or who were unable to complete their education. It gives them an opportunity to improve their education during non-regular school hours (Taiwan Ministry of Education, 2003). Cram schools also offer programs that provide supplementary education to persons with special needs (Her, 1977). The initial goals of cram schools was to provide schooling for those who had no access to regular education, as well as to offer supportive and complementary programs for people with learning difficulty (Her, 1977; K. M. Huang, 1993; Y. Y. Huang, 1995).

With the growing importance of competitive of entrance examinations in gaining admission to prestigious senior high schools and universities, however, the services and functions of cram schools changed along with the transformation of social structure. In particular, the most prevalent service of cram schools is to provide a supplementary academic program for those who desire to have high scores on the entrance examinations (H. P. Huang, 2002; L. F. Wu, 1993).

Along with this, long working hours have kept parents from returning home early enough to look after their children. They worry about their children lingering around and squandering precious time after school. For example, Chen (1978) and Wang (1983) pointed out that most students tended to hang out at places such as video arcades. To prevent them from becoming juvenile delinquents, parents prefer sending their children to cram schools which provide a learning environment. Hence, cram schools not only serve as a place for learning, but also a safe heaven for children to keep them from going astray.

2.2 *Types of cram schools*

Services provided by cram schools are meant to satisfy the needs of both parents and students. They are determined by the market demand. Among the great variety of cram schools in Taiwan, four distinctive types can be identified (J. S. Hsieh, 2001; Yeh, 1989). (1) *"bu shi ban"* (*bu xi ban*, 补习班): This is a group of students with a teacher who provides instruction in subjects taught in school; (2) "Un Chin Class" (*Un Chin Class*, 安亲班): This is more or less like a day-care center with an adult looking after a group of children with tuition charged. Homework supervision is part of this service. The material taught in the two kinds of cram schools above are closely related to the school syllabus. Hence, they can also be categorized as academic-oriented cram schools; (3) "Special class for specific subject" (特殊才艺班): This is also known as "Talent-and-skill class" (*Talent-and-skill class*, 才艺班) and this is a group of students with a teacher providing a program designed for a specific subject, such as foreign language, calligraphy, essay writing, art, music, dance, sports, mental calculation, and calculation on an abacus. Most of the knowledge taught in a "Talent-and-skill class" is not related to the school curriculum. So, it is categorized as a non-academic-oriented cram school. (4) Private tutoring: This is one-to-one instruction. Depending on the needs of the students, private tutoring can be academic or non-academic-oriented.

In academic-oriented cram schools, all compulsory subjects for the examination are included in the programs. Because mathematics is recognized as important for applied science and is a required subject in entrance examinations for higher education in Taiwan, it is always the predominant subject in cram schools for primary and middle school children, in particular.

Among the various kinds of cram schools, academic ones are the most popular and have the highest attendance, while few students would opt for private tutoring. L. F. Wu (1993) investigated the attendance of elementary school age children in various types of cram schools around Taiwan. Subjects were permitted to indicate multiple types of cram schools they attended. The results demonstrated that about 80% of the children attended cram schools; 54% of those who attended cram schools were engaged in academic programs and 18% in other programs; and approximately 40% attended non-academic cram schools. Wu also found that 81% of those who were going to enter junior high schools attended academic cram schools. The role of cram schools can be explicitly considered as an academic-mender following the regular schooling, particularly for higher graders.

2.3 *The instructional approach in cram schools*

Aiming to help students obtain higher scores and gain greater confidence on tests, direct instruction is considered the most effective instructional approach used in cram schools. In other words, teacher-centered lecturing is commonly used in cram schools.

"Working harder will lead to improved performance" is the maxim of cram schools. To improve students' proficiency in test-taking and to ensure they get high scores, the typical teaching process involves (1) lecturing and providing students with organized materials, (2) requiring students to practice with various types of problems and formats similar to those used in tests, and (3) repeated drills and tests (K. M. Huang, 1993; J. S. Hsieh, 2001).

In the case of mathematics learning, children memorize the content of organized materials and are taught strategies for solving problems like those in tests. Their basic skills in mathematical computation are enhanced through intensive training provided by cram schools. But this teaching/learning process will limit the children's development in creative thinking and the ability for flexible application of knowledge as well (K. M. Huang, 1993). Although the educational goals of cram schools are consistent with the Chinese belief of hard work and industriousness, the teaching approach adopted by cram schools has come under severe criticism for years.

2.4 *The trend of children's cram school attendance*

Children preferred academic-oriented cram schools to other types (L. F. Wu, 1993) before the educational reform movement. This can be attributed to the prevalent trend in the educational system as well as the intensely competitive entrance examinations for higher education (K. M. Huang, 1993).

   With the introduction of the reforms in mathematics education in the last decade and new admission requirements for senior high schools and universities, the trend of children attending cram schools seems to be changing. According to the study on primary school children's attendance of cram schools conducted by Taiwan Ministry of Education (2000), 54% of the primary school children attended cram schools. Furthermore, 27% of the children who attended cram schools were engaged in academic-oriented programs and approximately 26% attended non-academic-oriented cram schools. A comparison of the percentages of cram school attendance before and after the educational reform movement reveals that the number of children attending seems to be decreasing. H. P. Huang (2002) pointed out that there is a growing trend for elementary school children, lower graders in particular, to attend non-academic programs. More and more children are attending non-academic-oriented cram schools, although the academic-oriented ones are still preferred.

3 Parents' Influence on Children's Cram School Attendance

3.1 *The traditional value of academic success*

Far Eastern parents generally have higher academic expectations of their children and provide them with more learning opportunities than their foreign counterparts (Peng & Wright, 1994). This social phenomenon can be attributed to the importance of academic success emphasized in traditional Chinese thinking – for example, there is a saying that those who labor physically are governed by those who work with brain and mind from a famous literalist Liu Zongyuan (柳宗元) in Tang Dynasty (唐代）(B. I. Hsieh, 2002). Confucian beliefs about the role of hard work and ability in achievement, as well as emphasis on scholastic accomplishment, point to education as critical in the future of children (Stevenson, 1992; Stevenson et al., 1990; Xiang, 2002).

There is a long tradition of competitive examinations among the Chinese people. Xiang (2002) pointed out that this is a remarkably different heritage from that of western society. Since the introduction of a national examination system in China during the Sui Dynasty (隋代) in 600 A.D., examinations have been the main way for screening and identifying capable persons for public service. This examination system has endured for hundreds of years even though the social structure has changed drastically (K. M. Huang, 1993).

Seeking success through various examinations, including entrance examinations for education, is an important goal for students. Consequently, parents' expectations for their children drive them to enroll their children in extra programs to enhance their performance in examinations.

3.2 *Parents' belief about education*

Brought up in a culture with great emphasis on education and academic success, Chinese parents value scholastic achievement as their child's most important pursuit (Stevenson et al., 1990; Xiang, 2002). Stevenson et al. also found that once a Chinese child entered elementary school, the parents mobilized themselves to provide an environment conducive to achievement. Parents hold higher expectations and have great interests in their child's academic achievement. They tell their children explicitly that their primary task is to do well in school.

Previous research has demonstrated the influence that others have on children's academic development (Alexander & Entwisle, 1988;

Stevenson et al., 1990). For example, H. M. E. Huang and Ling (1993) found that a mother's belief about school learning was related to children's mathematics achievement. Parents' belief in the direct relationship between hard working and scholastic success is reflected in their greater willingness to send children to cram schools.

L. F. Wu (1993) investigated 1550 parents with lower (grades 1-2), middle (grades 3-4), higher (grades 5-6), and 7th graders from northern, central, and southern Taiwan. She found that 68% of the parents held the opinion that sending children to cram schools is necessary for getting better achievement, especially when children cannot understand the content taught in school. Moreover, H. P. Huang (2002) found that most parents who encouraged and sent their children to attend cram schools believe that "Stupidity can be remedied by diligence". K. H. Sun (1993) also pointed out that those parents who send their children to cram schools believe that higher achievement at young age means that the children are better prepared for entrance examinations to higher education.

3.3 *Parental level of education*

Parental level of education is another significant factor affecting parents' willingness to send children to cram schools. C. S. Sun and Hwang (1996) found that parents with a high level of education tend to provide more educational resources and supplementary assistance to their children and more likely to send their children to cram schools. On the other hand, K. H. Sun (1993) and J. S. Hsieh (2001) found that parents with a high level of education emphasize developing their children's talents; they favor specific programs, such as a foreign language, computers, the arts, music, and sports rather than academic subjects. This is more obvious for children in lower grades (Yeh, 1989). J. S. Hsieh (2001) and H. P. Huang (2002) proposed two reasons to account for such a phenomenon. First, because the school lessons are not too difficult, these highly educated parents are able to provide assistance to their children without the need to resort to outside help. Second, these parents believe that the more skills their children possess, the higher the opportunity for them to enter prestigious senior high schools and universities under the current admission system. Thus, they send children to "Talent-and-skill classes". Alternately, parents with a lower educational level are more likely to send their children to academic cram schools because they themselves are not in a position to assist their children in school work.

However, the percentage of children attending cram schools increases with age and grade. Children in higher grades, for example in 7th grade and above, are likely to attend academic cram schools (J. S. Hseih, 2001). In other words, the trend that parents prefer their children to attend non-academic cram schools to academic ones is reversed in higher grades. J. S. Hseih (2001) and H. P. Huang (2002) attributed this to the increasingly difficult school work where parent tutorial interventions may not prove sufficient. As children advance to higher grades, the school subjects become harder and parents see academic cram schools as the best alternative for their inadequate tutorial intervention.

4 Children's Reasons for Attending Cram Schools

With clear academic goals and enthusiastic support given by both the family and social culture, Chinese children are more motivated to pursue academic success and most of them focused more on doing well in school or going to college than American children (Stevenson, 1992). Stevenson also pointed out that Chinese children agreed with the general notions that any student can be good at math if he/she works hard enough and hard working will improve performance. The belief that achievement is dependent on diligence is the main reason why Chinese children are more willing to spend time on academic work through attending cram schools. L. F. Wu (1993) and H. P. Huang (2002) found that although most children who attended cram schools were compelled to by their parents, some eventually developed a positive attitude towards them.

H. P. Huang (2002) interviewed 41 higher graders from two elementary schools asking why they attend cram schools. The reasons provided by the children are discussed in the following.

4.1 *Achievement motivation and self-requirement*

Children with a high achievement motivation tend to place great emphasis on knowledge acquisition and competence (Slavin, 1997; Pintrich, Marx, & Boyle, 1993). Moreover, if a child performs well in mathematics, he/she is more likely to be labeled as a "clever" student. Furthermore, children are worried about competitive examinations in which academic success is determined by scores. Those who have failed examinations strive to get higher scores, so that they do not have to change their perception of themselves as good students (S. J. Wu, 1998). Previous research (H. P. Huang, 2002; J. S. Hsieh, 2001; L. F. Wu, 1993; Y. I. Wu, 1997) revealed that children believed that their academic performance would be enhanced by attending cram schools.

4.2 *Peer pressure*

Studies of elementary school age children have indicated that low peer popularity leads to poor utilization of academic ability (Schmuck, 1962). Research by Ladd and Price (1987) revealed that the social dimension of the peer group is especially important in the primary grades. During middle childhood, children begin to evaluate themselves in comparison to others and students in higher grades, in particular, tend to compare their academic abilities and skills with those of others (Slavin, 1997). Moreover, S. J. Wu (1998) demonstrated that children who perform poorly in school mathematics are at risk for developing low academic self-image and subsequent poor peer relationships. Children are aware of the fact that peer relationships would be impaired if their mathematics achievement is lower than the average of their classmates.

Previous studies (J. S. Hseih, 2001; H. P. Huang, 2002) found that children attend cram schools for two main reasons, as follows: First, it is to maintain a positive self-image and to be accepted among peers. Some children expect to make advances in mathematics performance through attending cram schools, thus they can have better peer acceptance and higher status within the peer group, especially for higher graders. Children feel honored if they are high achievers. Second, it is to acquire the ability to successfully demonstrate solutions to problems before classmates whenever called on by their teachers. Moreover, in a small cooperative group, everyone is supposed to contribute ideas and solve problems. Children hope to have the ability to offer and share ideas with peers actively rather than passively, while accepting opinions from others in group work.

In addition, H. P. Huang (2002) found that children who attended cram schools demonstrated that they learned the material in advance and acquired something new from extracurricular programs; they were able to show and share what they learned with peers. Previous research illustrated that to be able to propose different perspectives and show something new to classmates is a source of academic self-confidence (Slavin, 1997).

5 Children's Perception of the Relationship between Cram School Attendance and Mathematics Learning

Previous studies (H. P. Huang, 2002; J. S. Hsieh, 2001; Wang, 1983; L. F. Wu, 1993) indicated that children believe that cram schools offer students the opportunity to learn more after school, which in turn helps them obtain higher mathematics achievement in school.

Furthermore, small group problem-solving is more emphasized in post-reform teaching practice; however, too much time spent in group discussion leaves too little time for teachers to complete the syllabus (H. M. E. Huang, 2002). Children who attended cram schools revealed that they are able to understand more through previewing the mathematics lessons at cram schools. Moreover, school teachers tend to encourage students to present their solutions in an open problem-solving discussion. This puts the lower achievement children at a disadvantage because they might become confused by too many choices given in class. In cram schools, children have opportunities to ask questions to clarify what confuses them and to understand the best solution from direct instruction.

6   Primary School Teachers' Perception of the Interaction among Cram School, School-based Mathematics Learning and Instruction

Schools have the responsibility to teach the content of the curriculum and to implement the constructivist-based mathematics reforms. The mode of school mathematics instruction has been changed through teachers' inservice educational programs and the role of teacher has thus been radically reformed (Chung, 2000; Chung & Chu, 2001). The mode of student-centered instruction used in school mathematics is different from the teacher-centered lecture used in cram schools. It is worthwhile to explore how teachers view cram school education and its influence on their teaching practice. For the purpose of extracting more information from teachers' views, interviews using open-ended questions were conducted.

6.1 *Data collection*

Forty-four teachers from public elementary schools in Taipei city and county were interviewed (see Appendix). The interview contains questions probing how teachers perceive the impact of cram school attendance on different aspects of mathematics learning. These aspects include computation skills, homework completion, understanding mathematical concepts, self-confidence in mathematics, and teaching practices. The mean number of years of teaching experience was 12.4. Teachers' responses were categorized and frequencies were tabulated. Discussion was held between the two coders who reached a common consensus on how to categorize the opinions given. Inter-rater agreement was 95%. In addition, a content analysis of teachers' explanations was carried out to gain insight into the teachers' opinions of the impact of cram schools on mathematics learning and instruction.

6.2 *Results*

6.2.1. *Teachers' perceptions of the influence of cram schools on children's mathematics learning*

The analysis results showed that the percentage of children attending cram schools with mathematical programs was about 47%.

Table 1 shows how the teachers perceive the impact of cram schools on aspects related to school mathematics learning. As can be seen, 82% and 70% of the teachers reported that cram schools were of much help to children's mathematical computation skills and homework completion, respectively, while 7% and 5% thought that cram schools have a negative influence, respectively.

Table 1
Teachers' Views about the Influence of Cram Schools Attendance on Children's Mathematics Learning.

Aspect of school mathematics learning	Positive influence	Negative influence	No influence	No comments
Mathematical computation skills	82%	7%	2%	9%
Mathematical homework completion	70%	5%	-	25%
Understanding mathematical concepts	16%	52%	9%	23%
Self-confidence in mathematics learning	64%	4%	7%	25%

However, some teachers held the opinion that whether a child could benefit from cram school education depends on how much effort he/she invested. Two percent of the teachers did not think that cram schools have an influence on children's computation skills, while 9% and 25% of them did not comment on the relationships between cram schools and children's mathematical computation skills and homework completion, respectively.

Teachers also reported that children performed better on computation and homework through the training of cram schools, which in turn enabled them to gain more self-confidence in mathematics learning. While 64% of the teachers expressed the view that extra learning in cram schools boosts children's self-confidence in mathematics learning, 4% felt otherwise.

Subsequent interviews revealed the reasons why teachers felt that attending cram schools had a negative influence on children's self-confidence in mathematics learning. The responses frequently given included the following: "Some children have good skills in computation but poor understanding of the mathematical concepts, they cannot explain the mathematical reason behind their computation"; "Only doing well in calculation is insufficient for enhancing one's self-confidence in mathematics"; "Some children attended cram schools pre-learned the lessons, giving them a false impression about their mathematical competence; thus they tended to be less attentive or were frequently distracted. Consequently, they were unable to perform well in class eventually. The impression of their mathematics ability produced by cram school attendance would impair children's confidence in mathematics".

However, 7% expressed the view that cram school attendance seemed to have no relationship with children's self-confidence in mathematics learning and 25% did not have any comments about the relationship. Teachers expressed their view that self-confidence in mathematics learning depends on the children's ability and daily mathematical performance as well as the level of difficulty of the mathematical content, rather than cram school attendance. For example, children in lower grades are more likely to have greater self-confidence in mathematics learning because of the relatively less difficult mathematics content.

As seen in Table 1, 16% of the teachers reported that cram school attendance had a positive influence on children's understanding of mathematical concepts, but 52% felt otherwise. Two reasons can account for such opposing views. First, cram schools place emphasis on "short-cut" and "effectiveness", and focus solely on producing the correct answers to problems rather than exploring the systematic structure of mathematical concepts. Children frequently fail to solve problems that look novel to them. They just learn to mechanically apply a formula when solving problems through drill and practice. Such rote practice may enhance their homework performance or term tests that cover only content retention, but may weaken their meaningful construction of mathematical knowledge.

Nine percent of the subjects thought that cram school attendance is not related to children's understanding of mathematical concepts and 23% did not have any comments on this aspect. Teachers perceive that understanding mathematical concepts is more closely related to a child's ability and whether he/she pays attention when learning in class rather than cram school attendance.

Regarding the effect of cram schools on teaching practices, the results revealed that 59% of the subjects reported that cram schools have no impact on their teaching practice, while 41% of them thought that cram schools had only a slight influence on their teaching practice. Explanations offered by teachers are as follows.

    a. The instructional approach in schools is quite different from that used in cram schools. Understanding mathematical concepts through the process of observation, manipulation, operations, and discussion is emphasized by school teachers. Compared to the drill and practice in cram schools, the instructional approach and practice used in schools are meant to provide meaningful learning. Teachers commonly ask leading questions and guide the whole class through the conceptual development in a systematic and coherent way, rather than by rote.

    b. Apart from textbooks, materials, content, and activities designed and used in schools are relatively different from those in cram schools. School mathematics instruction stresses sharing and illustrating one's own thinking in an open classroom discussion. Furthermore, for the purpose of fostering children's creativity and applying mathematics knowledge in solving daily problems, school programs and projects are frequently provided by teachers.

    c. Teachers benefit from the homework supervision provided by cram schools. This can save time in checking assignments and help to keep them teaching on schedule. Furthermore, some low achieving children can catch up with other students through extra programs in cram schools. This tends to narrow the gap of individual differences among the students with mixed achievement levels, thus enabling a smoother teaching schedule.

d.   School teachers with a good knowledge of mathematics and children's cognition in mathematics are able to probe and diagnose children's misconceptions in class. Equipped with a better understanding of the pedagogical content, a greater variety of teaching strategies and more experience with children, school teachers know which approach may be most effective in a particular situation, and are sometimes able to correct misconceptions students develop in cram schools.

The reasons given why teachers considered that their teaching practice was slightly affected by cram school are as follows:

a.   Children's attitudes toward school learning may not be earnest owing to previous lessons in cram schools; that is, students presume they already know what was taught, so they tend to pay less attention and sometimes disturb the discussion and exploration process in class. This behavior may also cause class management problems.

b.   There is a need for teachers to spend time clarifying the concepts and misconceptions that children get from lessons in cram schools. Because the quality of cram school teachers varies greatly, they frequently cause misconceptions or inappropriate information.

c.   Some teachers complain that they have to "negotiate" with students concerning their reports and discussions, because some cram schools offered too much homework; that is, because children tend to spend much time in completing the exercises required by cram schools, they may complete school tasks or reports in a perfunctory manner.

To summarize the findings mentioned above, approximately half of the children of elementary school age attended cram schools with mathematical programs. Teachers have both positive and negative perceptions about cram schools, with respect to mathematics learning and teaching. Most teachers agreed that cram schools have merit in improving children's computation skills, supervising homework completion, and boosting self-confidence in mathematics. Homework supervision provided by cram schools, especially the Un Chin Class, saves or reduces the time spent by parents and teachers in checking assignments. This benefits most of those parents who do not have the ability and time to assist in their children's homework. Furthermore, under the supervision of cram schools, children perform better in their homework, which in turn enhances their self-confidence in mathematics. Opposing ideas about cram schools are often embedded in views on rote learning and its negative influence on understanding mathematical concepts as well as children's negative attitudes toward school learning.

7 Conclusion

This chapter explores the role of cram schools in Taiwan, as well as how parents and children perceive them. The major function of cram schools is to provide supplementary education, especially academic programs for compulsory subjects in entrance examinations. However, the service provided by cram schools is also changing in order to meet the needs and expectations of parents and children. The trend of cram school attendance, among children in lower grades, in particular, is gradually shifting to non-academic programs.

The benefits children can have from attendance at cram schools remain controversial. The growing popularity of attendance can be attributed to the influence of parents and certain children's factors. Parents tend to have high expectations for children's academic success, which is greatly emphasized in traditional Chinese values. Parental level of education also significantly affects their decision to send children to different kinds of cram schools. Besides being encouraged by parents, some children with higher achievement motivation and those who desire to maintain a positive self-image and acceptance among peers tend to seek academic supplement by attending these schools. With respect to learning mathematics, the popular belief held by many parents and children is that children may acquire academic proficiency through learning more and more substantive mathematics, which in turn improves school mathematics achievement.

Primary school teachers seemed to perceive positive effects of cram schools on children's mathematics learning. These include improved computation skills, homework completion, and greater self-confidence in mathematics. On the other hand, teachers did not agree that the cram schools' emphasis on rote-learning is so good, thinking that these schools fail to foster children's conceptual development. The influence of cram schools on children's understanding of mathematical concepts as well as flexible application of knowledge is deemed negative. However, some teachers argued that enrolling in extra programs does not ensure high achievement in mathematics because children tend to apply the algorithms and effective strategies learned in cram schools with limited understanding of the mathematical concepts behind them. Furthermore, children's distractions and negative attitudes toward learning, and the need to correct the misconceptions learned in cram school, pose problems for teachers in classroom teaching. School teachers recommend that parents should seriously consider the quality of the teachers when choosing a school.

Overall, cram schools have merit in satisfying the needs of parents and students. Although the intensive repetitive daily practice offered by cram schools helps foster children's academic abilities, in some ways it fails to develop creative thinking (H. P. Huang, 2002; K. M. Huang, 1993) and understanding of mathematical concepts.

Competence in such domains as mathematics rests on the children's ability to develop and link their knowledge of concepts and procedures. Rittle-Johnson, Siegler and Alibali (2001) suggested that the two essential types of knowledge that children should acquire are conceptual understanding and procedural skills. In order to help children become better learners, cram schools should focus more on promoting conceptual development in mathematics and fundamental cognitive processing, instead of great emphasis on drill. Furthermore, teachers think that children's ability and effort are more important mediators in mathematics learning than rote learning. At the same time, school teachers should also design and offer programs different from those provided by cram schools to avoid the problem of children getting distracted in class.

Furthermore, the quality of cram school teachers needs to be ameliorated through pedagogical programs. Mayer (2000) pointed out that changing views of mathematics learning can be a driving force in curricular reform, particularly in the teaching of prerequisite cognitive processes in school mathematics. The value of teaching cognitive processing has been pinpointed as a perquisite for basic academic achievement and as a means of promoting mathematical ability. It is necessary, therefore, to provide teachers in these schools with educational training to improve their teaching effectiveness. And to also help them be more consistent with the instructional approach in regular schools.

Acknowledgements

The author would like to thank Dr. Jerry P. Becker, Dr. Wong Ngai-Ying, and Dr. Fan Lianghuo for their helpful comments.

References

Alexander, K. L., & Entwisle, D. R. (1988). Achievement in the first 2 years of school: Patterns and processes. *Monographs of the Society for Research in Child Development, Serial No.218, 53*(2).

Chen, L. S. (1978). To consider more in the education of cram schools [In Chinese 取缔 补习教育的再商榷]. *Min Chu Chao* [In Chinese 民主潮], *28*(6), 9-11.

Chung, J. (2000). School-based teacher improvement as an effective support for mathematical curriculum reform. *Proceedings of the National Science Council (Part D): Mathematics, science, and technology education, 10*(2), 71-89.

Chung, J., & Chu, T. C. (2001). One teachers' professional growth during the implementation of the new mathematics curriculum. *Proceedings of the National Science Council (Part D): Mathematics, science, and technology education, 11*(2), 51-65.

Grow-Maienza, J., Hahn, D.-D., & Joo, C.-A. (2001). Mathematics instruction in Korean primary schools: Structures, processes, and a linguistic analysis of questioning. *Journal of Educational Psychology, 93*(2), 363-376.

Her, F. T. (1977). Study of Taipei short term cramming education, I [In Chinese 台北市短期补习班教育之研究(一)]. *Kuo Chiao Yueh Kan* [In Chinese 国教月刊], *24*(11), 10-13.

Hsieh, B. I. (2002). *Gu wan gwan jr* [In Chinese 古文观止]. Taipei: Sun Min Shu Ju.

Hsieh, J. S. (2001). The effect of cram schools on students' mathematics achievement. *Journal of National Taipei Teachers College, XIV* (Sept. 2001), 313-338.

Huang, H. M. E. (2001). Teaching mathematical problem solving in Taiwan elementary Schools. In E. Pehkonen (Ed.). *Problem solving around the world* (pp. 75-81). Finland: University of Turku.

Huang, H. M. E. (2002). Relationship between teachers' knowledge of school mathematics and their views of mathematics learning and instructional practices: A case study of Taiwan. *Journal of the Korea Society of Mathematical Education Series D: Research in Mathematical Education, 6*(1), 1-28.

Huang, H. M. E., & Ling, M. J. (1993). Mother's beliefs about ability and effort in school learning and child's learning achievement [In Chinese 母亲的儿童学习信念及其与儿童学业成就相关之探讨]. *Journal of Education & Psychology* [In Chinese 教育与心理研究], *16*, 413-458.

Huang, H. P. (2002). *The research on contributory factors to math tutoring after the school hours and effects on math learning for the senior schoolchildren* [In Chinese 国小高年级学童参加校外补习之背后因素与对数学学习影响之研究]. Unpublished master's thesis, Graduate School of Education, National Tai-Tong Teachers College.

Huang, K. M. (1993). Discussing cram school [In Chinese 谈补习]. *Shiann Dai Chiao Yu* [In Chinese 现代教育], *8*, 145-151.

Huang, Y. Y. (1995). Should children participate cram school? [In Chinese 学生一定要补习吗?]. *Chiao Shy Jy Yeou* [In Chinese 教师之友], *36*(4), 32-34.

Ladd, G. W., & Price, J. M. (1987). Predicting children's social and school adjustment following the transition from preschool to kindergarten. *Child Development, 58*, 1168-1189.

Mason, J., & Waywood, A. (1996). The role of theory in mathematics education and research. In A. J. Bishop, K. Clements, C. Keitel, J. Kilpatrick, & C. Laborde (Eds.). *International handbook of mathematics education* (pp.1055-1089). The Netherlands: Kluwer Academic Publication.

Mayer, R. E. (2000). Intelligence and education. In R. J. Sternberg (Ed.). *Handbook of intelligence* (pp. 519-533). Cambridge, MA: Cambridge University Press.

Peng, S. S., & Wright, D. (1994). Explanation of academic achievement of Asian American students. *Journal of Educational Research, 87*(6), 346-352.

Pintrich, P. R., Marx, R. W., & Boyle, R. A. (1993). Beyond cold conceptual change: The role of motivation beliefs and classroom contextual factors in the process of conceptual change. *Review of Educational Research, 63*(2), 167-199.

Rittle-Johnson, B., Siegler, R. S., & Alibali, M. W. (2001). Developing conceptual understanding and procedural skill in mathematics: An iterative process. *Journal of Educational Psychology, 93*(2), 346-362.

Schmuck, R. (1962). Sociometric status and utilization of academic abilities. *Merrill-Palmer Quarterly, 8*, 165-172.

Slavin, R. E. (1997). *Educational psychology-theory and practice* (5th ed.). Needham Heights, MA: Allyn & Bacon.

Stevenson, H. W. (1992). Learning from Asian schools. *Scientific American, 267*, 32-40.

Stevenson, H. W., Lee, S. Y., Chen, C., Stigler, J. W., Hsu, C., & Kitamura, S. (1990). Contexts of achievement. *Monographs of the Society for Research in Child Development, Serial No.221, 55*(1-2).

Sun, C. S., & Hwang, Y. J. (1996). Shadow education, cultural capital and educational attainment [In Chinese 补习教育、文化资本与教育取得]. *Journal of Taiwan Society* [In Chinese 台湾社会学刊], *19*, 95-139.

Sun, K. H. (1993). The situation and causes of cram school in elementary school and junior high school in Kaohsiung [In Chinese 高雄县市国民中小学学生之课外补习实况与成因之调查研究]. *Chiao Yu Tzu Liaw Wen Chai* [In Chinese 教育资料文摘], *31*, 135-153.

Szendrei, J. (1996). Concrete materials in the classroom. In A. J. Bishop, K. Clements, C. Keitel, J. Kilpatrick, & C. Laborde (Eds.). *International handbook of mathematics education* (pp. 411-434). The Netherlands: Kluwer Academic Publication.

Taiwan Ministry of Education. (1993). *Curriculum standards for elementary school in Taiwan* [In Chinese 国民小学课程标准]. Taiwan: Author.

Taiwan Ministry of Education. (2000). *The first – ninth grades curriculum alignment curricula guide in mathematics* [In Chinese 国民中小学九年一贯(第一学习阶段)暂行纲要]. Taiwan: Author.

Taiwan Ministry of Education. (2003). *Supplementary education* [In Chinese 补习教育]. Retrieved July 25, 2003, from http://www.edu.tw/statistics/multi/status-e6.htm

The China Post Staff. (2000, December 7). Taiwan's students top world league in science. *The China Post*, 19.

TIMSS-Forum. (2003). *TIMSS results*. Retrieved April 28, 2003, from http://nces.ed.gov/timss/search-result.asp

Wang, C. L. (1983). Does "Bushiban" help students' academic work?! [In Chinese 补习班-升学的救星?!]. *Ta Hsueh Tzar Jyh* [In Chinese 大学杂志] , *169*, 16-20.

Wong, N. Y., & Wong, K. M. (1997). The mathematics curriculum standards in ten regions [In Chinese 十地区数学教育课程标准]. *Mathmedia* [In Chinese 数学传播], *82*, 28-44.

Wu, L. F. (1993). Analyzing students' questionnaire in BiXiBan in elementary school [In Chinese 国小学生补习状况问卷分析]. *Jen Pen Chiao Yu Cha Chi* [In Chinese 人本教育札记], *43*, 12-18.

Wu, S. J. (1998). *The relationship among elementary school children's self-conception, motivation of mathematics learning and mathematics achievement* [In Chinese 国小学童自我概念、数学学习动机与数学成就的关系]. Unpublished master's thesis, Graduate School of Education, National Ping-Tong Teachers College.

Wu. Y. I. (1997). *Causal mechanism affecting elementary school student's academic achievement: A comparison between Tai-Tung county and Taipei municipality* [In Chinese 影响国小学童学业成就的因果机制 – 以台北市和台东县作比较]. Unpublished master's thesis, Graduate School of Education, National Tai-Tung Teachers College.

Xiang, P. (2002). Chinese children's self-perceptions of ability in physical education. *Journal of Research in Childhood Education, 17*(1), 97-105.

Yeh, Y. S. (1989). Study of the correlation among attending talent-and-skill cram education outside schools, children's academic achievement, ability of creation, self-conception and peer relationships [In Chinese 校外才艺补习教育与同龄儿童学业成就、创造力、自我概念及同侪关系之相关研究]. *Yan Shyi Tzy Shiunn* [In Chinese 研习咨讯], *54*, 28-30.

Appendix
(Translated from Chinese)

Questions on how primary school teachers view the effect of cram schools on school-based mathematics learning and instruction.

1. How many children are there in your class? How many children in your class attend extra mathematics programs or cram schools with mathematics classes?
2. According to your perception and observation in teaching practice, how does cram school education affect children's mathematics learning in aspects such as computation skills, mathematical homework completion, understanding mathematical concepts, and self-confidence in mathematics?
3. Would children's cram school attendance influence your teaching in school-based mathematics? Why?

☐ No influence on my teaching practice in school-based mathematics.
☐ Some influence on my teaching practice in school-based mathematics.

Reasons:

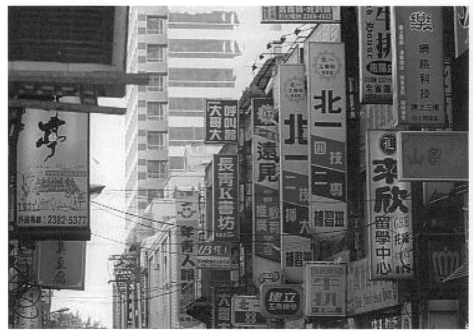

Figure. "Cram school street" in Taipei

Note. Photo provided by Prof. N. Y. Wong.

Section 3

PEDAGOGY AND LEARNING PROCESSES

Chapter 12

Teaching with Variation: A Chinese Way of Promoting Effective Mathematics Learning

GU Lingyuan   HUANG Rongjin   MARTON Ference

This chapter consists of two parts. First, based on a longitudinal experiment aiming at effective mathematics teaching and learning in China, a theory, called teaching with variation, is summarized by adopting two concepts of variation, i.e. conceptual variation and procedural variation. Secondly, it is demonstrated that the Chinese theory is strongly supported by several well-known Western theories of learning and teaching. Particularly, the Marton's theory offers an epistemological foundation and conceptual support for the Chinese theory. Moreover, the authors argue that the teaching with variation characterizes the mathematics teaching in China and by adopting teaching with variation, even with large classes, students still can actively involve themselves in the process of learning and achieve excellent results.

Key words: teaching with variation, conceptual variation, procedural variation, Chinese mathematics classroom, paradox of Chinese learners

1 A Paradox of Chinese Learners

1.1 *Contradictory view on Chinese mathematics learning*

Since the 1980s, many international comparative studies on mathematics achievement, which included Chinese students at primary and secondary schools, have repeatedly shown contradictory results:

On the one hand, a number of studies have shown that Chinese students outperformed their counterparts in the Western countries in both comparative mathematics achievements studies and at the International Mathematical Olympiad (Beaton et al., 1996; Lapoite, Mead, & Askew,

1992; Mullis, Martin, et al., 2000; Mullis, Michael, et al., 1997; Stevenson, Chen, & Lee, 1993; Stevenson & Stigler, 1992). On the other hand, many Western researchers have found that the learning environment in China did not seem conducive to "good learning"[1]. For example, with regard to teaching method, it was described as "passive transmission" and "rote drilling" (Biggs, 1991; Ginsberg, 1992; Kember & Gow, 1991). Ginsberg (1992), in particular, characterized teaching in China as student's passive learning under teachers' domination, by pointing out that this form of teaching is rather equivalent to a respected senior transmitting knowledge to an obedient younger student. It therefore appears that the teaching of mathematics in China is quite traditional and conservative.

This contradictory situation was called the "paradox of the Chinese learner" (Marton, Dall'Alba, & Lai, 1993) which has, internationally, attracted the interest of the researchers in mathematics education and cross-cultural psychology (Biggs, 1994; Biggs & Watkins, 1996, 2001; Leung, 1995, 2001; Morris et al., 1996; Watkins & Biggs, 2001).

1.2 *Interpretations of the paradox*

Logically, these two opposite observations cannot be seen to be simultaneously valid. Since many international comparative studies have shown that Chinese students outperformed their counterparts in the West, researchers have recently and thoroughly investigated mathematics teaching in China from different perspectives in order to interpret the paradox. The following section will discuss three relevant studies.

1.2.1 *Understanding knowledge from multiple perspectives: A comparative study on understanding mathematics knowledge of primary teachers in China and the United States*

Ma (1999) found that Chinese teachers normally received 10 to 12 years of formal schooling including teacher training while US teachers

---

[1] This also applies very much to other Confucian Heritage Communities such as Chinese Taiwan, Korea, Japan, and Singapore (Biggs & Watkins, 1996; Marton, Dall'Alba, & Lai, 1993).

received 16 to 18 years of schooling. However, the Chinese teachers were better equipped with knowledge of mathematics as a subject and were able to use more effective methods to teach it. The Chinese teachers emphasized the understanding of concepts from multiple perspectives, while the American teachers paid great attention to the procedural knowledge. For example, the American teachers usually emphasized how to calculate but without understanding the underlying rationale in depth, while the Chinese teachers not only required students to master computation fluently but also paid attention to the ability to select a proper and effective method to operate. It is obvious that these aims cannot be achieved by rote-drill. Stressing multiple methods and different understandings was argued as "an important feature of Chinese mathematics teaching" by Zheng (2001).

1.2.2 *Unfolding teaching progressively: Studies on the Chinese model of teaching and teacher induction education*

In the early 1990s, Paine (1990), basing her findings on the results from her fieldwork during 1986-87, described the "virtuoso model" of teaching in China. The characteristic of the virtuoso model is that lessons are dominated by teacher-talk in an expository and explanatory format, the students constituting the audience. According to Paine, teaching in Chinese classrooms involves transmission of knowledge progressively to students in a precise and elegant language. It resembles an artistic performance when a lesson is unfolded progressively. Recently, on the grounds of a qualitative study on teacher induction in Shanghai, Paine (2002) argued that studying the "focal points" (重点), "difficult points" (难点), and "hinges" (关键) of teaching materials through a collaborative and joining community of in-server teacher education practice could contribute to the "profound understanding of mathematics" (Ma, 1999) by Chinese mathematics teachers.

1.2.3 *Searching for different ways to solve a problem: Comparisons of mathematics classrooms in the Eastern countries and Western countries*

In the 1980s, a research group led by Harold Stevenson at the University of Michigan conducted a series of cross-cultural studies comparing the mathematics achievement of Chinese, Japanese and American students. It was found that students from Japan, Taiwan, and Mainland China attained significantly higher levels of mathematics competency than the American students. These studies were based on classroom observations of 800 mathematics classes in elementary schools from Beijing, China; Sendai, Japan; Taipei, Taiwan; and Minneapolis and Chicago in the United States, by using systematic time sampling and narrative observations (Lee, 1998). The following conclusions were reached with regard to students' thinking and understanding:

- The practice of presenting one mathematical concept in a number of different ways in East Asian classrooms is more common than in American classrooms.
- In Chinese and Japanese classrooms, the teachers' role is more like a coordinator than a judge.
- Japanese and Chinese teachers are more likely to provide learning experiences with concrete operations followed by abstract concepts. American teachers do so to a lesser extent.
- The quality of the mathematical thinking in which the student is engaged depends on both how the student responds to the questions and how the teacher asks the questions. It was found that American teachers were less likely to use any of the techniques that facilitated students' constructive thinking and conceptual understanding of mathematics than those in East Asia (Lee, 1998; Stevenson & Lee, 1995; Stevenson & Stigler, 1992).

To summarize, in the East Asian mathematics classroom, students are actively involved in learning tasks. They have opportunities to think mathematically. Teachers also apply their own teaching strategies to lead students to construct mathematical concepts. Although the stereotypical Asian education system places a strong emphasis on drilling procedural skills, the data illustrate that East Asian students also have frequent classroom experiences that facilitate their conceptual understanding of mathematics (Lee, 1998; Stevenson & Lee, 1995).

The TIMSS Video Study, in which a total of 231 randomly selected mathematics lessons were video-recorded in Germany, Japan, and the US, described three different patterns of mathematics lesson in the three locations (Stigler & Hiebert, 1999). One of their main findings was the rather sharp contrast between a prototypical American lesson and a prototypical Japanese one:

> In a typical Japanese lesson, after having reviewed the previous lesson, the teacher introduces the problem of the day, a problem complex enough to be used as a framework for the entire lesson and for elaborating different ideas and procedures. The students then work on the problem individually, as a rule, in a number of different ways. This is continued by work in groups. The teacher — and the students as well — comment on the strengths and weaknesses of different approaches. The teacher summarizes the work at last and points to the most powerful ideas that have come up during the lesson.
>
> In a typical American lesson, the teacher also starts with reviewing the previous lesson. Then the teacher may introduce definitions, terms, and above all, a method for solving certain kinds of problems. After the demonstration, the students are given a relatively large number of problems to practice on. After that, another type of problems may be introduced, the method for solving that kind of problems are then demonstrated by the teacher, and the students are given a further set of problems of this second kind to practice on.

The teaching strategy to search for multiple methods to solve a problem in the Japanese classroom can be often found in the Chinese mathematics classroom which is strikingly different from the United States.

The above studies showed some of the characteristics of mathematics classroom teaching in China, such as multiple understandings of concept and principle and multiple methods to solve a problem, which are opposite to the observations of passive learning and rote-drill. It is necessary to investigate Chinese mathematics teaching in depth in order to interpret the "paradox of Chinese learner".

1.3 *Focusing on teaching with variation*

These contradictory observations may be attributed to the different understanding of learning and teaching in different cultures, apart from cultural bias and limitations of outsiders. For example, some Western scholars argued that the fact that Chinese learners were regarded as "rote-learners" might be due to the exclusive dichotomy of memorization and understanding and juxtaposing the repetition learning and rote learning equally in the West. However, the repetition learning with certain variations could be meaningful (Marton & Booth, 1997; Marton, Dall'Alba, & Tse, 1996).

Marton, having reviewed some mathematics comparative studies (Stevenson & Stigler, 1992; Stigler & Hiebert, 1999), argued that "a main difference between Japanese and American classrooms is that in the Japanese classrooms the students work with few problems, consisting of many elements, while in the American classroom the students work with many problems consisting of few elements" (Marton et al., 2004).

According to the theory of variation derived from the phenomenography (Bowden & Marton, 1998; Huang, 2002; Marton, 1999; Marton & Booth, 1997; Rovio-Johansson, 1999), the different patterns of variation may be pertinent to uncover the paradox of Chinese mathematics learning, which also help us to understand mathematics teaching in China.

In the following sections, first, based on the "*Qingpu experiment*" which aimed to study and implement the notion of "teaching with variation" (变式教学), concepts and characteristics of "teaching with variation" will be described. Then, the Chinese concept of "teaching with variation" will be justified and theorized with connection to several Western theories. After that, the paradox of Chinese learners will be examined from the notion of "teaching with variation". Finally, it is also hoped to explore the characteristics of mathematics teaching in China and establish the Chinese theory of teaching with variation.

2 Experimental Foundations

In China, "teaching with variation" has been applied consciously or intuitively for a long time. Employing the previous experience and experiment, L. Gu (1981) systematically analyzed and synthesized the concepts of teaching with variation. He identified and illustrated the two forms of variations: "conceptual variation" and "procedural variation".

2.1 *Conceptual variation: Understanding concepts from multiple perspectives*

Teaching with variation is

> An important teaching method through which students can definitely master concepts. It intends to illustrate the essential features by demonstrating different forms of visual materials and instances or highlight the essence of a concept by varying the nonessential features. It aims at understanding the essence of object and forming a scientific concept by putting away nonessential features (M. Gu, 1999).

Traditionally, conceptual variation refers to the following two ways of creating variation: one refers to varying connotation of concept, called concept variation and the other refers to varying instances which confuse the connotation of concept, termed non-concept variation such as illustrating by counterexamples. These two types of variations make up "conceptual variation", which aims at providing students with multiple perspectives of experiencing concepts. The functions of both variations will be illustrated below.

2.1.1 *Inducing concepts by varying visual and concrete instances*

Abstractness is one of the fundamental features of mathematical concept. However, many concepts can be derived from the real world with physical background. It is important to allow students to have a concrete and visual experience in order to connect the abstract concept with its concrete embodiments.

Take the teaching of the "non-coplanar line" where two lines are not on the same plane. Based on the experience, the difficulties for learning the concept are: First, it is not easy to understand the concept due to its abstract nature; secondly, the concept belongs to three-dimensional space so that the distorting of the visual perception is inevitable when using two-dimension of diagram representation. The objects of this concept (i.e., extension) are thus not easily discernible. To solve the two difficulties, a experienced teacher would prefer to make use of the following two variations: One is to make use of concrete materials in daily life offering students sensory experience and helping them clarify the meaning of the concept (see Figure 1 (1)); The other is to provide different figures to diagrammatize the concept and transfer the visual perception to abstract concept. By means of the second variation, students will be helped to generalize their perception from concrete to abstract and understand the basic features of the concept figures and master the set of extension of the concept (Figure 1 (2)).

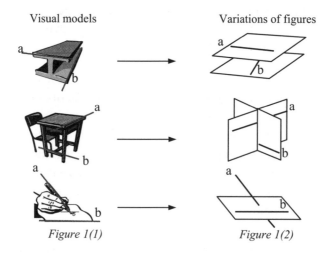

Visual models   Variations of figures

Figure 1(1)   *Figure 1(2)*

However, it must be pointed out that, at the inducing stage of a concept, the main purpose of using this variation is to help students establish the connection between concrete experience and abstract concept. Moreover, as the essence of a mathematical concept is abstract, the visual background of a concept must be disconnected in due course so that a concept is upgraded to an abstract level.

In addition, there are different levels of abstraction of mathematical concepts. It is relative whether one concept is abstract or concrete. For example, in order to illustrate the essence of the concept "equation", namely, "an expression containing unknowns and the equal sign", the following variations of concepts should be helpful:

$$2x = 1, \quad \frac{x}{3} + 1 = 2, \quad 4x - 3 = 5, \quad 3x + 4y = 12, \quad x^2 - 1 = 0, \quad x^2 + y^2 = 1$$

Even though these variations are abstract algebraic expressions, they are concrete in comparison with the concept of "equation".

2.1.2 *Highlighting the essence of concept by contrasting non-standard figure*

Since mathematics concepts consist of a clear set of extension, mastering a concept refers to distinguishing whether an object belongs to the set of extension or not. An effective way of teaching concepts is to highlight the essence of the concepts by classifying the varying objects of the extension in terms of their invariant features.

In the set of extension of concept, although logically all the objects are equivalent, certain objects have special positions. For example, a certain figure is the standard representation for the relevant concept due to the visual perception or initial awareness for the learners, as shown in Figure 2:

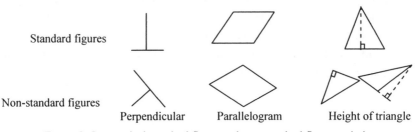

Standard figures

Non-standard figures

Perpendicular   Parallelogram   Height of triangle

Figure 2. Geometrical standard figure and non-standard figure variation

It is helpful to make use of standard figure for mastering concepts accurately, but the standard figure also limits the flexibility of thinking and even narrows the extension of the concepts. An effective way to overcome the disadvantage of use of standard figures is to highlight the essential features of the concepts through varying unessential features by providing different non-standard figures.

2.1.3 *Non-concept variation*

Connotation and denotation (extension) of a concept are two opposite yet complementary aspects. If the connotation is clarified, the extension is defined and vice versa. Therefore, teaching concepts should emphasize clarifying the connotation and differentiating the boundary of the set of objects in the extension. There are relationships among different concepts as shown in Figure 3.

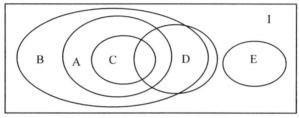

Figure 3. Relationship among concepts

The figure illustrates the relationships among different concepts. For example, B is the superordinate concept of A, C is the subordinate concept of A, A and D are intersected, while A and E are contradictory. Thus, it is necessary to clarify the differences between a concept and its relevant concepts in order to clarify the connotation of the concept.

Using "non-concept variation" can effectively achieve this aim. For instance, in two-dimensional geometry, through comparing non-concept figure and concept figure, the essence of a concept can be clarified and highlighted visually, as shown in Figure 4.

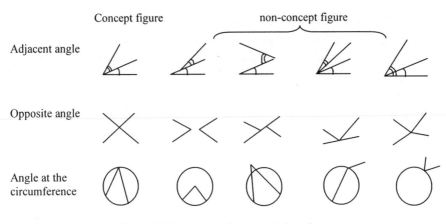

Figure 4. Non-concept figure variations for
discerning the essence of concepts (L. Gu, 1981)

There are many forms of non-concept figure variations. Demonstrating counterexamples is one commonly used method of non-concept figure variations, as illustrated in Figure 5.

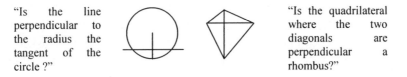

"Is the line perpendicular to the radius the tangent of the circle ?"

"Is the quadrilateral where the two diagonals are perpendicular a rhombus?"

Figure 5. Counterexamples

The left clearly demonstrates that the line perpendicular to the radius is not necessarily a tangent of the circle, while the right convincingly indicates that the quadrilateral where the two diagonals are perpendicular is not necessarily a rhombus.

2.2 *Procedural variation: Progressively unfolding mathematics activities*

Mathematics teaching consists of two types of activities. One is teaching declarative knowledge (i.e., concept). The other is teaching procedural knowledge (i.e., process). Since the procedural knowledge (problem solving and meta-cognitive strategies) is dynamic, using the conceptual variation which is static does not enable to enhance learning process. Thus, L. Gu (1981) adopted "procedural variation" to broaden the concept of variation so as to tackle teaching of procedural knowledge.

It is a fundamental fact that there is a hierarchical system in unfolding mathematics activities, which includes different steps to arrive at a solution or different strategies to solve problems. By procedural variation, the students can arrive at solutions to a problem and form connections among different concepts step by step or from multiple approaches. The functions of procedural variation are illustrated below.

2.2.1 *Enhancing the formation of concepts*

When the concept is regarded as a static object, the conceptual variation is used as an effective way of teaching. However, a concept is formed through a certain process of development which is also an important aspect of understanding the concept. To master a concept, it is helpful to allow students to experience the process of the formation of the concept and in particular to realize the need of introducing the new concept. Take as an example the teaching of the concept of "equation". There are two difficulties in learning the concept: one is the idea of "balance" and the other is the meaning of "unknown". If students are just asked to memorize the definition of an equation: "the expression which includes unknowns and the equal sign is called an equation", and then to discern the same equations from a set of expressions, the students might give correct judgment on whether an expression with an equal sign is an equation or not, understand the extension formally, but not understand the essence of the equation properly. An experienced teacher may adopt "procedural variation" to help students establish the concept progressively as follows:

Scaffolding 1: Representing the unknown by concrete things.

For example, "James pays 2 \$D for buying three rubbers and the seller gives him 2 coins in change (1/10 \$D). How much is for each rubber?" The following expression can present the question visually.

$$2D \ - \ \boxed{\diamond}\ \boxed{\diamond}\ \boxed{\diamond}\ = 2C \qquad \text{or} \qquad 2D \ - \ 3\boxed{\diamond}\ = 2C \qquad (1)$$

Scaffolding 2: Symbolizing the unknowns.

$$2D - 3x = 2C \qquad (2)$$

or

$$20 - 3x = 2 \qquad (3)$$

To some extent, the three expressions above represent the three stages of development of the algebraic symbol system: iconic algebra, simplified algebra, and symbolic algebra. By doing this, it not only helps students experience the simplicity of using symbol to represent numbers, but also provides a concrete model of the "equation" concept. But at this stage, the understanding of unknown is still associated with concrete objects. For example, the students might associate the x in (2) and (3) with a concrete price of rubbers, but not as a general symbol. In order to develop the abstract concept of x, it is helpful to set the further scaffolding:

Scaffolding 3: Replacing unknown x with symbolic "□".

$$20 - 3\square = 2 \qquad (4)$$

Although the equation (4) is far removed from the form of equation than the equation (3) in terms of the appearance, in fact, the "□" in equation (4) is of more general meaning than the x in equation (3). It can be imaged as a box for numbers; the students are furthermore asked to find the numbers, which make the equation tenable. In this way, it enables the students to understand that the number is the value of the unknown. Thus, equation (3) is a special case of equation (4). Moreover, it might help students to understand that the x in equation (3) not only symbolizes the particular object but presents a symbol which can be replaced by any number as the "□" in equation (4). Through working with this game, students not only understand the essence of "unknown" but also experience the basic idea of balance.

There is an essential difference between procedural variation and conceptual variation. The former aims at providing a process for formation of concept stage by stage, while the latter serves as an understanding of concept from multiple perspectives.

2.2.2 *Scaffolding for problem solving*

The fundamental principle of solving problems is to convert unsolved problems into solved problems, complicated problems to simple ones (Pólya, 1945). Since there is no clear relationship between unsolved (complicated) problems and solved simple problems, it is necessary to pave certain ways for implementing this transformation. It can be demonstrated in the following diagram:

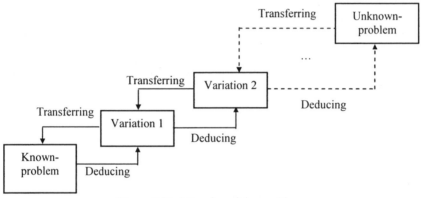

Figure 6. Variation for solving problems

It is a crucial phase in helping students to solve problems by using variation as the scaffolding of transferring problems in China. Students' experience in solving problems is manifested by the richness of varying problems and the variety of transferring strategies. The following is an example of application of procedural variation in problem solving.

As shown in Figure 7, *ABCD* is a trapezium and *BC//AD*. If the areas of $\triangle AOD$ and $\triangle BOC$ are S_1 and S_2, it is to be proved that the area of the trapezium *ABCD*, $S = S_1 + 2\sqrt{S_1 S_2} + S_2$.

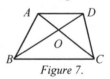

Figure 7.

In order to solve this problem, it is necessary to find the relationships between the area of trapezium and the areas of two given triangles. Moreover, as the trapezium can be separated into four triangles, the original problem therefore can be converted into finding the relationships between the areas of $\triangle$AOB and $\triangle$COD and the given areas of triangles S_1 and S_2. Thus, the key to solve the problem is to create the variations of problem which are related to the area relationships between given triangles and unknown triangles. The analysis of the following diagrams will offer the scaffolding for solving the original problem[2].

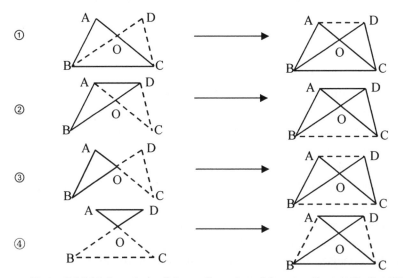

Figure 8. Multiple analysis of the configuration of the same diagram (L. Gu, 1981)

It was found that multiple analyses of the configuration of a problem not only helps students clarify the process of solving the problem and the structure of the problem, but is also an effective way of experiencing problem solving and enhancing the competency of solving other problems (L. Gu, 1994).

2.2.3 *Establishing a system of mathematics experience*

The purpose of creating the procedural variation is to develop the variety of methods of doing activities and the hierarchy of unfolding activities.

---

[2] Take Figure 8① for example, it is easy to find that the area of $\triangle AOB$ is equal to the area of $\triangle COD$. Let $S^* =$ area of $\triangle AOB$, then $S^*/S_2 = AO/OC$ and $S^*/S_1 = CO/AO$. Thus, $(S^*)^2/S_2\,S_1 = 1$, namely, $(S^*)^2 = S_2\,S_1$. Considering $S = S_1 + S_2 + 2S^*$, the result will be proved immediately.

Every mathematics activity consists of one or a series of procedural variations, which include steps and strategies for transferring/exploring. All these variations are made up of a system of experiences and strategies hierarchically and could be internalized into an important part of cognitive structure.

The knowledge system (i.e., concept system) consists of the logical structure of concepts/proposition, while the activity system (i.e., process) reflects the learner's own subjective experiences in problem solving. The cognitive structure includes concept knowledge and process knowledge. The richness and effectiveness of the process system are important for upgrading cognitive structure.

The variations for constructing a particular experience system (i.e., process ability) are derived from three dimensions of problem solving: (1) varying a problem: varying the original one as a scaffolding or extending the original problem by varying the conditions, changing the results and generalization, (2) multiple methods of solving a problem by varying the different processes of solving a problem and associating different methods of solving a problem, and (3) multiple applications of a method by applying the same method to a group of similar problems.

To be concise, in the process of the formation of concepts, the procedural variation reveals the logical, historical, and psychological processes of formation of concepts and therefore enhances students' learning stage by stage. During the process of solving problems, procedural variation manifests a series of concepts or propositions for scaffolding or the strategies and experiences for doing activities, thus fostering students' methods of solving problems with multiple stages or multiple options; in the process of the formation of cognitive structure, a hierarchical system of experience or strategies is formed by creating the procedural variation; the separated activity experience is therefore re-organized into an integration.

In other words, the purpose of the procedural variation is to form a hierarchical system of experiencing process through forming concepts or solving stages of problems. This teaching therefore is definitely not a "rote drill".

2.2.4 *An Empirical study on procedural variation*

Based on the previous analysis, the features and functions of conceptual variation and procedural variation are different. The former is static, emphasizing the comparison of different objects, thus the essence of concept and its extensions are highlighted and clarified by comparing the concept objects and non-concept objects. The latter is dynamic, emphasizing the connections among different processes, therefore the previous knowledge and the new knowledge are connected by providing proper scaffolding based on deliberately separating the mathematics activities into parts progressively. Thus, regarding procedural variation, it is a crucial issue how to design the procedural variation as scaffoldings in order to set an appropriate distance between the previous knowledge and the new knowledge. In order to measure how distant the to-be-explored problem is from the *anchoring part of knowledge,* (i.e., previous knowledge underpinning learning of the new knowledge and the exploration of the new problems), based on a teaching experiment conducted from 1987 to 1988 in *Qingpu*, the concept of "*potential distance*" was introduced and discussed (L. Gu, 1994).

In this experiment, 180 students in grade 8 were tested twice. The purpose of these tests was to examine the relationship between the "potential distance" and the problem solution. The two tests showed that there were different distances between the to-be-explored problem and *anchoring knowledge*, which affected the solving of the problem. Take the first test for example. In the test, the students were required to judge the relationship between two circles, based on the exploration of the relationship between the radii of the two circles and the distance of the centers of the two circles, as shown in Table 1.

The table shows that there are great differences between different grades concerning the potential distance when exploring the relationship between the two circles. At Junior 1, the students just learnt the length of segments without learning geometry formally, the potential distance is the longest; at Junior 2, students had learnt the triangles, the distance was shortened a little; and at Junior 3, the students had learnt the relationship between line and circle, the potential distance is then the shortest. Thus, with the increase of the grade, the students' knowledge is enriched progressively, and hence the potential distance becomes shorter stage by stage.

Table 1
"Potential Distances" for Students of Different Grades

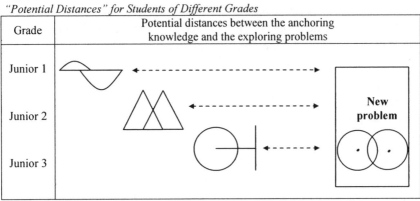

Grade	Potential distances between the anchoring knowledge and the exploring problems
Junior 1	
Junior 2	
Junior 3	

The experiment shows that the more distant the previous knowledge is from the new problem, the more difficult the task is. That means the knowledge and experience constitute the basis for solving a new problem. A shorter potential distance is helpful for students to understand and master the new knowledge, while a longer potential distance is useful for developing students' exploring competency. A successful teacher is adept at working within appropriate "potential distance" related to the learners' previous knowledge and experience and able to consider a suitable arrangement which can promote learning. That is the soul of the effective teaching (L. Gu, 1994).

The "potential distance" experiment is helpful for the understanding of procedural variation. It could be concluded that in the hierarchically organized procedural variation in teaching, by organizing proper *pu dian*[3]

---

[3] The meaning and function of scaffolding will be explained in Section 2 of this Chapter. There are two Chinese words which mean the same thing as scaffoldings. One is *pu dian* (铺垫) which is rooted in China and means a certain kind of support by which someone can do what s/he can't achieve without the support. For example, if a child wants to get something higher than his height, a block or a ladder is used for helping him/her to get it. The other is *jiao shou jia* (脚手架) which is translated from the scaffolding directly. Since *jiao shou jia* is more vivid than *pu dian*, recently, the former is used more common than the latter. However, we adopt *pu dian* because of its culture origin.

(铺垫, i.e. scaffolding), the potential distance between the previous knowledge and the new knowledge can be adjusted so as to make the teaching either inquiry-oriented or acquisition-oriented. This is a critical point for reforming traditional teaching methods.

3 Theoretical Interpretations

In the previous sections, based on experience and experiment, teaching with variation, with its classifications and applications in teaching, was discussed in detail. The rationale of teaching with variation will now be argued from a point of view of the psychology of education and the theory of mathematics learning.

3.1 *Meaningful learning*

There are different understandings and descriptions of learning from different perspectives. For instance, the radical constructivists argue that knowledge can not be transmitted from teacher to students and it can only be developed through students' own experiences. Yet, the social-constructivism, however, suggests that students can learn something from their own experiences and interaction between peers aided by the help of teachers within the zone proximal development (ZPD) (Gredler, 2001). Since traditional mathematics teaching in China emphasized transmission of subject matter knowledge and constructing of subject knowledge systematically, Ausubel's (1968) theory of meaningful learning was selected as the point of departure for the analysis of this study. Ausubel asserts that meaningful learning takes place only when the non-arbitrary and substantive relationship is established between learners' prior knowledge and the new knowledge.

This relationship substantiates the connection between the new knowledge and certain special aspects of the pre-knowledge, such as a figure, a symbol or a concept and an example in the cognitive structure of the learners. The question then arises as to how to help students establish the internal relationship, and how one can judge if the students have established this kind of relationship. The following discussion attempts to address these issues.

3.1.1 *Conceptual variation and the substantial connection*

By using "conceptual variation", the students can learn concepts from multiple perspectives: from concrete to abstract, from special to general, highlighting the essential features and clarifying the connotation of concept by excluding the obstruction of backgrounds. Thus, through conceptual variation, students could be helped to understand the essence of concepts and establish the substantial relationship.

3.1.2 *Procedural variation and nonarbitrary relationship*

By creating "procedural variation", the students can understand the origins of the knowledge and in which way and where it can be applied. Well-structured knowledge would thus be constructed. By creating this variation, it can help students to form concepts, solve problems, construct a system of activity experience, and further help students to comprehend different components of knowledge and upgrade the structure of knowledge; in the meantime, a non-arbitrary relationship between new knowledge and previous knowledge is built.

3.1.3 *Assessing meaningful learning*

How can one judge if students have established the substantive relationships between the new knowledge and previous knowledge? One effective way is to provide students with a group of variations of problems and the necessary knowledge to solve these problems. If the students can solve these kinds of problems correctly, then it can be concluded that the students understand the essence of these concepts.

3.2 *Relationship between the two variations*

3.2.1 *Duality of mathematical object*

According to Sfard (1991), many mathematical concepts can be conceived in two fundamentally different ways: structurally — as objects, and operationally—as processes. Seeing a mathematical entity as an object means being capable of referring to it as if it was a real thing—a static structure, existing somewhere in space and time. In contrast, interpreting a notion as a process implies regarding it as a potential rather than actual entity, which comes into existence upon request in a sequence of actions. Thus, whereas the structural conception is static, instantaneous, and integrative, the operational is dynamic, sequential, and detailed. These two approaches, although ostensibly incompatible, are in fact complementary (Sfard, 1991). She argued that usually the model of learning can be refined as follows: "if the conjecture on operational origins of mathematical objects is true, then first there must be a process performed on the already familiar objects, then the idea of turning this process into an autonomous entity should emerge, and finally the ability to see this new entity as an integrated, object-like whole must be acquired" (p. 18). Moreover, a mathematical concept is a node of a series of concepts: a concept is the operational result of the sub-concepts —structural object, or the operational material for forming its super-concepts. The following section will demonstrate that seeing a concept both as a process and as an object is indispensable for a deep understanding of mathematics.

3.2.2 *Mathematization and situationalization*

One method of learning concept is by formalizing a mathematical concept through manipulation of physical objects. We can examine learning division with residual as an example (Figure 9). Usually, the learning of this concept can be divided into two phases: formalizing and searching for the meaning.

The teacher can introduce the "residual" and "division with residual" by using children' experience in distributing beans. For example, if seven beans are distributed into three plates evenly, how many beans are in each plate and how many are left? Then, the remainder is the residual, and the trial of putting beans in each plate is regarded as "trial quotient", …. In this way, the transformation from the physical objects to the arithmetical form is referred to as a formalizing process, while the process from the arithmetical form to interpretation is called "searching for meaning". Furthermore, mathematizing[4] is the scaffolding among concrete, semi-concrete, semi-abstract, and abstract, and is also shifted between physical objects and arithmetic forms. Experiencing the process of mathematizing, not only enhances students' understanding of "division with residual" but also benefits students' searching for the rules in the arithmetical forms. For example, when students are asked to find the relationships among the dividend, divisor, quotient, and residual, they could say that "divisor time quotient plus the residual is equal to the dividend" and could also explain that the reason why "the residual is less than the divisor" is that "if the residual is larger than the divisor, then the number of the remaining beans is larger than the numbers of plates, thus, each plate can be allocated at least one bean".

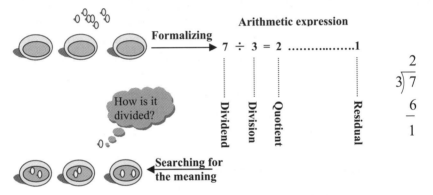

Figure 9. Formation and application of division with residual

There is a big gap between the physical and arithmetic form. It is crucial whether or not teachers can build a bridge between them in their teaching. A experienced teacher might utilize the following processes: first, the teacher demonstrates the ways of distributing beans concretely, then, the students are asked to contemplate the process of distributing beans, when the beans and plates are moved away. After repeating this process, the gap might be filled automatically. This way of dealing with "division with residual" can be illustrated by the following diagram

---

[4] Please refer to the relevant explanation of the "mathematization" in "Revisiting Mathematics Education: China Lecture", by H. Freudenthal, 1990.

(Figure 10) which manifests the three forms of representation suggested by Bruner (1964), namely, enactive, iconic, and symbolic. Moreover, the iconic representation is an important medium for realizing the transformation from active representation to symbolic representation.

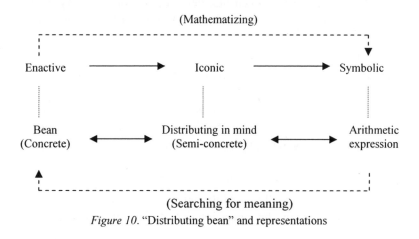

Figure 10. "Distributing bean" and representations

3.2.3 *Cognitive conflict and logical development*

In order to solve the cognitive conflict caused by the operations within existing concepts, a new concept has to be introduced. One example of this is the introduction of irrational number.

- *Introduction and trial.* If students master the rational number concept, they are asked to construct an isosceles right-angled triangle with leg 1 and measure the length of the hypotenuse (denoted as $\sqrt{2}$).
  Fist of all, the students try to estimate with decimal fraction stage by stage as follows:
  $1 < \sqrt{2} < 2, 1.4 < \sqrt{2} < 1.5, 1.41 < \sqrt{2} < 1.42$, and so on, *ad infinitum.*.
- *Conflict.* It seems that the length of the hypotenuse cannot be represented by a rational number. However if it is a rational number, it can be represented as a ratio of two whole numbers without any common factors. Thus $\sqrt{2} = \dfrac{m}{n}$ (there

are no common factors between m and n).

Squaring: $m^2 = 2n^2$.

The m is then definitely an even number, thus $m = 2k$ and therefore, $(2k)^2 = 2n^2$, namely, $2k^2 = n^2$.

Then, n is also an even number. This is contradictory to the assumption that there are no common factors between m and n.

Hence, $\sqrt{2}$ is not a rational number.

- *Constructing irrational number.* What do we mean by $\sqrt{2}$? It is necessary to define the new object and therefore the irrational number has to be introduced. The irrational number can for instance, be defined by Dedekin partition or Cauchy rational sequence and so on.

It was argued that a mathematical concept is a node of a series of concepts: a concept is the operational result of the sub-concepts — structural object — or the operational material for forming its super-concepts.

To summarize, the mathematical learning objects can be conceived as both operational processes and structural objects. The former presents the features of development of a mathematical object, while the latter manifests the essential features of a mathematical object.

First of all, creating *conceptual variation* is helpful for students to uncover the essential features of the concept, define the connotation of the concept, and further understand the concept. That is to say that it could help students understand the structural aspects of the concept. Creating *procedural variation* is then helpful for students to establish the connection between the new knowledge and previous knowledge and construct a suitable structure of knowledge. By creating the two variations, we thus enhance the understanding of the two aspects of a mathematical object: operational process and structural object; the two aspects of a mathematical object are meanwhile complementary.

3.3 *Theory construction*

Conceptual variation and procedural variation are two fundamental teaching strategies. The conceptual variation aims at helping students understand concepts from multiple perspectives while the procedural variation helps students to establish the internal connection between what they know already and the object of learning. Thus, these two aspects are critical and complementary. In fact, the two types of variations, which are based on the analysis of experiences of and experiments with mathematics teaching in China, can be supported and interpreted by certain Western theories such as Dienes' theory of mathematics learning (Dienes, 1973), Marton's theory of variation (Bowden & Marton, 1998; Marton & Booth, 1997), and the scaffolding theory (Bruner, 1985; Wood, Bruner, & Ross, 1976). The following sections examine these theories and further justify the rationale of the two variation strategies.

3.3.1 *Diene's theory of mathematics teaching and learning*

Drawing heavily on Piagetian theory (Piaget, 1952) and having worked with Bruner on an experimental mathematics project at Harvard, Dienes has developed a theory of mathematics learning. According to Dienes, mathematics is about structural relationships between concepts connected with numbers (pure mathematics) together with their applications to problems arising in the world (applied mathematics). The learning of mathematics means to apprehend such relationships together with their symbolization and to acquire the ability to apply the resulting concepts to real situations.

Dienes (1973) suggested four principles of mathematics learning: (1) Dynamic principle, (2) Constructivity principle, (3) Mathematical variability principle, and (4) Perceptual variability principle. In particular, he further explained the last two principles as follows:

According to mathematical variability principle, concepts involving variables should be learnt by experiences involving the largest possible number of variables. To give the maximum amount of experience and structures to encourage the growth of the concept, it seems *a priori* desirable that all possible variables should be made to vary while keeping the concept intact. For example, in order to learn the concept of a parallelogram, it will be helpful to vary the shape by changing the angles and lengths of the opposite sides and the positions, as long as we keep the opposite sides parallel. Clearly, a set of congruent parallelograms placed in the same position would not be a suitable set of experiences for the growth of the concept.

With respect to perceptual variability, by providing tasks which look quite different but have essentially the same conceptual structure, it is assumed that there will be a separation of the structure of concept from its different embodiments. In other words, it will be desirable to vary the perceptual representation while keeping the conceptual structure invariant. For example, parallelograms can be drawn on paper, made out of two congruent wooden triangles, traced with pegs on pegboard, found in wallpaper patterns, and so on. Learners learn what there is in common among these different representations and it is this common feature which is the mathematical concept.

3.3.2 *Marton's theory of variation*

3.3.2.1 Meaning of learning

This theory - still being developed - has grown over three decades of research on learning in different fields. Steps in its development are described in more detail by Marton and Booth (1997) and Marton et al. (2004). A central idea of the theory is how we act in the world is a function of how we see the world. So if we want to enable our students to act in the world in powerful ways, we have to enable them to see the world in powerful ways. To see something in a powerful way amounts to discerning its critical features and focusing them simultaneously. "Critical features" are critical in relation to what the learner is trying to achieve. Whether or not the learners can discern critical features and learn to discern critical features in a certain situation depends on what varies and what is invariant in that situation; the reason being that we can only discern that which varies.

We would not be able to see the "greenness of green" or grasp the idea of color if we lived in a world where everything had the same green color. We would not able to feel our happiness if we were equally happy all the time. We would not be able to experience what distinguishes a wine from other wines if it was the first glass of wine we had. We would only experience what distinguishes wine from other kind of drinks we had previously. Drinking the first glass of wine and always drinking the same wine is incidentally the same from this particular point of view.

The reason is, according to the theory, that we do not notice people, things, or characteristics of people or things, and so on, but we notice differences between people, things, or differences in the characteristics of people or things. We might think that being dark, tall, bright, for example, are characteristics of a certain individual, but what we actually notice is the way in which this particular individual differs from other individuals. If everybody were equally dark, tall, and bright, these qualities would simply disappear. When we see certain qualities in someone we meet the first time, we really feel that this individual has these or those qualities, but what we actually see is how this particular individual differs from all other individuals that we have come across earlier in our lives. This is exactly why we see, experience the same people, things, and situations differently: We notice how they differ from the people, things, and situations we have come across earlier and we, as people, have certainly not come across exactly the same people, things, situations even if just now we happen to look at the same person, thing, or situation.

This is why you can never teach a child what three is, without making him aware of what is *not* three, e.g., one, two, or four, etc. A necessary condition for learning any number in a certain situation is that there is a variation in numbers in that situation. (We are very well aware of the fact that children learn numbers across situations and there is always sufficient variation in numbers in our surroundings.) Numbers have two critical features: "many-ness" (corresponding to their cardinality) and sequential position (corresponding to their ordinality).

Each number represents a certain value in these two dimensions; characteristic for three is its "threeness" and its "thirdness". But such qualities are (experientially) not inherent in any single number; they reflect how every single number differs from other numbers. We cannot thus consider a single number in isolation and sense its "many-ness" and serial position; in themselves, they have none. We have to be aware of the other numbers simultaneously in order to firstly sense "many-ness" and sequential position as dimensions of variation and secondly to sense the specific values in those dimensions ("threeness" and "thirdness") by means of contrast with any other single number.

What the theory suggests is that for any specific capability that we might wish to develop in students, they must experience a certain pattern of variation/invariance in order to develop that capability. If such a pattern is present in the class, it is still no guarantee that every student will experience it. But if it is absent, it is guaranteed that none of them can possibly experience it. (That is due to what can be experienced during a certain lesson or a certain sequence of lessons. The students can, however, experience this pattern of variation/invariance derived from what they have encountered during and outside of the lessons.)

Every situation has, of course, its pattern of variation/invariance and every teacher makes use of such patterns all the time. It can, however, be done in different ways and done more or less consciously. What the present theory can possibly be used for is a more conscious and thus hopefully more rational use of variation/invariance.

The basic idea is, of course, that different patterns of variation make different things possible for the students to experience. It is assumed that the students will be more likely to learn what is possible to learn than what is not.

Here, we briefly characterize some common patterns of variation/invariance.

3.3.2.2 Patterns of variation/invariance

1. The most common pattern is probably what we might call *generalization*. What is invariant is a concept (parallelogram, "3", etc.), a method of solution, and so on. What varies are the different instances of the concept (e.g., "three apples," "three cups", "three cats", etc.) or different cases to which the method of solution is applied (e.g., finding the unknown side in a right-angled triangle by using Pythagoras theorem when the other two sides are known). In such cases, the focus is on that which is invariant (concept or method of solution) and the idea is to separate what is critical for the concept or solution method in question from what is irrelevant (other features of instances on cases).

2. In the opposite pattern of variation/invariance, the one which is highlighted in the theory discussed here, what is to be discerned and what is figural, is that which varies and what is invariant is background. We call this *separation,* because two or more aspects are separated by letting some vary, while others remain invariant. One example of this is the discernment of "many-ness" and serial positions discussed above. They can not be experienced without experience variation in number (and hence variation in "many-nesses" and serial positions). In order to grasp them not only do the numbers have to vary, but other features have to be invariant. If a child always saw two pigs, three cats, four cows, and never the other way around, he or she would not be able to separate "pig-ness" from "two-ness", "cat-ness" from "three-ness", and "cow-ness" from "four-ness". But if she compares two pigs with three pigs and four pigs, both "many-ness" and serial positions can easily be separated from the irrelevant fact that it is pigs we are counting.

   In a similar way in order to grasp the idea of "method of solution", there must be more than one method for solving the very same problem. If the students encounter one method only for every kind of problem, they cannot possibly separate the "method of solution" from "the kind of problems". It is only possible for them to do so if the former varies, while the latter is invariant. Otherwise, they are bound to see the way of solving the problem that they are engaged in as *the* method of solution and not as *a* method of solution. An example of this was given above with reference to Japanese and Chinese classrooms.

3. By means of the pattern of variation/invariance, two or more aspects (or dimensions of variation) are separated from each other. The focus is on the aspect that varies (or the aspects that vary). But we may be interested in different aspects of certain instances or cases, or in specific "values" in the dimensions of variation under consideration (such as 1, 2, 3, ... as regarding "many-ness" and sequential positions or a particular method of solution as regarding "methods of solution for a certain kind of problems"). Here an instance or a case is compared with one or more instances or cases where what is invariant recedes to background, while that which varies becomes

visible. The pattern of variation/invariance might be exactly the same as in the case of "separation" above, but the focus here is not on the dimension of variation, but on a particular value in that dimension (such as on "three-ness" and "third-ness" instead of "many-ness" and serial positions and on a particular method of solving a certain kind of problems instead of on "methods of solving a certain kind of problems"). This we call *contrast*.

3.3.3 *Dienes and Marton's theories and conceptual variation*

Dienes theory seems to focus mainly on the pattern of variation/invariance, identified as *generalization* by Marton. In addition, the patterns of separation and contrast in Marton's notions resemble "highlighting the essences of concept by contrasting non-conceptual figures" discussed early. Therefore, both Dienes and Marton elaborated the *conceptual variation* from different perspectives. Although in Dienes' theory, the process of forming concepts was emphasized as a "dynamic principle", in L. Gu's theory, the process of developing concepts and solving problems was treated as *procedural variation*. Thus, L. Gu's theory seems to broaden the concept of variation. It is quite interesting that these three theories derived from different cultures but concerned with relatively similar notions of variation for fostering mathematics learning and teaching. It may imply that the notion of variation is a crucial aspect of mathematics learning and teaching.

3.3.4 *Scaffolding theory and procedural variation*

Vygotsky describes learning by using the concept zone of proximal development (ZPD), which was defined as follows:

> The distance between the actual developmental level as determined by independent problem solving and the level of potential development as determined through problem solving under adult guidance or in collaboration with more capable peers (Vygotsky, 1978, p. 86).

In particular, he emphasizes the role of support by adults and the exchanges among more capable peers in establishing and widening the zone of proximal development and finally enhancing the development of learners' potential ability. It was the attention given to how teachers help students to develop the potential ability that resulted in the establishment of the theory of scaffolding.

3.3.4.1 The view of teaching inherent in "scaffolding theory"

Based on the ZPD theory, Wood et al. (1976) adopted the word "scaffolding" to describe how children learn under the guidance of the adult. By offering scaffold, the components of a task which require the capability beyond the scope of learners are controlled by the adult and the children can focus on those parts of the task which can be solved by their own efforts. Therefore, learners can complete the task, which require a high cognitive demand. They can achieve the performance which is impossible without the guidance of adults. According to Bruner (1985), scaffolding in teaching means a process: a more capable person helps children to progress from the current level to the potential level.

As a tool of teaching, scaffolding is durative and temporary. In the process of teaching, when the children have made enough progress within the scope of scaffolding, the scaffolding is unnecessary and needs to be moved away. On the other hand, with the requirement of learning new knowledge, new scaffolding needs to be built in a proper position within ZPD. The scaffolding, which assists students in building new knowledge and developing creativity, not only enlightens students in their understanding, but also guides them to move toward the particular answers, which are expected by the teachers.

3.3.4.2 "Scaffolding" and procedural variation teaching strategy

The notions of scaffolding emphasize how teachers establish appropriate and dynamic "scaffolding" to enhance student's development within the ZPD, and suggest relevant teaching strategies. Although this theory just provides general descriptions and suggestion, it can be also used for justifying the *procedural variation*. There are two different types of scaffoldings in terms of the functions of teaching: one is affective and the other is cognitive. Regarding the cognitive function, it mainly reduces the difficulties, clarifies the critical points, focuses on and demonstrates the process of solving problems.

One concept is worthy of note: *pu dian* (i.e., procedural variation), which is commonly used in Chinese classroom teaching and similar to the scaffolding in the West. Similar to the word scaffold, the word *pu dian* is derived from the description of daily life. For example, by putting blocks or stones together as a *pu dian*, a person can pick fruit from a tree which cannot be reached without the *pu dian*. The implication for teaching is by establishing *pu dian*, the students can complete the tasks which cannot be done without the *pu dian*. In this sense, there is fairly close similarity between the theory of scaffolding in the West and *pu dian* in China. However, the procedural variation pays much attention to the process and hierarchy.

3.3.5 *Basic ideas of teaching with variation*

Based on the previous discussions, "teaching with variation" can be summarized by way of examining the following aspects:

3.3.5.1 Meaningful learning and two types of variations

The previous discussions have attempted to argue that through the strategies of variation, students would be helped to understand the essential features of mathematical objects and establish the substantive connection between the new object of learning and previous knowledge. If meaningful learning is to establish non-arbitrary and substantive connection between the new knowledge and previous knowledge, then teaching with variation can foster meaningful learning.

3.3.5.2 Internal relationship between the two variations

Each of the two variations serves each aspect of duality of a mathematical object respectively. Conceptual variation aims at constituting a space of variation for students to experience critical aspects of the object of learning, and enhancing the understanding of the essential feature of the object, while the procedural variation intends to pave the way to help students establish the substantive connections between the new object of learning and the previous knowledge. The duality of the mathematics object can be seen when the two variations serve different aspects of the object complementarily and different strategies serve different purposes in the light of the different situations.

3.3.5.3 Implication for teaching

There are two strategies to implement teaching with variation: conceptual variation teaching and procedural variation teaching. By conceptual variation strategy is meant the aim of constituting a space of variation which focuses on the critical aspects of the objects of learning. Through procedural variation strategy, students are helped in the establishing of the substantive connections between the new object of learning and the previous knowledge by providing certain scaffoldings and further improving their development within ZPD.

4 Implication and Discussion

4.1 *Rethinking Chinese mathematics classrooms*

As demonstrated above, the teaching with variation, a popular mathematics teaching method in China caters for two objectives of mathematics teaching: First, understanding mathematics objects (concepts and principles) from multiple perspectives by adopting conceptual variation, secondly, unfolding the mathematics activities progressively by using procedural variation. In line with this point of view, the features of Chinese mathematics classrooms are examined below.

In Chinese classrooms where emphasis is placed on constructing subject knowledge systematically (Zhang, S. Li, & J. Li, 2003), it is critical to set a suitable "potential distance" and space of variation in order to implement effective teaching. Probably, the superficial phenomena such as large size of classrooms in China, where the teacher controls the class activities and prefers to explain the content clearly and effectively, would induce the Western researchers to characterize

Chinese classrooms as being teacher-centered with students learning passively. However, when investigating how the lessons are organized and how students involve themselves in the process of learning, it was found that by adopting teaching with variation, even with large classes, students could still actively involve themselves in the process of learning and achieve a meaningful learning. Moreover, it is possible to avoid rote learning by adopting a certain strategy of variation. Thus, the "paradox of Chinese learners" might originally be a misperception by Western scholars due to the limitation of their philosophies and theories (Biggs & Watkins, 2001).

4.2 *Discussion*

Based on the analysis of Chinese classrooms from the perspective of teaching with variation, some characteristics of Chinese mathematics classrooms were identified and a paradox of Chinese learners was revisited. However, we would argue that it is the teaching with variation that makes the mathematics teaching meaningful in Chinese classrooms if it is used properly, yet also makes the mathematics teaching passive and rote-oriented if it is used improperly.

One could argue, of course, that the approach to teaching mathematics was developed in a particular part of China and therefore hardly representative for what we might refer to as "Chinese Pedagogy". But, we should remember that this theory was developed mainly inductively and hence it is more an attempt to characterize — rather than prescribe — good practice in Chinese mathematics teaching. Furthermore, Ko and Marton (2004) argue that what is considered good practice in the Chinese context must necessarily include the constitution of necessary patterns of variation/invariance. Otherwise, the students would not be able to learn what they are expected to learn and what they actually learn in reality.

By making explicit principles used (not always consciously) by successful educators, others can learn and develop their capabilities to teach further.

4.2.1 *Concerning exploration: Setting proper potential distance*

In the traditional Chinese classrooms, the systematic subject knowledge is emphasized and the teacher also plays a key role in the teaching. It was found that through certain strategies of variation, students could understand and master subject matters systematically and effectively. However, some internationally comparative studies showed that although Chinese students always performed excellently in solving routine problems, compared with their counterparts in the West, it is not necessarily the case when solving daily life situations involving open-ended problems (Cai, 2001). One should be aware that if teaching with variation is not used appropriately, such as inadequate scaffolding being offered too slowly, students' learning would not be challenged and possibly become passive. Thus, it is important to stress the process of exploring knowledge and solving everyday life and open-ended problems. From the perspective of teaching with variation, these attempts can be implemented in the process of teaching. Through designing a far more potential distance or larger stages of scaffoldings, learning could be made more challenging, and teaching could creatively foster the ability of problem solving by providing more open-ended problems.

4.2.2 *Concerning experience: Constructing appropriate space of variation*

"The space of learning" (Marton et al., 2004) consists of different dimensions of variation in critical aspects of the objects of learning that constrain and make learning possible. The richness of this space will affect the extent and degree of understanding the objects of learning. If the space is too small, it may provide students with incomplete conditions resulting in a narrowness of understanding. On the other hand, if the space is too broad, which students may be able to explore extensively, it is also possible to distract students' attentions from understanding and mastering of the essence of the concept. Therefore, in the teaching with variation, the space of learning constituted jointly by the teacher and students is of crucial importance for understanding what the students learn and what they cannot possibly learn (cf N. Y. Wong,

Marton, K. M. Wong, & Lam, 2002).

In general, in order to prepare students for future involving varying conditions, we have to create opportunities for them during their school years to encounter conditions that vary in critical respects.

Acknowledgements

Ference Marton's participation in the writing of this chapter was financially supported by the Swedish Research Council and The Bank of Sweden Tercentenary Foundation.

References

Ausubel, D. P. (1968). *Educational psychology: A cognitive view*. New York: Holt, Rinehart & Winston.

Beaton, A. E., Ina, V. S. M., Michael, O. M., Eugenio, J. G., Dana, L. K., & Teresa, A. S. (1996). *Mathematics achievement in the middle school years: IEA's Third Mathematics and Science Study (TIMSS)*. Chestnut Hill, MA: TIMSS International Study Center, Boston College.

Biggs, J. B. (1991). Approaches to learning in secondary and tertiary students in Hong Kong: Some comparative studies. *Educational Research Journal, 6,* 27-39.

Biggs, J. B. (1994). What are effective schools? Lessons from East and West (The Radford Memorial Lecture). *Australian Educational Researcher, 21,* 19-39.

Biggs, J. B., & Watkins, D. A. (1996). The Chinese learner in retrospect. In D. A. Watkins & J. B. Biggs (Eds.), *The Chinese learner: Cultural, psychological, and contextual influences* (pp. 269-285). Hong Kong: Comparative Education Research Center, The University of Hong Kong; Melbourne, Australia: Australian Council for Education Research.

Biggs, J. B., & Watkins, D. A. (2001). Insight into teaching the Chinese learner. In D. A. Watkins & J. B. Biggs (Eds.), *Teaching the Chinese learner: Psychological and pedagogical perspectives* (pp. 277-300). Hong Kong: Comparative Education Research Center, the University of Hong Kong; Melbourne, Australia: Australian Council for Education Research.

Bowden, J., & Marton, F. (1998). *The university of learning*. London: Kogan Page.

Bruner, J. S. (1964). Some theorem on instruction illustrated with reference to mathematics. In E. R. Hilgard (Ed.), *Theories of learning and instruction* (pp. 306-335). Chicago, IL: University of Chicago Press.

Bruner, J. S. (1985). Vygotsky: A historical and conceptual perspective. In J. V. Wertsch (Ed.), *Culture, communication and cognition: Vygotsky perspective* (pp. 21-34). Cambridge, UK: Cambridge University Press.

Cai, J. (2001). Improving mathematics learning: Lessons from cross-national studies of U.S. and Chinese students. *Phi Delta Kappan, 82*(5), 400-405.

Dienes, Z. P. (1973). A theory of mathematics learning. In F. J., Crosswhite, J. L. Highins, A. R. Osborne, & R. J. Shunway (Eds.), *Teaching mathematics: Psychological foundation*(pp. 137-148). Ohio: Charles A. Jones Publishing Company.

Freudenthal, H. (1990). *Revisiting mathematics education: China lectures*. Dordrecht, The Netherlands: Kluwer Academic Publishers.

Ginsberg, E. (1992). Not just a matter of English. *HERDSA News, 14*(1), 6-8.

Gredler, M. E. (2001). *Learning and instruction: Theory into practice* (4th ed.). Columbus, OH: Merrill Prentice Hall.

Gu, L. (1981). *The visual effect and psychological implication of transformation of figures in geometry* [In Chinese 演变图形在几何教学中的直观效果和心理意义]. Paper presented at annual conference of Shanghai Mathematics Association.

Gu, L. (1994). *Theory of teaching experiment: The methodology and teaching principle of Qingpu* [In Chinese 青浦实验的方法与教学原理研究]. Beijing: Educational Science Press.

Gu, M. (1999). *Education directory* [In Chinese 教育大辞典]. Shanghai: Shanghai Education Press.

Huang, R. (2002). *Mathematics teaching in Hong Kong and Shanghai: A classroom analysis from the perspective of variation*. Unpublished doctoral dissertation, The University of Hong Kong, Hong Kong.

Kember, D., & Gow, L. (1991). A challenge to the anecdotal stereotype of the Asian student. *Studies in Higher Education, 16*(2), 117-128.

Ko, P. Y., & Marton, F. (2004). Variation and the secret of the Virtuoso. In F. Marton, A. B. M. Tsui, P. P. M. Chik, P. Y. Ko, M. L. Mok, I. A. C. Mok, et al. (Eds.), *Classroom discourse and the space of learning*. Mahwah, NJ: Lawrence Erlbaum.

Lapointe A. E., Mead, N. A., & Askew, J. M. (1992). *Learning mathematics*. Princeton, NJ: Educational Testing Service.

Lee, S. Y. (1998). Mathematics learning and teaching in the school context: Reflections from cross-cultural comparisons. In S. G. Garis & H. M. Wellman (Eds.), *Global prospects for education: Development, culture, and schooling* (pp. 45-77). Washington, DC: American Psychological Association.

Leung, F. K. S. (1995). The mathematics classroom in Beijing, Hong Kong and London. *Educational Studies in Mathematics, 29*, 197-325.

Leung, F. K. S. (2001). In search of an East Asian identify in mathematics education. *Educational Studies in Mathematics, 47*, 35-51.

Ma, L. (1999). *Knowing and teaching elementary mathematics: Teachers' understanding of fundamental mathematics in China and the United States*. Mahwah, NJ: Lawrence Erlbaum Associates.

Marton, F. (1999, August). *Variatio est mater studiorum* [Variation is the mother of learning]. Opening address presented at the 8th EARLI conference, Göteborg, Sweden.

Marton, F., & Booth, S. (1997). *Learning and awareness.* Mahwah, NJ: Lawrence Erlbaum Associates, Publishers.

Marton, F., Dall'Alba, G., & Lai, K. T. (1993). *The paradox of the Chinese learner (Occasional Paper 93.1).* Melbourne, Australia: Educational Research and Development Unit, Royal Melbourne Institute of Technology.

Marton, F., Dall'Alba, G., & Tse, L. K. (1996). Memorizing and understanding: The keys to the paradox? In D. A. Watkins & J. B. Biggs (Eds.). *The Chinese learner: Cultural, psychological, and contextual influences.* Hong Kong: Comparative Education Research Center, The University of Hong Kong; Melbourne, Australia: Australian Council for Education Research.

Marton, F., Tsui, A. B. M., Chik, P. P. M., Ko, P. Y., Lo, M. L., Mok, I. A. C., et al. (2004). *Classroom discourse and the space of learning.* Mahwah, NJ: Lawrence Erlbaum Associates.

Morris, P., Adamson, R., Au, M. L., Chan, K. K., Chang, W.Y., Ko, P. Y., et al. (1996). *Target oriented curriculum evaluation project (interim report).* Hong Kong: INSTEP, Faculty of Education, The University of Hong Kong.

Mullis, I. V. S., Martin, M. O., Gonzalez, E. J., Gregory, K. D., Garden, R. A., O'Connor, K. M., et al. (2000). *TIMSS 1999 internal mathematical report: Findings from IEA's report of the Third International Mathematics and Science Study at the eight grade.* Cherstnut Hill, MA: TIMSS International Study Center, Boston College.

Mullis, I. V., Michael, O. M., Albert, E. B., Eugenio, J. G., Dana, L. K., & Teresa, A. S. (1997). *Mathematics achievement in the primary school years: IEA's Third International Mathematics and Science Study (TIMSS).* Cherstnut Hill, MA: TIMSS International Study Center, Boston College.

Piaget, J. (1952). *The child's conception of number.* London: Educational Supply Association Ltd.

Paine, L. W. (1990).The teacher as virtuoso: A Chinese model for teaching. *Teachers College Record, 92* (1), 49-81.

Paine, L. W. (2002, April). *Learning to teach through joining a community of practice in Shanghai: Curriculum control and public scrutiny of teaching as context for teacher learning.* Paper presented at the American Education Research Association Annual Meeting, New Orleans, USA.

Pólya, G. (1945). *How to solve it.* Princeton, NJ: Princeton University Press.

Rovio-Johansson, A. (1999). *Being good at teaching: Exploring different ways of handling the same subject in higher education.* Sweden: ACTA Universitatis Gothoburgensis.

Sfard, A. (1991). On the dual nature of mathematics conception: Reflections on processes and objects as different sides of the same coin. *Educational Studies in Mathematics, 22*(1), 1-36.

Stevenson, H. W., Chen, C., & Lee, S. Y. (1993). Mathematics achievement of Chinese, Japanese, and American children: Ten years later. *Science, 25*(9), 53-59.

Stevenson, H. W., & Lee, S. Y. (1995). The East Asian version of whole-class teaching. *Education Policy, 9,* 152-168.

Stevenson, H. W., & Stigler, J. W. (1992). *The learning gap: Why our schools are failing and what we can learn from Japanese and Chinese education.* New York: Summit Books.

Stigler, J. W., & Hiebert, J. (1999). *The teaching gap: The best ideas from world's teachers for improving education in classroom.* New York: The Free Press.

Vygotsky, L. S. (1978). *Mind in society: The development of higher psychological processes. Cambridge,* MA: Harvard University Press.

Watkins, D. A., & Biggs, J. B. (2001). The paradox of the Chinese learner and beyond. In D. A. Watkins & J. B. Biggs (Eds.), *The Chinese learner: Cultural, psychological, and contextual influences* (pp. 3-26*)*. Hong Kong: Comparative Education Research Centre, The University of Hong Kong; Melbourne, Australia: Australian Council for Education Research

Wong, N. Y., Marton, F., Wong, K. M., & Lam, C. C. (2002). The lived space of mathematics learning. *Journal of Mathematical Behavior, 21*(1), 25- 47.

Wood, D., Bruner, J. S., & Ross, G. (1976). The role of tutoring in problem solving. *Journal of Child Psychology and Psychiatry, 17*(2), 89-100.

Zhang, D., Li, S., & Li, J. (2003). *An introduction to mathematics education* [In Chinese 数学教育导论]. Beijing: Higher Education press.

Zheng, Y. (2001). *Mathematics education: From theory to practice* [In Chinese 数学教育: 从理论到实践]. Shanghai: Shanghai Educational Press.

Chapter 13

Cracking the Paradox of Chinese Learners: Looking into the Mathematics Classrooms in Hong Kong and Shanghai

HUANG Rongjin   LEUNG Koon Shing Frederick

This chapter presents the findings of a study on the mathematics classrooms in Hong Kong and Shanghai in an attempt to explore a so-called Paradox of Chinese Learners. Eight Hong Kong lessons and eleven Shanghai lessons in which Pythagoras' theorem was taught were examined in great detail from the perspective of variation. It was found that in both cities the teachers (1) tended to emphasize exploration of the theorem, (2) seemed to emphasize exercises with variation, and (3) controlled the classroom activities but they still encouraged students to engage well in the process of learning. The findings suggest that good teaching seems to take place in the Chinese classrooms despite their large class size, and further challenge the very idea of the paradox of Chinese learners. Furthermore, they demonstrate that exploration of Chinese mathematics pedagogy should be done with caution because of intra-cultural differences.

Key words: paradox of Chinese learner, perspective of variation, Chinese mathematics classroom, classroom interaction

1 Background

The paradox of the Chinese learners that their seemingly unfavorable learning environment produces students who outperform their counterparts in the West has been well recognized (Biggs & Watkins, 1996; Gu, Huang, & Marton, this volume; Marton, Dall'Alba, & Lai, 1993), and the paradox has been explored by researchers from various perspectives (Lapointe, Mead, & Askew, 1992; W. O. Lee, 1996; Leung,

1995, 1998, 2001; Stevenson, Chen, & S. Y. Lee, 1993; Stevenson & Stigler, 1992; Watkins & Biggs, 1996). It is suggested that factors such as cultural beliefs, curriculum, and teacher competence all play different roles in students' academic success or failure (Leung, 1998; Ma, 1999; Stevenson & Stigler, 1992; Wong, 1998).

Both teachers and classroom settings play an important role in helping students construct their mathematical concepts. In order to explore the paradox mentioned above, this study attempts to look at what really happened in mathematics classrooms by investigating the ways Pythagoras' theorem was handled basing on a theory of learning. This theory was proposed by Gu et al. (this volume) on the basis of experiments and theoretical reflection. Gu et al. suggest that teaching by creating certain dimensions of variation is a feature of mathematics classrooms in China which may be helpful for understanding the effective teaching despite the large class size. According to this theory, discernment is a fundamental constituent of learning and students can never discern anything without experiencing a certain necessary pattern of variation (see section 2.1 for details). This research focuses on the following two questions:

1. What patterns of variation do mathematics teachers in Hong Kong and Shanghai create for students to experience?
2. How do mathematics teachers in Hong Kong and Shanghai help students involve in the process of learning?

2 Theory and Methodology

2.1 *Theory of variation*

Based on the experience and some longitudinal experiments in China and heavily influenced by cognitive theory and constructivism, a theory of mathematics teaching/learning, called Theory of Variation, has been developed (Bowden & Marton, 1998; Huang, 2002; Gu, 1994; Gu et al., this volume; Marton & Booth, 1997). According to this theory, meaningful learning is to enable learners to establish a substantial and non-arbitrary connection between the new and their previous knowledge

(Ausubel, 1968), and classroom activities are to help students establish this kind of connection by experiencing certain dimensions of variation. This theory suggests that two types of variation are helpful for meaningful learning (Gu et al., this volume). One is called "**conceptual variation**", and the other is called "**procedural variation**".

Conceptual variation consists of two parts. One part is composed of varying the connotation of a concept: standard variation and non-standard variation. The other part consists of highlighting the substantial features of the concept by contrasting with counterexamples or non-conceptual diagrams. The function of this variation is to provide learners with multiple experiences from different perspectives.

Procedural variation is concerned with the process of forming a concept logically or historically, arriving at solutions to problems (scaffolding, transformation), and forming knowledge structure (relationship among different concepts). The function of **procedural variation** is to help learners acquire knowledge step by step, develop learners' experience in problem solving progressively, and form well-structured knowledge. Furthermore, these notions are supported by Dienes' (1973) theory of mathematical learning, Vygotsky's (1978) notion of zone of proximal development, and Sfard's (1991) duality of mathematical concept. According to this theory, the **space of variation** consists of different dimensions of variation in the classroom, and they form the necessary condition for students' learning in relation to certain learning objectives. For the teacher, it is critical to consider how to create a proper space of variation focusing on critical aspects of the learning object through appropriate activities. For the learner, it is important to experience the space of variation through participating in constituting the space of variation. In this study, we will focus on what and how the space of variation is constituted.

2.2 *Participants*

In this study, the Chinese cities of Hong Kong and Shanghai were selected as two cases to be investigated. Within each setting, several lessons were purposefully selected, as discussed below.

2.2.1 *The Hong Kong lessons*

The Hong Kong videos from the TIMSS 1999 Video Study on the teaching of Pythagoras' theorem were collected. Thus, the Hong Kong data for the present study consists of the following: (1) eight CDs of the sampled lessons, (2) questionnaires for understanding teachers' background, instructional practices, attitude, and professional development, and (3) sample of students' work in the lessons: samples of text pages, worksheets and other materials used in the lessons, and samples of tests that the teachers used to evaluate students' understanding of the concepts learnt.

2.2.2 *The Shanghai lessons*

Correspondingly, adopting the procedure of videotaping designed by the TIMSS 1999 Video Study, eleven Shanghai lessons from nine different schools were videotaped. Supplementary documents like those in Hong Kong were collected as well. The background of the teachers and the lessons in the two cities is described in Table 1.

Table 1
Background of the Videotaped Lessons in Hong Kong and Shanghai

		Hong Kong	Shanghai
Total number of lessons		8	11
Average duration of lessons		39	43
Average number of students		36	48
Background of schools	High	2	2
	Medium	1	4
	Low	5	5
Background of teachers	Bachelor's degree	62.5%[1]	36%
	Years of teaching	7	10

[1] According to "Education Indicators for the Hong Kong School Education System in 1999 Abridged Report" (Education Department, 2000), the average class size and the average duration of the lessons in Hong Kong were 37.8 students per class and 40 minutes per lesson respectively, and the bachelor's degree ratio was 84.3% (referring to highest degree teachers hold"); while according to "Shanghai Education Yearbook 2002" (Shanghai Municipal Education Commission, 2003), the average class size in Shanghai was 46.6 students, the average duration of lessons was 45 minutes, and the bachelor's degree ratio was about 36%.

2.3 *Data analysis*

2.3.1 *Transcription*

The CDs of the Hong Kong lessons and relevant multimedia database with English transcripts from LessonLab, Inc. of Los Angeles were already available to the researchers. For Shanghai, all videos of the lessons were digitized into CDs. The teachers who delivered the lessons respectively transcribed the CDs verbatim in Chinese and the data analysis mainly depended on the Chinese transcripts and the original CDs. During the process of data analysis, the CDs were referred to from time to time to ensure that the description represented the reality as closely as possible.

2.3.2 *Coding*

The coding focused on the following aspects:

- Approach and dimension of variation
- Classroom interaction

Since the coding of the first aspect is more inductive in nature, it will be illustrated in the relevant Results sections in this chapter and will not be described here.

Regarding classroom interaction, different dichotomies of patterns of interaction were found, for example, traditional approach versus constructivist approaches (Cestari, 1998), funneling versus focusing (Wood, 1994, 1998; Voigt, 1995), and univocal versus dialogic (Wertsch & Toma, 1995). According to Cestari (1998), in the traditional approach, the teacher tends to make more frequent use of statements, encourage students to memorize by imitation and repetition drill, and emphasize the final product and the correctness of students' answers; whereas the teacher using a constructivist approach tends to make use of students' questions and feedback for the subsequent teaching, encourage students to find the solutions by their own efforts, emphasize the process of achieving the solutions, and value student's mistakes as a suitable condition for learning. In the funnel pattern of interaction in Wood's

(1998) classification, students' thinking focuses on trying to figure out the response that the teacher wants instead of thinking mathematically for himself. On the other hand, in the focusing pattern of interaction, students learn as they participate more equally in the dialogue, in which a high level of interaction between teacher and students creates opportunities for the latter to reflect on their own thinking. According to the previous descriptions of different dichotomies on the patterns of interaction, it was found that these dichotomies essentially described a similar scenario: one refers to knowledge transmission, while the other refers to knowledge construction. Hence, in this study, the researchers adopted the vivid metaphor of funneling versus focusing.

3 Results

The findings will be presented in two parts. The first part is concerned with the patterns of space of variation for students to experience Pythagoras' theorem and the second part focuses on the patterns of classroom interaction.

3.1 *Patterns of variation*

After a close look at all the sampled lessons, it was found that the lessons in both cities included the following stages: introduction, justification and practicing (see Huang, 2002, for details). The dimensions of variation created at each stage will be illustrated below.

3.1.1 *Introduction of the theorem*

3.1.1.1 Approaches to discovery

Two main approaches for exploring the theorem were found: discovering the side relationship directly (D1) and discovering the side relationship via the area relationship (D2). Within each approach, some dimensions of variation were created, as shown in Table 2.

Table 2
Ways of Exploring Pythagoras' Theorem

Category of exploration of the theorem		Frequency*	
		Hong Kong (8)	Shanghai (11)
Approach D1	Making conjecture on side relationship through calculating triplets.	2	6
Approach D2	Deducing the side relationship via examining the area relationship through manipulating puzzles	4	1
	Discovering and proving the theorem at the same time via investigating area relationship	1	1

* The sum of frequency of approach of exploration is not equal to the total of the teachers because there are teachers who just told the theorem as a fact to students directly. This direct approach is excluded from this count.

The striking difference between Hong Kong and Shanghai is that the teachers in Hong Kong preferred approach D2 (63%), while the teachers in Shanghai preferred approach D1 (55%). The typical approaches to discovering the theorem in the two cities will be illustrated below.

3.1.1.2 The typical Hong Kong approach

In four lessons, the theorem was explored through playing very similar games as follows:

Given a bag containing five pieces of puzzles and a diagram as shown on the right, students are asked to

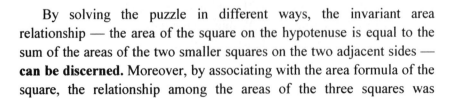

- fit the 5 pieces into square C in the diagram in the shortest time;
- rearrange the above 5 pieces into two smaller squares A and B in the diagram

By solving the puzzle in different ways, the invariant area relationship — the area of the square on the hypotenuse is equal to the sum of the areas of the two smaller squares on the two adjacent sides — **can be discerned.** Moreover, by associating with the area formula of the square, the relationship among the areas of the three squares was transformed into the relationship among the lengths of the three sides of the right-angled triangle, which is Pythagoras' Theorem.

3.1.1.3 The typical Shanghai approach

There were five lessons in which Pythagoras' theorem was explored by investigating special triplets. There were two key steps for making a conjecture on the side relationship among the three sides of a right-angled triangle. One is the creation of the triplets and the other is the use of the triplets. Take lesson SH04 for example. In the lesson, students were asked to draw several right-angled triangles given two adjacent sides and they were asked to measure the hypotenuses:

1. Given that two adjacent sides are 3cm and 4cm respectively, measure the hypotenuse;
2. Given that two adjacent sides are 6cm and 8cm respectively, measure the hypotenuse;
3. Given that two adjacent sides are 5cm and 12cm respectively, measure the hypotenuse.

After completing these activities, the students were asked to give their answers aloud. Then the teacher summarized that in any right-angled triangle, if the two adjacent sides were given, then the hypotenuse could be found. Thus three triplets (3, 4, 5), (6, 8, 10) and (5, 12, 13) were created through the activities.

Essentially, the purpose of examining the side relationship from different triplets is to discover the invariant relationship: the square of the hypotenuse is equal to the sum of the squares of the adjacent sides. However, how the class activities were conducted for discovering this relationship in the lessons was different. In some lessons, students were asked to make conjectures after group discussion and check their conjectures by examining the triplets. In other lessons, teachers demonstrated this special relationship with different triplets and induced the conjectures.

How does the difference in the two typical ways of discovering the theorem contribute to students' learning? This issue will be discussed below.

3.1.1.4 Geometrical representation versus numerical operation

In the typical Hong Kong approach, students can discern and separate the area relationship (the sum of the areas of the squares constructed from the two adjacent sides is equal to the area of the square constructed from the hypotenuse in a right-angled triangle) by manipulating the puzzles differently (different ways of fitting by different groups). By creating this dimension of variation, i.e., different ways of fitting the puzzle, it is possible for students to discover the area relationship. Then through appropriate transformation of the area relationship into the side relationship, it is possible to find out the side relationship, namely, Pythagoras' Theorem. Essentially, what the students experienced differently is the variation in area relationship, which actually is the geometrical representation of the theorem.

In contrast, what Shanghai students experienced differently is the variation in side relationships, which was discovered by investigating different Pythagoras' triplets numerically. Thus, the numerical aspect is the focus in this approach.

So the Hong Kong teachers attempted to explore the theorem from a *geometrical aspect*, while the Shanghai teachers attempted to explore the theorem from a *numerical aspect*. Therefore, it could result in different spaces of variation. For Hong Kong students, the theorem was manifested not only in a mathematical formula but also in a visual geometrical presentation. For Shanghai students, the theorem might not be associated with any geometrical presentation.

3.1.2 *Justification of the theorem*

This part mainly focuses on the way in which Pythagoras' theorem is justified in Hong Kong and Shanghai classrooms. Justification refers to providing reasons why the theorem is true. The validity of a proof does not depend on a formal presentation within a more or less axiomatic-deductive setting, not on the written form, but on the logical coherence of conceptual relationships that are not only to convince others that the theorem is true, but also to explain why it is true (Cooney, Brown, Dossey, Schrage, & Wittmann, 1996; Hanna, 1990, 1998, 2001). "Proof" in this study is grouped into two categories. One is called *mathematical proof*, in which the theorem is proved deductively and logically by using geometrical properties and theories or the operations of algebraic expressions. The other is called *"verification"*, in which the theorem is shown to be true by using certain evidences such as solving a puzzle or demonstrating some cases.

3.1.2.1 Approaches to justification

The approaches to justification can be summarized in Table 3.

Table 3
Distribution of the Ways of Justification

Ways of justification		Frequency*	
		Hong Kong (8)	Shanghai (11)
Visual verification	Playing games	5	0
	Demonstration using diagrams	1	0
Mathematical proof	Single proof	2	3
	Multiple proofs	1	8

* The sum of the ways of justification is not equal to the total of the teachers since there are some teachers who gave different kinds of way of justification.

The most prominent difference between these two cities regarding justification is that the Shanghai teachers paid considerable attention to the introduction of **mathematical proofs.** On the contrary, the Hong Kong teachers seemed to hold different attitudes toward justification. Six out of the eight teachers tended to **verify the theorem** either through exploring activities for discovering the theorem or certain other activities for verifying the theorem once it was found (see Table 3).

3.1.2.2 Verification versus mathematical proof

According to Table 3, the typical way of **justification** in Hong Kong is visual verification (six out of the eight teachers), while the typical way of justification in Shanghai is **mathematical proof** (all the teachers), especially multiple proofs (eight out of the eleven teachers). The following illustrates these two types of justification.

The typical Hong Kong way — verification

If we consider certain exploring activities as verification, it was found that six out of the eight teachers verified the theorem visually (some teachers did not justify the theorem at this stage, but they verified the theorem by exploring the theorem at the previous stage). The typical way of verification was demonstrated in section 3.1.1, which serves as both discovering and verifying.

The typical Shanghai way — mathematical proof

All the Shanghai teachers introduced mathematical proof. In particular, nine of them introduced multiple mathematical proofs. At this stage, three dimensions of variation were identified. Firstly, in the heuristic approach (procedural variation), a special case was investigated as a trial first and then the general situation was investigated. Secondly, a diagram, which was crucial for the introduction of the proof, was either taken with its structure and orientation for granted or justified visually and logically. Thirdly, multiple proofs were introduced. Since these three dimensions are interrelated, some of them appeared simultaneously in some lessons. The following section illustrates how these dimensions of variation are constituted in a lesson (SH09).

3.1.2.3 Procedural variation: from special to general

There were three lessons in which the teacher intentionally organized activities for investigating the cases from **special to general** for students to explore the proof progressively.

In lesson SH09, after students had made conjectures on the side relationship based on group activities, they were asked to prove the conjecture by examining a special case and then exploring the proof in the general situation.

Firstly, the teacher divided the class into groups of four and students were asked to put some congruent **isosceles right-angled triangles** into a square. After that, they were asked to project their diagrams on the screen as shown in Figures 1(1) and 1(2). Based on students' calculations on the areas of the squares in two diagrams, the special relationship: $2a^2 = c^2$, i.e., $a^2 + a^2 = c^2$ was found, where a is the adjacent side and c is the hypotenuse of the isosceles right-angled triangle.

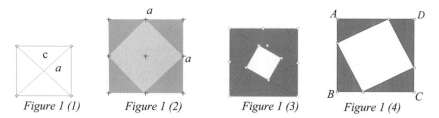

| Figure 1 (1) | Figure 1 (2) | Figure 1 (3) | Figure 1 (4) |

Secondly, the students were asked to play a similar game with **four congruent right-angled triangles**. After finishing this activity in groups, two diagrams were projected on the screen by students (Figure 1(3) and Figure 1 (4)). Students also gave their explanations of the figures.

The teacher constituted two dimensions of variations for students to learn the proofs. One was the heuristic approach: **investigating the cases from special to general.** This approach could not only help students discover the theorem easily but also, more importantly, provide an opportunity for students to experience an important way of mathematical thinking. Another was introducing **multiple proofs.** Two different proofs were discussed. By introducing two different proofs, it was possible for students to separate a strategy, *dissecting area method*, from the two particular proofs, according to the theory of variation.

3.1.2.4 Does the same proof mean the same thing?

To a certain extent, the Hong Kong teachers also paid attention to the introduction of mathematical proof (three out of the eight lessons). In order to understand what really happened when a proof was introduced in mathematical classrooms in Hong Kong and Shanghai, a proof, which was introduced by the teachers in both cities, was examined in detail. In this proof, the students were required to find the area of a square by the method of dissecting area, simplifying the expression, and finally deducing Pythagoras' Theorem. It was found that only two teachers from Hong Kong introduced this proof, while ten out of the eleven Shanghai teachers introduced the same proof. From each city, a lesson (HK4 and SH02) in which the proof was introduced in the same way is discussed in detail below.

The teacher in lesson HK4 introduced the proof by following a semi-structured worksheet as follows:

Consider a square *PQRS* with side $a + b$ and prove Pythagoras' Theorem by finding the area of *PQRS* with two different methods.

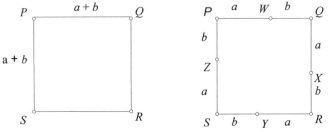

Method 1: Find the area of *PQRS* directly.
Method 2: Hint: Join *WX*, *XY*, *YZ*, and *ZW*. *PQRS* is divided into
          four __ , and, one _____ *WXYZ*.
          Let the hypotenuse of the right-angled triangle *WPZ*
          be *c*, then Area of *PQRS* = _____ .

The Shanghai teacher's approach is as follows:

The students were asked to fit the squares together by using four congruent right-angled triangles. Then, they were asked to calculate the areas of the squares, and think about the proof of the theorem in groups. After that, students were encouraged to verbalize the steps of calculating the area of a square by using different methods, and the teacher wrote the proof on the blackboard:

$S_{\text{large square}} = S_{\text{small squares}} + 4\,S_{\text{triangles}}$

$$(a+b)^2 = c^2 + 4 \times \frac{1}{2}ab$$

Simplifying: $a^2 + b^2 = c^2$

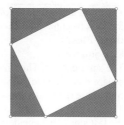

From a mathematical point of view, the two methods of the proof are the same in essence. However, it may make differences in students' learning when the proof is introduced differently. Firstly, the following excerpts, Table 4, demonstrate the kind of classroom interactions when one method of calculating the area of the square was introduced.

Table 4

Excerpts of a Hong Kong Lesson (HK4) and a Shanghai Lesson (SH02)

HK4	SH02
The first method (namely, calculating the area of *PQRS* directly) was discussed. After the students have found that the square *PQRS* was divided into four congruent right-angled triangles (see figure 2(1)), the discussion then moved on to the following episode.	After students created a figure by using four given congruent right-angled triangles, the teacher presented the diagram on a small blackboard (see figure 2(2)). Then the students were asked to calculate the area of the diagrams with different methods, as shown below.
1. T: Congruent. Right. So you may say, *PQRS*, now this time, after you joined the four sides, you will have to divide it into four congruent right-angled triangles. 2. T: So *PQRS* is divided into four congruent right-angled triangles and also, **another figure, *WXYZ*, that's a?** 3. Ss: **Square.** 4. T: Square. So now, this is the second method. The second method in finding about the area of this square with the side *a* plus *b*, so now, **this time, how to find about its area?** 5. T: There are four congruent triangles. [They are] **Right-angled triangles with the side, base is *a*, height is?** 6. Ss: **I.**	1. T: This is what he put. He cut a big square outside and a small square inside. Then put the big one on the small one. Ensure that the vertexes of the small square are on the four sides of the big one. **Would you please prove it?** (Nominating a student) 2. S*: Sorry, I can't.* 3. T: You have put it (together), but you can't prove it? Who can? ***You, please.*** 4. S: (Coming to the front and proving on the blackboard) $S_{\text{large square}} = (a+b)^2$. 5. T: How do you know that this side is *a*? 6. S: Because the two triangles are congruent. 7. T: How to prove they are congruent?

7.	T: b. You know the area *ab* over two for each triangle. **And then four of them. Plus?**		Don't be nervous.
8.	Ss: *c* **square.**	8.	**S: I've forgotten.**
9.	T: *c* square, right. The smaller square that is inside. So you may find, there're two *ab* plus *c* square. Two *ab* plus *c* square. How about the last step? By considering the two different methods in **finding the area of the same square, what do you find?**	9.	T: He's forgotten. Please give him a hand. Go back to your seat, please. Tao Li.
		10.	S: I've forgotten.
		11.	T: You've all forgotten. How to prove? **Liu Wenju, would you please prove it?** Be brave.
10.	T: Method one, you find a square plus two *ab* plus *b* square. How about the second one? Method two you find two *ab* plus *c* square. So what do you find?	12.	S: There's one that is equal. $\angle 1 + \angle 2 = 90°$, $\angle 1 + \angle 3 = 90°$, $\angle 2 = \angle 3$.
		13.	**T: What's the reason?**
		14.	S: (Together) the complementary angles are equal.
11.	T: Oh, both sides there're two *ab*, so you cancel this, and finally **you find a squared plus *b* squared is *c* squared.** Is it?	15.	S: We can get congruence according to ASA.
		16.	T: With the same reason, we can get the four triangles equal. Now continue, please.
		17.	S: $S_{\text{large square}} = (a+b)^2$.

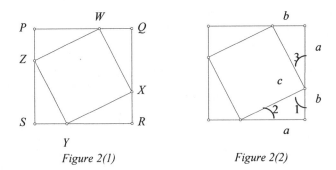

Figure 2(1)   *Figure 2(2)*

Space of variation. There are two critical aspects in this proof as stated in the worksheet. One aspect is to dissect the square into one smaller square and four congruent right-angled triangles. Another aspect is to calculate the area of the square by two different methods and simplify the expression of an area relationship into a side relationship.

Regarding the first aspect, in the Hong Kong lesson, the students got used to following the teacher's instructions and the worksheet seemed to limit students' thinking. Furthermore, the teacher did not provide justification as to why the central figure was a square. However, in the

Shanghai lesson, the students were not only asked to present the diagram, but also to justify the statement on the diagram. In this sense, a dimension of variation for experiencing the diagram was created: **taking for granted and justifying the diagram logically.**

Regarding the second aspect, basically the Hong Kong teacher stated the relevant formulae and simplified the expression on his own. Thus, the students were seldom given a chance to express their own understanding and thinking. On the contrary, the Shanghai teacher always let the students express verbally the formula and the relevant transformation. In this regard, the Shanghai lesson seemed to have created more **space for students to verbalize the process of deductive reasoning.**

3.1.3 *Practicing or applying the theorem*

3.1.3.1 Distribution of problems

According to Gu (1994), problems can be classified according to three basic elements. The initial status (A) is the condition of the problem. The process of solving the problem (B) is the transition of approaching the conclusion based on existing knowledge, experience, and the given conditions. The final stage (C) is the conclusion. A problem is considered as a prototype if it consists of an obvious condition, conclusion and solving process familiar to the students. The prototypes can be transformed by removing one or two of the three components or introducing components which obscure students' perception. Such transformed exercises are called closed and open variation respectively. Furthermore, Gu (1994) simplifies Bloom's taxonomy of teaching objectives (i.e., knowledge, comprehension, application, analysis, synthesis, and evaluation) into three types of objectives based on an experiment with 3,000 students of the same grade in secondary schools. The three types of objectives are memorization (including knowledge and calculation), interpretation (including comprehension and application), and exploration (analysis and synthesis and evaluation). Moreover, it has been found that the three types of teaching objectives can be achieved by providing students with three kinds of problems respectively. Based on the purposes of the problems, they can be classified exhaustively into three different categories: *memorization, interpretation, and exploration.* However, after looking at all the lessons in Hong Kong, it was found that there was no problem at the memorization level, but there were some problems which did not belong to any of the three categories. These were problems which served the purpose of preparing for the learning of Pythagoras' Theorem, such as problems in calculating square roots etc. This kind of problems was entitled *prerequisite* problems in this chapter. The frequencies of the problems used in the sampled lessons in the two cities are shown in Figure 3.

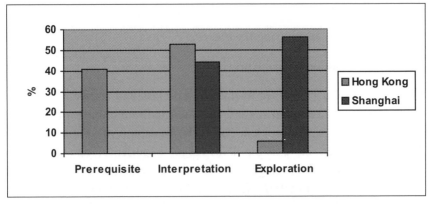

Figure 3. The distribution of problems at different levels

The above figure shows that, in the Hong Kong lessons, more than 40% of the problems are at the prerequisite level, more than half of the problems are at the interpretation level (called "basic level"), and fewer than one tenth of the problems fall into the exploration level. In the Shanghai lessons, there is no problem at the prerequisite level and more than half of the problems are at the exploration level. It seems that the Hong Kong teachers tended to practice at the prerequisite and basic level while the Shanghai teachers prefer to practice at the basic level and higher level.

3.1.3.2 Feature of practicing: Explicit variation versus implicit variation

In this study, the researchers adopted an implicit-explicit distinction to differentiate between the ways of varying problems. If the changes from a prototype problem (in which the learnt knowledge can be applied directly) to its variations are identified visually and concretely (such as variations in numerical values, positions of figures etc., but the conditions for applying the relevant knowledge still are explicit), then this kind of variation is regarded as explicit. On the other hand, if the changes from the original problem to its variations have to be discerned by analysis abstractly and logically (such as variation in parameter, subtle change or omission of certain conditions, or change of contexts, or reckoning on certain strategies etc., thus the conditions or strategies for applying the relevant knowledge are implicit), then this kind of variation is characterized as implicit. This implicit-explicit distinction is illustrated below.

Suppose the students were just taught Pythagoras' theorem and they encountered the application of the theorem for the first time. The following exercises would illustrate the two types of variations.

Explicit variation:

In the following right-angled triangles, the lengths of two sides are given. Find the length of the third side and put the answer in the appropriate brackets.

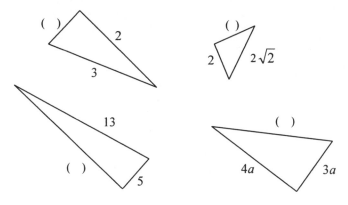

Implicit variation:

(1) In a right-angled triangle, if two of its sides are 3 and 4, find the length of the third side.

(2) An army of soldiers wants to attack a castle, which is separated from them by a river and a wall. The river is 15 m wide and the wall is 20m high.

    a) How can the soldiers reach the top of the wall (if they cannot fly over the wall by any means)?

    b) What is the shortest distance to get to the top of the wall?

It was found that in both cities, exercises of both types of variation were used. However, the Hong Kong teachers tended to use explicit variation in the exercises, while the Shanghai teachers seemed to prefer providing implicit variation in the exercises

3.1.4 *Patterns of teaching*

The patterns of teaching in terms of space of variation constituted in these sampled lessons are shown in the following diagram.

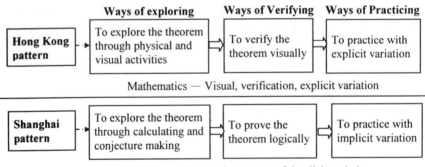

Figure 4. Two approaches to handling Pythagoras' Theorem

A model of the Hong Kong lesson consists of the following stages:

- Deducing the side relationship via investigating the area relationship by solving puzzles (physical, geometrical, visual);
- Justifying the findings by different methods (mathematical proof or visual verification);
- Assigning class work with explicit variation (varying in numerical values and orientations).

It seems that in the Hong Kong lessons, the nature of mathematics is perceived as intuitive and subject to verification and it can be mastered by drilling exercise with explicit variation.

On the other hand, a model of the Shanghai lesson includes the following stages:

- Making a conjecture on the relationship among the three sides of right-angled triangles by investigating special Pythagoras number triplets (numerical manipulation);
- Proving the conjecture mathematically (integration of geometry and algebra);
- Providing well-structured exercises with implicit variation (broad coverage and internal connections).

It seems that in the Shanghai lessons, the nature of mathematics is perceived as abstract and logical and mathematics can be mastered by drilling exercise with implicit variation.

3.2 *Pattern of classroom interaction*

When looking at the way of constituting the space of variation, the pattern of classroom interaction can be classified into two types: focusing pattern and funnel pattern. From the lessons observed in this study, it is found that the former pattern was more prevalent in Hong Kong than in Shanghai. Using the two lessons (HK4 and SH02) in section 3.1.2 as examples, we can see that in the Hong Kong lesson, the teacher attempted to funnel students towards the teacher's expected answer by asking a series of simple and convergent leading questions (2,

5, 7 of Table 4). Even though the teacher posed one open-ended question (4), in the end, it was broken down into several convergent questions (5, 7). Meanwhile, the teacher gave clear explanations (9-11) when answering the questions he had raised. Based on the above analysis, the pattern of interaction in that Hong Kong classroom should be characterized as a **funnel pattern** as defined by Wood (1998).

In the Shanghai lesson (SH02), through a series of soliciting questions which were mainly open-ended (1, 13), the teacher encouraged students to focus on the critical aspects and express their own explanations. Even though some students encountered difficulties in answering the questions, the teacher would ask another student for an answer until a desired answer (3, 8, 11) was given. Thus, the pattern of interaction in that lesson can be characterized as the "**focusing pattern of interaction**" (Wood, 1998).

Using this same method of analysis, the sample in Hong Kong all seemed to adopt the "funnel pattern" of interaction while the sample in Shanghai attempted to adopt different approaches of classroom interaction. Four out of the eleven teachers in Shanghai tried to employ the "focusing pattern" in which students were encouraged to construct their own knowledge through well-designed activities and open-ended questions.

On the whole, although the teachers in both cities emphasized their roles in organizing classroom activities and encouraging students to engage in the process of learning, the Shanghai teachers seemed to pay more attention to students' explanation than the Hong Kong teachers did.

4 Findings and Discussion

4.1 *Summary of the findings*

The ways of teaching Pythagoras' Theorem in Hong Kong and Shanghai portrayed in the previous sections show some similarities and differences. The main similarities are (1) **Emphasizing the exploration of the topic**, (2) **Emphasizing exercises with variation**, (3) **Teacher dominance and student active engagement in the mathematics classroom**. Meanwhile, some differences were observed: (1) **Numerical**

operation versus physical manipulation. In the activities for exploring the theorem, the teachers in Shanghai tended to encourage students to make a conjecture based on numerical operations, while the teachers in Hong Kong preferred to help students discover the theorem based on manipulative operations. (2) **Proof versus verification.** Either in the activity for exploring and proving the theorem or in applying the theorem, the teachers in Shanghai tended to use abstract or symbolic presentation, while the teachers in Hong Kong tended to employ visual and concrete presentation. Furthermore, the teachers in Shanghai preferred to prove the theorem mathematically, while the teachers in Hong Kong tended to verify the theorem visually.

4.2 *Interpretation of the findings*

It has been argued that *conformity* is the essence of the Chinese culture which has enabled the Chinese people to grow and prosper for thousands of years (Abraham, 1989; Chang, 1957). By citing the Chinese dictum "without rule and compasses, no square or circle could be drawn", Y. Zheng (2002) argued that although conformity has the implication of rule abiding, it is in fact a prerequisite to implement various innovations and it may have a fundamental influence on the Chinese pedagogy of mathematics, particularly in Mainland China. From this point of view, it is understandable why a unified curriculum is advocated and public examination is so long-standing in China. Even nowadays, Shanghai and Hong Kong still have their respective uniform syllabuses and examination systems. When looking at the classroom practice in detail, some similarities observed might be traced to a common cultural tradition. On the other hand, the differences observed may be attributed to the history of Hong Kong, as it was a British colony for more than one and a half centuries. The main findings will be interpreted as follows:

4.2.1 *Emphasizing exploring*

The finding that the teachers in both cities emphasized the exploration of the theorem seems to be contradictory to many of the observations in other studies. For example, Chinese classroom learning is described as rote learning or passive learning (Biggs & Watkins, 1996; Morris et al., 1996), and teaching strategy in Mainland China is characterized as "refined lecture and extensive exercise" before the 1980s (Zhang, S. Li, & J. Li, 2003). But in this study, the students made their own findings based on certain activities.

This might have resulted from the efforts in the reform of classroom teaching in the past decades. For example, in Hong Kong, under the influence of the New Math movement in the 1970s, the activity approach to teaching has been advocated and many activities designed by the authorities and the teachers are available (Wong, 1993). In Shanghai, the new geometry textbook was divided into three stages. At the first stage (grades 1-6), the stage of "visual geometry", the main purpose is to recognize different geometric figures and simple properties and calculation. The second stage (grades 6 –7), the stage of "experimental geometry", aims to develop proper arguments based on transformation and experiment dealing with reasoning implicitly. The third stage (grades 8-9), the stage of "deductive geometry", introduces deductive proof (Cheng, 2000). The textbook developed according to this design has been in use since 1990. Since the teaching in both cities is textbook-oriented (Biggs & Watkins, 1996), the observed emphasis on activities (or experiment) may be due to these recent changes.

Another reason may be due to the specificity of the topic. For this topic, certain exploratory activities were presented in the textbooks in Hong Kong and Shanghai. Also there were some reference materials which provided various activities such as playing games and fitting figures. Thus, it is easy to design exploring activities if the teachers emphasize this kind of activities.

4.2.2 *Emphasizing practice*

The stereotype of teaching in China has been that it emphasizes repetitive drills. However, this study suggests that the teachers in the two cities emphasize practicing with varying problems. It might be interpreted from the following aspects.

First, in ancient China, the general meaning of "learning" (学) or "knowing" (知) accounted for learning (学 习) while "practice" (drill/exercise) (习) meant acquisition by practicing. According to Xu Shen (许慎, 1981), "to learn means to be awaken from ignorance " (学, 觉悟也); and "to practice means repeated trial flights by the young bird" (习, 数飞也). Thus, practicing is a necessary part of learning. As Confucius (1956) said, "Is it not a pleasure, having learned something, to try it out at due intervals?" (学而时习之, 不亦说乎?) (*Analects,* I. 1). A widely accepted axiom, "practice makes perfect" (熟能生巧), may also reflect this philosophy of learning in China.

Secondly, the long history of an examination culture in China may aggravate the importance of practice in learning and affect the mathematics teaching to a certain extent (P. Y. Lee, Zhang, & Z. Zheng, 1997). In Hong Kong and Shanghai, individual examination syllabuses exist. The public examination, which must be subject to the same examination syllabus, has been conducted year after year. But the test paper must avoid overlapping in terms of the test items. Therefore, the problems in the test paper always varied with different contexts or forms in the same mathematical content. In order to help students achieve high performance in those examinations, teachers have to try their best to provide different kinds of problems in certain contents extensively so that students are able to tackle various problems confined to certain domains without feeling strange. This belief is echoed by the Chinese saying "remaining essentially the same despite all apparent changes" (万变不离其宗). That is to say, it will enable students to solve the problems with the same content regardless of the contexts in which the problems are embedded if the students master the knowledge and skills by practicing with extensive variation of exercises focusing on the same content. This may be the reason why the teachers in both cities pay so much attention to exercise with variation.

Thirdly, with regard to varying the problems, it seems that the teachers in Shanghai attempt to vary the problems implicitly, while the teachers in Hong Kong prefer to vary the problems visually and explicitly. This difference may reflect the difference in teachers' beliefs in teaching mathematics. Western teachers believe that learning can be made meaningful if the teaching is connected to concrete models, while Mainland Chinese teachers believe that abstract representation can develop students' critical thinking and logical reasoning ability (An,

Kulm, & Wu, 2002; Becker, Sawada, & Shimizu, 1999; Cai, 2002). It may be reasonable to assume that the teachers in Hong Kong tend to accept the Western beliefs in this aspect. In this sense, it is understandable why the teachers in Hong Kong employed an explicit variation of problems, in which the numbers and orientations of diagrams were varied.

4.2.3 *Teacher dominance and student active engagement in the mathematics classroom*

When looking at the classroom interaction, an apparently contradictory scene appears in the mathematics classroom in both cities. On the one hand, the teachers organized the lesson and controlled the transaction of classroom activities, so that lessons proceeded smoothly. On the other hand, the students engaged themselves in the process of learning by well-designed activities and a series of leading or open-ended questionings.

Teachers dominating teaching in Chinese classrooms was well documented by many previous studies, and was often associated with teacher-centeredness and passive student learning from the perspectives of Western researchers (Biggs & Watkins, 1996; Morris et al., 1996; Paine, 1990). Nevertheless, recent studies have shown that teacher-controlled teaching might not necessarily result in teacher-centered and student passive learning. Rather, there were many elements of student-centeredness in Chinese classrooms (Mok & Morris, 2001; Cortazzi, 1998; Cortazzi & Jin, 2001). According to the Western theories, teachers dominating the teaching would impede students' motivation to learn and produce low achievement. The question is: How can teacher dominance and student-centeredness coexist and work well in the Chinese mathematics classrooms? It may be due to some unique cultural values or beliefs in China. The following discussion tries to interpret this feature in the Chinese mathematics classrooms.

First, as argued by Stigler and Heibert (1999), the reason why there were disruptions in the US classrooms which were seldom found in Japanese lessons might be due to different beliefs about the classroom. The Japanese believe that the classroom is wholly for student learning without being disrupted by others, but the Americans might not hold similar beliefs. It was often found that there were less discipline problems and disruptions in Chinese classrooms than in the counterparts in the West (Leung, 1995; Stevenson & Stigler, 1992). It may be because Chinese and Japanese were influenced by the Confucian tradition so that they share a similar belief about the classroom. This assumption can be echoed by the Chinese aphorism "Rearing without education is the fault of the father, teaching without strictness is the negligence of the teacher" (子不教父之过,教不严师之惰). It means that the teacher should take the responsibility to teach students strictly when they come to school or the classroom.

Secondly, it may reflect the evolution of the mathematics classroom in China. In the past two decades, especially in Shanghai, authorities and educators have paid much attention to improving classroom teaching by learning from Western theories and practices, which emphasized more student-centered learning. It is very important to note that in the Chinese setting, while learning from the West, the essence of its own tradition has still remained. As argued by Y. Zheng (2002), the evolution of modern education in China "is primarily a process of assimilation. That is to say, rather than being alienated by foreign factors, the foreign values were absorbed and assimilated into the Chinese culture". This notion was supported by the famous slogan of the self-strengthening movement in the early twentieth Century, "Chinese learning for basic principle, Western learning for practical use" (Y. Zheng, 1999, p.195). Moreover, Y. Zheng (2002) argued that there is "a basic feature of Chinese mathematics education". Instead of going to the extremes, Chinese mathematics educators prefer to strike a balance between various extremes in education, which is the central idea of *zhong yong* (中庸之道) in the sprit of the Chinese culture (Chang, 1957).

Thus, it can be argued that through assimilation of student-centered teaching strategies into the traditional teacher-centered strategies, a unique teaching strategy consisting of both teacher's control and students' engagement in the learning process emerges in the Chinese classrooms.

Thirdly, how can the teacher and the students work effectively in the classroom? It may be that the teacher and the students share certain norms about the teacher's roles and the students' responsibilities. In particular, Cortazzi and Jin (2001) offered an explanation of the uniqueness of the Chinese classrooms from a learning perspective by adopting the two concepts of "listening-oriented learning" and "learner-trained learning". "Learner-trained learning" means that students know the procedures and react promptly to teachers' cues so that the teachers can switch activities smoothly and without disruption. By "listening-oriented learning", it means that when students listen to the teacher's lectures and other students' discussions with question and challenge actively in their mind, they are learning from the teacher and their fellow students in their heads.

Finally, it may be that the dichotomy between student-centeredness and teacher-centeredness was originally too artificial to capture the subtle characteristics in the classroom. Particularly in China, whole-class teaching is still a dominating method of organizing the lesson, and group discussion seldom occurs. It is easy to characterize the teaching strategy to be teacher-centered based on superficial features such as the teacher's expository teaching and students' attentive listening. However, as demonstrated in this study and a number of other studies (Cortizzi & Jin, 2001; Mok & Ko, 2000), elements of student-centeredness often appear in the Chinese mathematics classroom. Thus, the researchers tend to challenge the validity of the dichotomy of student-centered and teacher-centered teaching as a way of describing teaching strategy, at least when it is used for the Chinese mathematics classroom.

4.2.4 *Abstract presentation and proof versus concrete presentation and verification*

It was found that the teachers in Hong Kong emphasized visual and concrete representation for exploring and practicing while the teachers in Shanghai preferred to use abstract representation. Correspondingly, the Hong Kong teachers emphasized visual verification of the theorem, while the Shanghai teachers emphasized mathematical proof. What are the possible explanations?

Firstly, it is argued that although the culture of Confucianism seemingly did not emphasize logical inference and deductive justification, the method of thinking is convergent, closed, and deductive in essence. Thus, mathematics is not emphasized in the Confucian culture, but Confucianism does not refuse and deny mathematics. In contrast, "the culture of evidential investigation" (考据文化) in the Ming and Qing Dynasty (1644-1911), which emphasized evidence and logical reasoning , gives logical reasoning legitimacy in mathematics. For example, "investigating for evidence" usually depends on "reduction to absurdity" (反证法), which enhances the development of "evidence and deduction" in mathematics education (Zhang, S. Li, & J. Li, 2003). Zhang (2002) argued that this might be a reasonable explanation for why Euclidean geometry (adapted from the *Elements*) has historically been valued so much in secondary schools in China although it was adopted from the West.

Secondly, even in the current mathematics curriculum in Shanghai, the emphasis is put on abstract presentation and logical deductive thinking. It is to be an expected phenomenon that when teaching geometry, particularly when teaching Pythagoras' Theorem, geometric proof is stressed since it is believed that geometric proof is a good way to develop students' logical reasoning ability. In the official textbook, two different proofs of Pythagoras' Theorem are introduced. Moreover, the teachers clearly manifested their emphasis on the proof in both the intended lesson plan and the implemented classroom practice.

Thirdly, in the textbooks used in Hong Kong, some visual exploring activities are presented and one proof is introduced as well. However, the teachers in Hong Kong seemed to pay more attention to verifying the theorem through exploring activities than proving the theorem explicitly.

4.3 *The paradox revisited*

As described above, the paradox is how East Asian classrooms can produce high achieving students in mathematics in a learning environment which is perceived to be unfavorable to students' learning. Based on the findings in this study, the following is a discussion of the paradox.

4.3.1 *Good teaching*

This study finds the following characteristics of mathematics classrooms in Hong Kong and Shanghai:

- The teachers emphasized exploring and constructing knowledge;
- The teachers provided exercises with variation;
- The teachers helped students engage in the process of learning.

Although the class size of the lessons investigated in this study was large (more than 40 students) and the teachers controlled the classroom activities, it is difficult to associate the above characteristics of mathematics classrooms with rote learning and passive learning. Some other studies also seemed to support these findings of this study (Mok & Ko, 2000; Stevenson & Stigler, 1992). For example, Stevenson and Stigler (1992) found that:

> The techniques used by Chinese and Japanese teachers are not new to the teaching profession nor are they foreign or exotic. In fact, they are ones often recommended by American educators. What the Chinese and Japanese examples demonstrated so compellingly is that when widely and consistently implemented, such practice can produce extraordinary outcomes (p. 198).

So it may be that the paradox itself is dubious.

4.3.2 *Misperceptions of Chinese teaching*

Biggs and Watkins (2001) further supported the observation here by pointing out that "any paradox would exist only if Chinese learners had been badly taught, and as far as the teaching we have visited in Mainland China and some Hong Kong classrooms is concerned, that is simply not true" (p. 290).They explained that the reason for the paradox was due to Western researchers' misperceptions caused by their theoretical considerations and perspectives. Different levels of observations were suggested in order to understand why the paradox was posed. If we look superficial characteristics of the classroom such as large class sizes, teacher led teaching, authoritarian teacher and poor resources, teaching in China would likely be conceived as poor teaching in the Western frame of reference. However, if we look at how teachers encourage students to engage in appropriate learning activities, it would be concluded that the teaching is more student-centered and there is a continuing desire to engage students more effectively. This is achieved through a collective and reflective practice, which might be "evolved and cohered to form a powerful script" (p. 290).

4.3.3 *Intra-cultural differences*

This study also shows some differences between Hong Kong and Shanghai in terms of the ways of handling Pythagoras' Theorem. For example, the Hong Kong teachers preferred to verify the theorem visually and vary problems explicitly, while the Shanghai teachers preferred to prove the theorem logically and vary problems implicitly. As discussed above, this may be due to some intra-cultural differences.

Some substantial differences in terms of the classroom interaction and in-service teacher education were pointed out by Biggs and Watkins (2001). Moreover, Mok and Morris (2001) mentioned that one should be cautious in using the term "an 'Asian' or 'Confucian' model of teaching". Thus, when comparing mathematics teaching between Hong Kong and Mainland China, the historical and political contexts should be taken into consideration in order to have a more thorough understanding of their differences.

5 Concluding Remarks

Starting from an interest to understand the paradox in Chinese mathematics classrooms (that the seemingly un-conducive learning environment in China produces unexpectedly high achievement in mathematics), the researchers have carried out this study, but an unexpected conclusion emerged from this study. The "paradox" does not exist because good teaching actually takes place in the Chinese mathematics classrooms. It is also interesting that there are some critical similarities found from a content free perspective while there are certain striking differences found from a content specific perspective. The most impressive findings are the students' active involvement in tackling mathematics contents and solving mathematics problems under teachers' skillful guidance in a large class, which is not easy for Westerners to understand according to the very different philosophies and theories. Is this phenomenon of teacher control with students' active engagement in the process of learning mathematics in the Chinese classrooms due to certain particular philosophy or cultural value in China? The answer to this question may provide an important clue to uncover the mystery of the teaching and learning of mathematics in China.

References

Abraham, W. R. (1989). *The role of Confucian and Jewish educational values in the assimilation of the Chinese Jews of Kaifeng, supplemented by Western observer accounts, 1605-1985.* Doctoral dissertation, Columbia University Teachers College. (UMI No. AAT 8913096)

An, S., Kulm, G., & Wu, Z. (2002). The impact of cultural difference on middle school mathematics teachers' beliefs in the U.S. and China. In K. D. Graf, F. K. S. Leung, & F. Lopez-Real (Eds.), *Mathematics education in different cultural traditions: A comparative study of East Asian and the West* (pp. 105-114). Hong Kong: Faculty of Education, The University of Hong Kong.

Ausubel, D. P. (1968). *Educational psychology: A cognitive view.* New York: Holt, Rinehart & Winston.

Becker, J. P., Sawada, T., & Shimizu, Y. (1999). Some findings of the U.S.-Japan cross-cultural research on students' problem-solving behaviors. In G. Kaiser, E. Luna, & I. Huntley (Eds.), *International comparisons in mathematics education* (pp. 121-139). London: Falmer.

Biggs, J. B., & Watkins, D. A. (1996). The Chinese learner in retrospect. In D. A. Watkins & J. B. Biggs (Eds.), *The Chinese learner: Cultural, psychological, and contextual influences* (pp. 269-285). Hong Kong: Comparative Education Research

Centre, The University of Hong Kong; Melbourne, Australia: Australian Council for Education Research.

Biggs, J. B., & Watkins, D. A. (2001). Insight into teaching the Chinese learner. In D. A. Watkins & J.B. Biggs (Eds.), *Teaching the Chinese learner: Psychological and pedagogical perspectives* (pp. 277-300). Hong Kong: Comparative Education Research Centre, The University of Hong Kong; Melbourne, Australia: Australian Council for Education Research.

Bowden, J., & Marton, F. (1998). *The university of learning*. London: Hogan Page.

Cai, J. (2002, April). *The development of U.S. and Chinese student's generalized and generative thinking in mathematics*. Paper posted at American Education Research Association Annual Meeting, New Orleans, LA.

Cestari, M. L. (1998). Teacher-student communication in traditional and constructivist approaches to teaching. In H. Steinbring, M. G. B. Bussi, & A. Sierpinska (Eds.), *Language and communication in mathematics classroom* (pp. 155-166). Reston, VA: National Council of Teachers of Mathematics.

Chang, C. (1957).*The essence of Chinese culture*. Taiwan, China: The China News Press.

Cheng, C. (2000). *A comparison and study on mathematics education* [In Chinese 数学教育比较与研究]. Shanghai: East China Normal University Press.

Confucius. (1956). Confucian Analects. (E. Pound Trans. and Introduced). London: Owen.

Cooney, T. J., Brown, S. I., Dossey, J. A. Schrage, G., & Wittmann, E. C. (1996). *Mathematics, pedagogy, and secondary teacher education*. Portsmouth, NH: Heinemann.

Cortazzi, M. (1998). Learning from Asian lessons: Cultural experience and classroom talk. *Education 3 to 13, 26*(2), 42-49.

Cortazzi, M., & Jin, L. (2001). Large class in China: "Good" teachers and interaction. In D. A. Watkins & J. B. Biggs (Eds), *Teaching the Chinese learner: Psychological and pedagogical perspectives* (pp. 115-134). Hong Kong: Comparative Education Research Centre, The University of Hong Kong; Melbourne, Australia: Australian Council for Education Research.

Dienes, Z. P. (1973). A theory of mathematics learning. In F. J. Crosswhite, J. L. Highins, A. R. Osborne, & R. J. Shunway (Eds.), *Teaching mathematics: Psychological foundation* (pp.137-148). Ohio: Charles A. Jones Publishing Company.

Education Department. (2000). Education Indicators for the Hong Kong School Education System in 1999 Abridged Report. Hong Kong: Education Department.

Gu, L. (1994). *Theory of teaching experiment –The methodology and teaching principle of Qinpu* [In Chinese 青浦实验的方法与教学研究原理]. Beijing: Educational Science Press.

Hanna, G. (1990). Some pedagogical aspects of proof. *Interchange, 21*(1), 6-13.

Hanna, G. (1998). Proof as explanation in geometry. *Focus on Learning Problems in Mathematics, 20* (2 & 3), 4-13.

Hanna, G. (2001). Proof, explanation and exploration: An overview. *Educational Studies in Mathematics, 44*(1-2), 5-23.

Huang, R. (2002). *Teaching mathematics in Hong Kong and Shanghai: A classroom analysis from the perspective of variation*. Unpublished doctoral dissertation, The University of Hong Kong, Hong Kong.

Lapointe A. E., Mead, N. A., & Askew, J. M. (1992). *Learning mathematics.* Prinerton, NJ: Educational Testing Service.

Lee, P. Y., Zhang, D., & Zheng, Z. (1997). Examination culture and the teaching of mathematics [In Chinese 考试文化与数学教学]. *EduMath, 4,* 96-103.

Lee, W. O. (1996). The cultural context for Chinese learners: Conceptions of learning in the Confucian tradition. In D. A. Watkins & J. G. Biggs (Eds.), *The Chinese learner: Cultural, psychological, and contextual influences* (pp. 25-42*)*. Hong Kong: Comparative Education Research Centre, The University of Hong Kong; Melbourne, Australia: Australian Council for Education Research.

Leung, F. K. S. (1995). The Mathematics classroom in Beijing, Hong Kong and London. *Educational Studies in Mathematics, 29,* 197-325.

Leung, F. K. S. (1998). The implications of Confucianism for education today. *Journal of Thought, 33,* 25-36.

Leung, F. K. S. (2001). In search of an East Asian identity in mathematics education. *Educational Studies in Mathematics, 47,* 35-51.

Ma, L. (1999). *Knowing and teaching elementary mathematics: Teachers' understanding of fundamental mathematics in China and the United States.* Mahwah, NJ: Lawrence Erlbaum Associates.

Marton, F., & Booth, S. (1997). *Learning and awareness.* Mahwah, NJ: Lawrence Erlbaum Associates.

Marton, F., Dall'Alba, G. & Lai, K. T. (1993). *The paradox of the Chinese learner.* (Occasional Paper 93.1). Melbourne, Australia: Educational Research and Development Unit, Royal Melbourne Institute of Technology.

Mok, I. A. C., & Ko, P. Y. (2000). Beyond labels – Teacher-centered and pupil-centered activities. In B. Adamson, T. Kwan, & K. K. Chan (Eds.), *Changing the curriculum: The impact of reform on primary schooling in Hong Kong* (pp. 175-194). Hong Kong: Hong Kong University Press.

Mok, I. A. C., & Morris, P. (2001). The metamorphosis of the "virtuoso": Pedagogic patterns in Hong Kong primary mathematics classroom. *Teaching and Teacher Education, 17,* 455-468.

Morris, P., Adamson, R., Au, M. L., Chan, K. K., Chang, W. Y., & Ko, P. K. (1996). *Target oriented curriculum evaluation project (interim report).* Hong Kong: INSTEP, Faculty of Education, The University of Hong Kong.

Paine, L. W. (1990).The teacher as virtuoso: A Chinese model for teaching. *Teachers College Record, 92* (1), 49-81.

Shanghai Municipal Education Commission. (2003). Shanghai Education Yearbook 2002. Shanghai: Shanghai Educational Publishing House.

Sfard, A. (1991). On the dual nature of mathematics conception: Reflections on processes and objects as different sides of the same coin. *Educational Studies in Mathematics, 22*(1), 1-36.

Stevenson, H. W., Chen, C., & Lee, S. Y. (1993). Mathematics achievement of Chinese, Japanese, and American children: Ten years later. *Science, 25*(9), 53-59.

Stevenson, H. W., & Stigler, J. W. (1992). *The learning gap: Why our schools are failing and what we can learn from Japanese and Chinese education.* New York: Summit Books.

Stigler, J. W., & Hiebert, J. (1999). *The teaching gap: The best ideas from world's teachers for improving education in classroom.* New York: The Free Press.

Voigt, J. (1995). Thematic patterns of interaction and sociomathematical norms. In P. Cobb & H. Bauersfeld (Eds.), *The emergence of mathematical meaning: Interaction in classroom culture* (pp. 163-201). Hillsdale, NJ: Erbaum.

Vygotsky, L. S. (1978). *Mind in society*. Cambridge, MA: Harvard University Press.

Watkins, D. A., & Biggs, J. B. (1996). *The Chinese learner: Cultural, psychological and contextual influences*. Hong Kong: Comparative Education Research Centre, The University of Hong Kong; Melbourne, Australia: Australian Council for Education Research.

Wertsch, J. V., & Toma, C. (1995). Discourse and learning in the classroom: A sociocultural approach. In L. P. Steffe & J. Gale (Eds.), *Constructivism in education* (pp. 159-174). Hillsdale, NJ: Lawrence Erlbaum.

Wong, N. Y. (1993). Mathematics education in Hong Kong: Development in the last decade. In G. Bell (Ed.), *Asian perspective on mathematics education* (pp. 56-69). Lismor, NSW: The Northern Rivers Mathematics Association.

Wong, N. Y. (1998). In search of the "CHC" Learner: Smarter, works harder and something more. In H. S. Park, Y. H. Choe, H. Shin, & S. H. Kim (Eds.), *Proceedings of the ICMI-East Asia Regional Conference on Mathematical Education* (Vol. 1, pp. 85-98). Korea: Korea Society of Mathematics Education.

Wood, T. (1994). Patterns of interaction and the culture of mathematics classroom. In S. Lerman (Ed.), *Cultural perspective on the mathematics classroom* (pp. 149-168). Dordrecht, The Netherlands: Kluwer Academic Publishers.

Wood, T. (1998). Alternative patterns of communication in mathematics classes: Funneling or focusing? In H. Steinbring, M. G. B. Bussi, & A. Sierpinska (Eds.), *Language and communication in mathematics classroom* (pp. 167-178). Reston, VA: National Council of Teachers of Mathematics.

Xu, S. (1981). *Etymology* [In Chinese 说文解字] (Y. Duan commented). Shanghai: Shanghai ancient book press.

Zhang, D. (2002). The culture of evidential investigation [In Chinese 考据文化]. *Science* [In Chinese 科学], *4*.

Zhang, D., Li, S., & Li, J. (2003). *An introduction to mathematics education* [In Chinese 数学教育导论]. Beijing: Higher Education press.

Zheng, Y. (1999). The status of Confucianism in modern Chinese education, 1901-1949: A curricular study. In G. Peterson, R. Hayhoe, & Y. Lu (Eds.), *Education, culture, and identity in twentieth-century China* (pp. 193-216). Hong Kong: Hong Kong University Press.

Zheng, Y. (2002). Mathematics education in China: From a cultural perspective. In K. D. Graf, F. K. S. Leung, & F. Lopez-Real (Eds.), *Mathematics education in different cultural traditions: A comparative study of East Asian and the West* (pp. 268-278). Hong Kong: Faculty of Education, The University of Hong Kong.

Chapter 14

Identifying a Pattern of Teaching:
An Analysis of a Shanghai Teacher's Lessons

LOPEZ-REAL Francis   MOK Ah Chee Ida

LEUNG Koon Shing Frederick   MARTON Ference

Does a national script exist? We have reservations about an affirmative answer to this question for two major reasons. First, it is dangerous to attempt to identify a teacher's "script" from a selection of "snapshot" lessons. Second, such a characterization may suggest implicitly that a teacher's approach is almost invariable from lesson to lesson. Our detailed analysis of a sequence of lessons by a teacher in Shanghai has shown that variation between lessons certainly does occur but, despite such variation, we can identify a "pattern" of teaching over time that characterizes a teacher's approach. We define a "pattern of teaching" to mean: *The identifiable features of a teacher's classroom practice, occurring in a repeated manner over a period of time, that together constitute the characteristics of the teacher's style.*

Key words: mathematics teaching, mathematics classroom practice, comparative studies

1 Introduction

The publication of the results of the Third International Mathematics and Science Study (TIMSS) in 1996 and of its follow up study (TIMSS-R) in 2000 has attracted much attention from the public as well as the education sectors worldwide (Law, 1996, 1997; Mullis et al., 2000). In these studies, students in Asian countries outperformed their counterparts in the West in mathematics. In recent years, the phenomenon referred to as "the Asian learner paradox" has been discussed by a number of authors (see, for example, Watkins & Biggs, 1996, 2001). Stated briefly, this is the apparent contradiction between the teaching methods/environment in Asian schools (i.e., large classes, whole class teaching, examination driven teaching, content rather than process oriented, emphasis on memorization, etc.) and the fact that Asian students have regularly performed better than their Western counterparts in comparative studies. The paradox lies in the fact that the above characterization of Asian teaching describes features that much research shows is not conducive to effective mathematics learning.

Following the TIMSS study, national norms for teaching practice were identified through the analysis of a statistically representative sample of videotaped eighth-grade mathematics classes in Japan, Germany and the United States and reported in the book "The Teaching Gap" (Stigler & Hiebert, 1999). The main thesis of this book is the claim that culturally-specific teacher "scripts" were identified by which the practices of teachers in the US, Japan, and Germany might be differentiated and studied. This is a powerful image, but does a national teaching script really exist? The first thing to note is that the Japanese lessons described in the video study certainly do not "fit" the Asian stereotype. In addition, our own experience of teachers in Hong Kong, and elsewhere in Asia suggests that the Japanese "image" as portrayed in "The Teaching Gap" is not at all typical. Our own impression of the popular pedagogy in Hong Kong is closer to the German model reported in "The Teaching Gap" where concepts are carefully explained but the "transmission" mode is still dominant (Lopez-Real & Mok, 2002).

Some disquiet has been expressed by a number of researchers about the methodology used in the TIMSS Video Study, particularly concerning the taping of just one lesson per teacher. With the hypothesis that the actions and associated attitudes, beliefs, and knowledge of students constitute a culturally-specific coherent body of learner practices, the Learner's Perspective Study (LPS), a new international project led by David Clarke at the University of Melbourne, is underway. The LPS project has confirmed a number of international partners to collect data at their own expense, namely, Australia, Germany, Japan, the US, South Africa, Sweden, Philippines, Israel, and China (Hong Kong and Shanghai). An important feature of the project is its documentation of the teaching of sequences of lessons rather than single lessons like the

TIMSS Video Study. Each class was recorded for a minimum of ten consecutive lessons. The documentation enables analysis to capture chains of association within a single lesson as well as across several lessons. Another important feature of the methodology is the attempt to record the lessons from multiple perspectives. Essential features of the recording are (i) the on-site mixing of the images from two video cameras to provide a split-screen record of both teacher and student actions and (ii) the use of the technique of video-stimulated recall in interviews conducted immediately after the lesson to obtain participants' reconstructions of the lesson and the meanings which particular events held for them personally. Two students were interviewed after each lesson. Each teacher participated in three video-stimulated interviews and completed two substantial questionnaires before and after videotaping, as well as a shorter questionnaire after each videotaped lesson. This design enables us to take both the teacher's and learners' perspectives into consideration in the post-lesson construal of the classroom practices (Clarke, 2002).

The Hong Kong team is responsible for collecting both the Hong Kong and Shanghai data and what is discussed in this chapter is taken from the Shanghai data. The three lessons discussed in detail were consecutive lessons taught by the same teacher. The teacher had more than 20 years of teaching experience, graduated in 1982, and was designated as a "First Class Teacher in Secondary School" (中学一级教师) by the Shanghai Academic Title Appraisal Committee (上海市职称评定委员会) in 1992. In this chapter, we focus on the teacher's perceptions. Drawn from the interview data, we compare this to the transcript and video data of the three lessons and finally we try to describe the teacher's pedagogical approach in terms of his "pattern" of teaching.

2 The Teacher's Perceptions

2.1 *General comments on teaching*

Three interviews were conducted with the teacher and these interviews were structured around viewing a taped lesson as described above.

However, apart from making specific comments on those parts of the lesson that the teacher considered important, he also frequently made more general comments about his own teaching style and the mathematical pedagogy advocated by his school. For example, at one point he claims:

"You (the interviewer) can see clearly that I have certain characteristics or a certain personal style. Basically I would set the situational questions and then allow the students to try solving them. They would learn the knowledge in the process. Basically this is the format, so I think it is very helpful in improving the ability of the students."

The mention of "situational" questions is further elaborated in another section of the interview where the teacher is explaining the school's position with regard to teaching mathematics:

"The first requirement is to create situational questions. So most of our lessons adopt this method, for it can stimulate the students into becoming more self-motivated, it can cultivate their interest to be more active to learn. The second requirement is that it can also build the foundation for future activities."

These dual features of situational questions, or problems, and the laying of foundations are often referred to by the teacher during his interviews. We shall discuss these two aspects in more detail later. In another section he very specifically refers to the theoretical basis for his and the school's approach. Here he tries to explain how he has tried to structure a particular lesson (on solving simultaneous equations) according to this theory:

"Actually I was practising what ... Mr. Gu[1] said in his book. .... So in this lesson, it had fulfilled every aspect that our school emphasized. For example, we had the situational aspect, that is

---

[1] Refers to Gu Lingyuan, a renowned professor in mathematics education, working in Shanghai Academy of Educational Sciences. He is also a co-author of Chapter 13 of this volume.

the first part in the five parts mentioned by Mr. Gu. The second part is the activities for the students to try. I applied it as well. The third part is to summarize and conclude. I asked the students to do the summary as well. ....The fifth one is reflection. When teaching the students, I got some messages through reflection ..... I would reflect at the appropriate time and correct the mistakes."

Despite the fact that the teacher refers to the five parts of the theory but actually mentions only four, this is perhaps less important than the fact that he is clearly trying to structure his lesson around a particular theoretical framework and that he claims that this is the mathematics teaching philosophy of the school. In order to put his comments into context, we explain here the 5-component framework for teaching identified by the Experimenting Group of Teaching Reform in mathematics led by Professor Gu in Qingpu County, Shanghai. This framework was based on a longitudinal empirical study and the five components are:

1. Using problems as a starting point for teaching;
2. Guiding students to develop exploratory activities;
3. Establishing variation in practice to raise the effectiveness of practice;
4. Summarizing to adopt into the knowledge structure; and
5. Modifying according to the fine categorization of teaching objectives.

(Experimenting Group of Teaching Reform in mathematics in Qingpu County, Shanghai, 1991)

As we can see, the component that the teacher omits is that concerned with the use of variation to enhance teaching. In fact, there is evidence in the lesson videos that he does use variation as a strategy but he never refers to this explicitly in the interviews. All the interview extracts above give us a picture of this teacher's general perceptions of his and the school's teaching approach. Let us now examine some specific illustrations given by the teacher with regard to the three lessons.

2.2 *Specific comments on lessons*

In the interviews, the teacher would stop the tape at points that he considered to be important in the lesson and give his reasons. Analyzing the second lesson on coordinates, the teacher first of all comments on his aims and the overall content:

> *"This lesson aimed at letting students know how to determine the location of a certain point based on its coordinates in a coordinate plane. This would let the students know there is a corresponding relationship between the points in the plane and the coordinates."*

The lesson he is referring to here is the second in a sequence on coordinates, the first having established the concept and how to describe a location with correct notation. At various points in this second lesson, the teacher highlights where he is trying to generate discussion and exploration among the students. For example:

> *"Here I gave a question for the students to discuss whether this was on the x-axis or the y-axis ... and what were the characteristics of the coordinates. During this discussion students could get the conclusion through observation. That was good for the students to learn from each other."*

> *"This example is not in the textbook. I put this one in myself. ..... By moving it, I have changed the location. I let the students investigate the coordinates of the vertex."*

> *"I asked the students to discuss the question first, discussing in small groups first, because this question was quite difficult. ...... Finally, when we exchanged ideas together, some students said they didn't think comprehensively, they thought of only one solution. By exchanging ideas among students, the question was solved comprehensively."*

> *"This lesson was conducted according to the method I use normally. I let students discuss when there is a difficulty, discussing in groups."*

We certainly have an impression here of a teacher who values the importance of peer discussion and is regularly giving students the opportunity to explore and discuss in groups. Moreover, we can also see that the teacher does not blindly follow the textbook but has used at least one example of his own in order to promote some investigation. We may also note his use of a problem that has more than one solution and that this fact emerges after the small group discussions.

In his comments on another lesson, concerning the development of the elimination method for solving simultaneous equations, the teacher first highlights his introductory activity. This lesson is also the second in a sequence. This time the sequence was on simultaneous equations and the first lesson concentrated on the concept of a system of equations in two unknowns. The teacher explains his approach and the students' response:

> *"Actually I set a situational question as it can increase the interest of the students. .... This question is different from the one we have in the book. ..... Judging from the answers of the students, they could easily get the results from the numbers I gave. They could find out easily, because in the second requirement of the question one more student ticket is added. So he knows that the two numbers (totals) should be subtracted. It helps to build a good foundation for the students about elimination by adding/subtracting."*

These comments reinforce the impression given before about his approach. Again, we may notice the emphases on structuring the problem in such a way that it lays a good foundation and on using a situational problem. And once more, it is interesting to note that he has used his own problem rather than that in the textbook. The implication is that he feels this problem serves his purpose better, perhaps for motivational reasons, perhaps for structural reasons, or indeed perhaps both. In another part of the interview, the teacher refers to a problem he set for the students at the end of the lesson in preparation for the next lesson:

> *"Given the equation $2x + 3y = 8$, I asked them to set a new equation so that it could become part of a system of equations. I*

hoped that the students would set equations which were related to the next lesson and the coefficients were multiples. Actually it fulfilled my intention ..... their results included coefficients being equal, or contrary (opposite sign), with no multiple or with multiples, or both of the equations have to be multiplied with a number to make the coefficients equal. This built a good foundation for the following lesson."

The most interesting feature about this comment is that he is again stressing the building of a good foundation for the next stage, but in this case it appears to come from quite an "open" situation where presumably he cannot be certain of the outcome. Nevertheless, as his next comments make clear, he can draw on his previous experience in structuring the sequence in this way:

"It is very seldom that the students would react in a surprising way. Why? Frankly speaking ... after years of teaching ..... I am very familiar with the content of the lessons and every time I would write down the problems in my notebook. When the time comes to prepare for the same lesson, I would have known what the problem might be, so it is very seldom that anything unexpected happens.

When one of the students changed the coefficients into the same or contrary, he multiplied by a fraction. Multiplying only one of the equations with a fraction would make the calculation a bit troublesome. This method is not mentioned in the textbook. ..... This student is creative, so I have encouraged him in the lesson. That's good, right! That was totally out of my expectation."

The reference to writing down problems in his notebook and using this when he next teaches the same content illustrates rather vividly that this teacher is not only drawing on the theoretical structure referred to earlier but is also combining this with his own experiences and reflections. It is also fascinating to see that, despite his initial claim that the unexpected very seldom occurs, he then goes on to describe a striking example of precisely this happening. One suspects that this event will also be written in his notebook and perhaps incorporated in some way into his future teaching.

We have tried to capture in all the above comments, the teacher's perceptions of his own teaching approach and also his perceptions of some of the particular lessons that were videotaped and what were the important elements of the lessons. In selecting these elements, he has tried to illustrate how his own approach, in his view, is actualized in the classroom. In the next section, we examine the lessons referred to in more detail from the observer's perspective. We relate this analysis to the teacher's perspective and propose a descriptive model of his pattern of teaching.

3 First Lesson on Coordinates

As we have described in the introduction, our study is concerned with the analysis of *sequences* of lessons taught by a number of different teachers. This is in contrast to the approach used by the TIMSS Video Study which was based on a large number of single lessons providing a series of individual "snapshots". In line with the Learners' Perspective Study, we strongly believe that it is impossible to capture a teacher's individual style and approach to teaching unless one can study his/her development of a topic over a sequence of lessons. This provides a picture of the teacher's "script" *across* lessons rather than *within* a lesson and each embedded lesson within the sequence contributes to the overall picture.

In the particular case we are concerned with in this chapter, the value of studying consecutive lessons is well illustrated by considering the first two lessons in the sequence on coordinates. We have quoted some of the teacher's comments on the second lesson in the previous section. Our own observations of the videotape of that lesson validate the comments given by the teacher concerning his regular use of small exploratory tasks which generate discussion among the students. However, let us now examine the first lesson on coordinates.

This lesson is the introduction to the concept of coordinates and focuses on the description of a point in the coordinate plane as the ordered pair (x, y). Throughout the lesson, the emphasis is on the importance of "correct" notation and procedures for describing a point. The lesson starts with showing a slide of a row of dots as shown here:

$$1 \quad \bullet \quad OA \quad \bullet \quad \bullet \quad OB \quad \bullet$$
$$\quad\quad 1 \quad 2 \quad 3 \quad 4 \quad 5 \quad 6$$

The students are then asked to describe the positions of dots A and B. There is no logical reason for the row to be labeled 1 and this fact is not mentioned. However, the reason becomes clear when the teacher (T) shows the next slide which illustrates a grid of 5 rows of 6 dots with two of the dots again labeled A and B. Once more, the task is to describe their positions.

```
5     •     ∘A    •     •     •     •
4     •     •     •     •     •     •
3     •     •     •     •     •     •
2     •     •     •     •     ∘B    •
1     •     •     •     •     •     •
      1     2     3     4     5     6
```

One of the students (Doris) answers:

Doris: A is at row 5, column 2. B is row 2, column 5.
T: Oh. Let's start indicating with columns.

The teacher's response is rather striking here and very indicative of the way the whole lesson will proceed. There is no comment on whether the student's answer correctly describes the position. There is no attempt to discuss the answer with the other students. There is simply the statement that we should start with the column without any explanation as to why. Doris goes on to give the "correct" description after which the teacher shows how this should be written:

T: Write a comma between the two numbers. Use a bracket for the pair of numbers. The first number 2 indicates the column, the second number 5 indicates the row.

Again, we note that there is no attempt to discuss with the students how we might write down the description; only the instruction concerning the conventional notation. The fact that this is simply a *convention* is also not mentioned at any time. The next student to describe a point uses the same order as Doris and states the row first. The teacher responds and goes on to discuss order:

> *T: Please sit down. Haven't I just said a sentence about that? We use the first number to indicate the column, the second number to indicate the row .... Right? .... There is an order for the two numbers. So we call such a pair of numbers an ordered pair.*

The choice on the part of the teacher to contrast A (2, 5) with B (5, 2) is presumably quite deliberate as it highlights the importance of order in eliminating any possible ambiguity in the description of a point. But again, the question of ambiguity is not mentioned or discussed. The emphasis is purely on following a convention. In the next stage of the lesson the teacher goes on to define the x, y coordinate axes and the common zero position of the two axes as the origin. This is actually a significant step from the grid arrangement of dots used previously where a zero label was, of course, not relevant. In fact, mathematically we have moved from a discrete model to a continuous one. We could say that there is an *implicit* identification of the previous dots in the first case with the intersection of grid lines in the second. However, this is not explicitly discussed in the lesson.

The students are next asked to draw the axes defining the rectangular coordinate plane on their own worksheets. After some minutes, the teacher shows a couple of the students' examples to the class and asks if they are correct or not. To one example the class responds (E = everybody):

> *E: Incorrect.*
> *T: Where's the mistake?*
> *E: The direction*
> *T: The direction is wrong. We've said the direction for y axis is that the part pointing up is positive. He points downwards, right? Wrong, okay.*

In the next stage, a series of points (A to F) is shown in the x-y plane and the teacher describes very precisely how the coordinates of point A can be found:

> *T: To find the column that the point belongs to, then we can draw a perpendicular line to x axis passing through point A. This perpendicular line is M indicating 3 on the x axis. .... In the following, we draw a perpendicular line to y axis passing through point A. The perpendicular line is N indicating 4 on the y axis.*

The students are then asked how to find the coordinates of the other points. Student Dana replies:

> *Dana: First, the perpendicular for point B is negative 3.*
> *T: What do you mean by perpendicular for point B?*
> *Dana: Um, downward perpendicular from point B.*
> *T: Downward perpendicular, passing through point B.*

It is very clear from this exchange that the teacher is not only concerned with the "correct" procedure but is also very insistent on precise language. After some further repetition of the precise language and procedure, the teacher asks the students about point C:

> *T: Let's say it together, point C.*
> *E: Perpendicular line passing through point C to x axis and perpendicular line passing through C to y axis, indicating negative two, negative three.*

The lesson continues in the same way when looking at the other points. The procedure and precise language is repeated many times by the teacher. At a later stage, he draws attention again to the written form:

> *T: Everybody, please pay attention. I've found that some classmates have missed the brackets. That is to say, for the coordinates of point A, there should be a comma in between the two values of the coordinate. We should add a pair of brackets at both ends.*

The lesson progresses with further examples but its tenor continues in the same way throughout. How would an observer characterize this lesson? It almost seems to epitomize a transmission mode of teaching with a heavy emphasis on "form" (e.g. conventional notation), on procedures, on repetition and practice, and on rote learning (including unison response). However, if we were to base our picture of this teacher on this one lesson, it would clearly give an unfair impression, since the next lesson follows rather a different pattern. We need to see this lesson in the context of its being one in a sequence. Indeed, it is clear from the teacher's own comments in his interviews (quoted earlier) that this lesson fits into his notion of the importance of laying a solid foundation. In fact, in a later part of the lesson, the students are confronted with the coordinates (0, −2.5) and (3.5, −1.5), neither of which seem to pose the slightest difficulty for them. From the teacher's point of view, this may be seen as a good justification for his very procedural approach to the start of the topic. In the following lesson, he demonstrates the other aspects of his theoretical framework by posing many small problems for the students to discuss and work on, sometimes in pairs or groups. We shall discuss these tasks in more detail in the next section.

4 Second Lesson on Coordinates

There are in fact many similarities between the first two lessons on coordinates, particularly in terms of their tight structure and the teacher's "control" over the objects of learning. Nevertheless, there are also some significant differences which we highlight here. The lesson begins with a familiar pattern, similar to that reported in Stigler and Hiebert (1999), of a quick revision of the previous lesson's conclusions. This is then followed up by the first new task:

> *T: So, now I have a question. If I tell you the coordinate of the point D is (3, 4), students, please find out the location of point D.*

The students work individually on this task for a short time and then student Emma is called on:

T: Okay, Emma, explain to the classmates how you find the location of point D.
Emma: Firstly I've obtained 3 on the x axis .... then, um .... then I obtained 4 on the y axis. From the two points, use a dotted line to extend upwards from the 3 on the x axis.
T: Use a dotted line to extend upward?
Emma: Um, to extend perpendicularly upwards.
T: On which axis?
Emma: Perpendicular on the x axis, then perpendicular to the 4 on y axis, the meeting point of the two lines is point D.

The task itself is, of course, the exact reversal of the skill learnt in the first lesson. Then, a point was shown in the plane and students had to determine its coordinates. Now, the coordinates are given and the students must determine the position. The short exchange above is rather typical of this lesson and, in contrast to the first lesson, there are a number of interesting elements to notice. In the first lesson all the questions asked by the teacher were "closed" questions. Here, the teacher does not simply ask the student for the answer but asks her to *explain* her procedure for getting the answer (i.e., the question is open in nature). In addition, the correct procedure established in the first lesson came *from the teacher*, together with many repetitions of the exact language to be used. However, here we see that the new procedure comes *from the student*. Moreover, the student's language is already quite precise and is clearly modeled on the language used in the first lesson. Perhaps this illustrates a further justification of the teacher's emphasis on laying a foundation.

Another interesting feature of this exchange is the teacher's opening phrase "So, now I have a question". Throughout the lesson, a similar phrase is used time and again and is a clear "signal" that the students will have to think about something new. This again is in contrast to the first lesson where many closed questions were asked but were never "signaled" in this way. For example, in the task just described, a previous point already shown in the plane is A (4, 3). The teacher now continues:

T: OK, so we've got the location of the point and now I have a question. Compare this (3, 4) with the first point A (4, 3). Why aren't they the same point? Both of them have 3 and 4 as the numbers. Why aren't the two points the same?

In fact, the concept of order had already been established in the first lesson but here we see the teacher raising it again, this time with a view to getting the students to articulate the reasons and necessity for the notation. In the next task, the students have to plot a series of points and this is followed by having to draw a triangle given the coordinates of its vertices. In these two tasks, there are three points that lie on the axes. This is clearly deliberate and we can see how the teacher follows up on this:

> *T: I have a question. In the exercise, points A and C are on the x axis. In this figure ... in the last exercise, point E is on the y axis. So I want to ask you all, in the coordinate plane, what are the characteristics for such a point? ...... Let's discuss. Discuss in groups of two.*

The students are now specifically asked to discuss this question and, although the focus of the enquiry is clearly very narrow, the emphasis is on the students coming up with their own description of the characteristics. This is followed up with some whole class discussion where the teacher suggests a slight modification to the students' description. For example, one student refers to the "latter" number being zero. The teacher asks what this latter number is called and the student then changes it to "vertical coordinate". But it is clear that the teacher is now working from the students' ideas and suggestions.

In the next task, a square is drawn and then the teacher translates the square to new positions, first by a downwards shift of 3 units and then by a shift left of 2 units. The students are asked to give the new coordinates of the vertices at each stage. This task is conducted purely as an exercise in describing the new positions but it can also be seen as laying a foundation for the next problem which involves some mental visualization. In this next task, the students are given just two points belonging to a square, A (5, 0) and B (5, –4), and are asked to determine the coordinates of the other two vertices C and D. Again, the teacher encourages the students to work in groups on this task:

> *T: I know only the coordinates of A and B. ..... But how about the square? We haven't finished drawing it, so where are points C and D? What are their coordinates? Four students in one group, try and draw, discuss and look into, and find out the coordinates of C and D.*

As the groups work, the teacher circulates and comments on the students' work. In some cases, he is correcting errors but, on at least two occasions, he is also encouraging them to think further than their original solution. For example:

> *T: Think about it again. Is this the only way to draw (a square)?*

Later the students are asked to present their solutions and the first one shown gives C as (1, 4) and D as (1, 0). The teacher asks if anyone found a different solution and Eliza answers:

> *Eliza: Our method of drawing is the same as that one, however its square is pointing to the right, while ours is pointing to the left.*
> *T: The square is pointing to the left?*
> *Eliza: Another side of the square. The side AB is drawn at the right hand side, CD is to the left hand side.*
> *T: Would you explain how to draw.*

The pattern of regular "mini-exploration tasks" has continued, with discussion among the students first, followed by presentation of solutions. We may notice once more the teacher's insistence that the students describe their work as precisely as possible. However, in contrast to the first lesson, here the teacher does not impose his own description but merely repeats the student's effort ("The square is pointing to the left?"). The implication is clear to the student who then attempts to be more precise in her description. This is followed by further elaboration and explanation of the solution.

The lesson finishes with a little more practice and then a reminder by the teacher, stated twice, of the new knowledge/skill acquired in the lesson:

> *T: Today we've learnt how ... we can use the coordinates of a point to find the location of the point in the rectangular coordinate plane.*

This was a regular feature of his pattern of teaching and the phrase "Today we've learnt ...." occurred in every lesson recorded.

The two lessons discussed thus far differ significantly when viewed from a de-contextualized, isolated perspective. However, seen as part of a sequence and in the light of the teacher's own philosophy, we can identify an overall coherence. A pattern begins to emerge that is a combination of foundation/consolidation and mini-exploration. Referring back to the teacher's interview comments, there is one aspect he emphasizes which is conspicuous by its absence in these two lessons. This is the setting of situational questions/problems. In order to examine this aspect of his teaching, in the next section, we analyze another lesson of the sequence.

5 First Lesson on Linear Equations

The topic of the lesson is "linear equations of two unknowns and solutions". The teacher begins by referring to a problem about stamps:

> *Wong Junior goes to the post office to buy several two-dollar and one-dollar stamps, at least one of each kind, costing a total of ten dollars. How many of each kind of stamps does he get?*

This is indeed a situational problem which creates a context for the students to think about possible solutions. The task itself is open in the sense that it has different possible solutions. However, it is so simple and straightforward that it does not give much opportunity for exploration. Without any prescribed methods, the students easily suggest different answers by trial and error and they end up with a table of four answers.

After this, the teacher guides the students to set up an equation in two unknowns to solve the problem and inspect the characteristics (the degree and the number of unknowns) of the equation:

> *T: Since we've learned about equations before, this question can be solved by using equations ... let's think about the unknowns before the equations are set. So what do you think of the question? How to set the unknown? How about setting more than one unknown? [Students thinking]*
>
> *T: Dan.*
>
> *T: Good. Set two unknowns. I can set two-dollar stamps as x, one-dollar stamps as y, so according to this question how should the equations be set?*
>
> *T: x plus y, right? x plus y equals ten, does everyone agree?*
>
> *E: No.*
>
> *T: Why don't you agree? [Students thinking]*
>
> *T: Felix.*
>
> *Felix: (...) x plus y is (equal to ten), x stamps plus y stamps equals ten, as well as, one is quantity, the other is money.*
>
> *T: Using ten, so what should be done?*
>
> *Felix: Two x plus y equals ten.*
>
> *T: Two x plus y equals ten, in this question we can set two x plus y equals ten, right? Okay, let us see. This equation and our linear equation in one unknown, from the number of unknowns, compare the power of the unknown x and see if there is any difference?*
>
> *T: Donald.*
>
> *Donald: Compare with the system of linear equations in one unknown, it has one more unknown.*
>
> *T: One more unknown, so how many unknowns are there now?*
>
> *Donald: Two unknowns.*
>
> *T: Two unknowns, right? Okay, please sit down.*
>
> *T: So how about the power of the unknown?*
>
> *E: One.*
>
> *T: One, right. So we call this kind of equations linear equations in two unknowns. Linear equation in two unknowns, if they consist of two unknowns and the power of each of the unknowns is one, we call this kind of equations linear equations in two unknowns.*

There are two very clear elements in this opening segment of the lesson. First, the teacher creates a context, or a "situation" in his own words, for the application of equations. After this concrete start and a discussion of the solutions, the teacher quickly moves to a generalized, abstract representation of the problem. Again, more discussion is generated about how to set up the equation and then the focus turns to inspecting the number and power of the unknowns. The teacher concludes the discussion by introducing the formal name "linear equation in two unknowns." Juxtaposing the two approaches, we observe a shift from an authentic context about stamps to a mathematical context about the characteristics of equations, establishing the definition of a linear equation in two unknowns formally in the latter. It is clear that the main purpose of the introductory situational problem, which is hardly challenging, is as a vehicle for considering a new mathematical concept.

Immediately following this, the teacher gives some exercises for consolidation of this newly learnt concept. He shows a slide with 6 equations and asks whether each is a linear equation in two unknowns or not:

$$1.\ 2x + 3 = 0 \qquad 2.\ x + 2y - 1 = 0 \qquad 3.\ 1/2\ x = 2/3\ y + 1$$
$$4.\ 2x + 5y = z \qquad 5.\ x^2 + 2y = 1 \qquad 6.\ 2xy = 5$$

The first 5 equations are simple cases and the students easily give the correct answers with supporting reasons. When they come to the last question "$2xy = 5$", the teacher asks the students to discuss in pairs before making a judgment. After a few minutes, the teacher resumes the whole class discussion again.

T: Does it belong to the system and for what reason? Okay, let us justify whether it belongs to the system or not, if you think it is, please raise your hands. [Some students raising their hands]
T: Okay. Anyone thinks it is not? We let those who disagree to explain. Why is it not? Franc.
Franc: It is because two xy, xy is an unknown.
T: x y is an unknown? [Students laughing]
T: Students laughed, is x y an unknown?
E: x y are two unknowns.

> *T: If you use this method to justify, of course your justification is wrong, right? What else? Freda .*
>
> *Freda: The power of each unknown should be one, while two x y is a unit, the power of it is two.*
>
> *T: The power of this single unit is two, so it is not. Does everyone agree?*
>
> *E: Agree.*
>
> *T: Please sit down, very good, everybody should note, to justify whether it is a linear equation in two unknowns, we have to look for the power of the unknowns, that is, we must examine the conditions of the system. That is to say the power of the unknown. The power of the term two x y is two. We know that the power of linear equations in one unknown is one. So this equation should not be a linear equation in two unknowns. In the six linear equations, we can say only question two and three are linear equations in two unknowns. Okay, this is our first exercise.*

The teacher's way of dealing with the sixth question is very different from the earlier part of the lesson. The question is relatively more complex than the others and the teacher is fully aware of this. This is why he encourages the students to discuss in pairs. In the later whole class discussion, he starts with a very open manner which is quite different from the earlier part of the lesson. He lets the students argue for both possibilities and peer comments are invited. A conclusion is drawn only after the class has come to a consensus on the degree and the number of unknowns in the equation.

In this lesson we observe a way of introducing a mathematical concept with a structural pattern: *situation-abstraction-consolidation-exploration*. The teacher starts from a problem, then shifts to a mathematical context formulating the mathematical concept by an abstraction from the situation created by the problem. This is followed with some consolidation exercise and then with a short exploration on a complex problem.

In the next part of the lesson, this pattern is repeated with a focus on the solutions instead of the characteristics of the equations. The teacher refers to the stamp problem for a second time and introduces the definition of solution. Following this, the class is again asked to do some consolidation exercises on a slide for which the students have to determine whether 5 given pairs of values of x and y are solutions of "2*x* + *y* = 3", or not. Following this, the teacher refers to the stamp problem for a third time. In this case, he asks the class to remove the equation from the context of the stamp problem and generates a whole class discussion on the number of solutions for an abstract equation:

> *T: Okay, so we can go back to the previous question. We have found there are four solutions to the question and I have a question for you. Since we supposed x and y are the numbers of the stamps and, according to this, we have four solutions. I ignore the actual meaning of buying the number of stamps and look directly into the equation. Let's consider whether two x plus y equals ten has only four solutions.*
>
> *E: No.*
>
> *T: So can you give me an example. [Students thinking]*
>
> *T: As you said no, can you give me an example? Set a pair of unknowns with values to be a solution of the equation. By the way, aren't we being inside it? Dabo.*
>
> *Dabo: x equals one over two, y equals nine.*
>
> *T: x equals one over two, y equals nine, so let us do the checking for him, right or not?*
>
> *E: Yes.*
>
> *T: It is a solution of the equation, but it is not an answer to the question, so can you give another example?*
>
> *S: x equals five, y equals zero.*
>
> *T: x equals five, y equals zero right? Right, sit down.*
>
> *T: You try again.*
>
> *S: x equals six, y equals minus two.*
>
> *T: x equals six, y equals minus two. Okay or not?*
>
> *E: Okay.*
>
> *T: Okay, good. So how many solutions are there?*
>
> *E: Infinite number.*
>
> *T: Infinite number. There are infinite numbers of solutions for this equation, so for any linear equations in two unknowns there are infinite numbers of solutions. So using a few solutions to infer all the solutions, we call this a set of solutions for the linear equations in two unknowns. [Showing slides]*

Although there is no pair work prior to this discussion, the discussion shares similar features to those we have already described in a mini-exploration, such as genuine invitation of different answers and peer comments. The teaching thus far in the lesson is for the purpose of understanding the meaning of some mathematical concepts, equations, and solutions. The development of the whole lesson evolves from the stamp problem which is visited three times and each time with a different aspect of the object of learning (the equation, the solution, and infinite number of solutions, respectively) being brought to the fore. The situation-abstraction-consolidation-exploration pattern is repeated in his way of teaching these concepts.

In the remaining part of the lesson, he teaches the students a procedure to solve an equation by rewriting one unknown in terms of the other, followed by substitution. As with the first lesson on coordinates, his questioning style changes to a very directive mode. There is no opportunity to discuss different ways of solving the equations and the students have no alternative except to follow the teacher's guidance closely. In addition, the teacher is very demanding in the students' oral representation of how to move the terms in the transformation of the equation and the oral representation is well supported with the teacher's writing on the board. This is repeated with another similar question. Then the students are asked to do some consolidation exercises in the textbook. Comparing this latter part with the earlier part of the lesson, it appears that the teacher's style changes when dealing with different kinds of content. He shows the situation-abstraction-consolidation-exploration pattern when teaching the meaning of a concept and is very directive when teaching a procedure.

6 Pattern of Teaching

The three lessons we have discussed above all have rather distinctive features and if we were viewing them as single "snapshots", we might well conclude that they represented three different teachers. This illustrates very clearly the danger of trying to characterize a teacher's style or "script" by a single lesson observation. The challenge, as researchers and observers, is to consider the lessons as part of a teaching sequence and to try to identify whether or not any teaching "pattern" emerges. However, before we continue, it is worth pointing out that the three lessons analyzed were in fact *consecutive* lessons, despite the topics perhaps appearing unrelated at first sight. The order was Linear Equations followed by the two Coordinate lessons. In the fourth lesson of this sequence the teacher begins with these opening comments:

> *T: In the previous lessons we've learnt about the ... concept of linear equations in two unknowns and also the ... concepts of the rectangular coordinate plane. We know that after setting up a rectangular coordinate plane, the points in the plane can be represented by pairs of ordered numbers. ..... So is there any connection between the two concepts? Let's use the equation 2x − y = 3 as an example for investigation.*

We can now see these lessons as forming part of a coherent and connected whole. In the same way, can we see the teacher's approach to teaching as part of a coherent pattern?

Before we attempt to describe such a pattern, let us briefly consider the characterizations of "typical" mathematics lessons in the US and Japan as described in Stigler and Hiebert (1999). The main features of the lessons in the US appeared to be demonstration and practice. That is, the teacher explained some new technique or concept to the class and this was followed up by demonstrating some examples and the students practising similar examples. The overall impression is one of very procedural mathematics and very directive teaching. In contrast, the main features of the Japanese lessons appeared to involve problem-solving and discussion. That is, the students were presented with a challenging problem to explore at the start of a lesson and after attempting the problem, individually or in groups, their solution attempts were discussed. We do not want to discuss whether or not these characterizations are valid here; indeed, Stigler and Hiebert themselves caution about the dangers of over-simplification. Nevertheless, they go on to remark "simplified descriptions provide an important starting point for complex activities" (p.26). Using the same principle, we suggest that the contrasting teaching approaches of "directive or transmission teaching" and "exploratory teaching" may provide a useful starting point for analyzing a particular teacher's methodology. In this sense, the US and Japanese "models" may be considered as close to the two extreme positions illustrated in Figure 1.

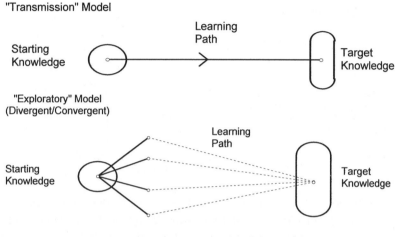

Figure 1. "Extreme" models of mathematics teaching

Viewed from this perspective, our analyses of the lessons in the previous sections point to some interesting conclusions. As we have illustrated, the first lesson on coordinates would place the teacher firmly towards the "transmission" end of our Directive/Exploratory contrast. But as we have seen from the analyses of the other two lessons, this would be a gross distortion of the teacher's methodological approach. Indeed, the second lesson on coordinates provides an immediate contrast. In this case, far more of the lesson is conducted in an exploratory mode and this is probably the dominant mode of the lesson. In a further contrast, the lesson on linear equations is characterized by having a fairly even balance between directive and exploratory teaching. If we consider the rationales behind his teaching, as professed by the teacher himself, it seems clear that he is using a very directive approach when he is "laying foundations" or "establishing new procedures". (In what follows we shall take "Foundations" to include new procedures.) It appears that he gives an equal importance in his teaching to both foundations and exploration, where the students have the opportunity to discuss and express their own ideas. Nevertheless, it is also clear that the overall direction of the learning is tightly controlled by the teacher and the explorations are never "large, open investigations" but rather "mini-explorations" The teacher's approach could be described as a "foundation & Exploration" model as shown in Figure 2.

"Foundation & Exploration" Model

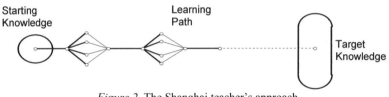

Starting
Knowledge

Learning
Path

Target
Knowledge

Figure 2. The Shanghai teacher's approach

It is important to point out that this "model" does *not* represent equally spaced out elements of foundation-laying and exploration, nor are these elements intended to be of equal duration. This is a model that represents the teacher's approach over a *sequence* of lessons. Thus, almost the whole of the first lesson on coordinates can be seen as a foundation element within the model, whereas the second coordinate lesson mostly consists of exploratory elements. We should also point out that this model is intended to broadly describe the *teacher's activity* during a sequence. Clearly there are other elements in a lesson that are not shown in this picture, for example, when the students are engaged in classroom practice. At such times, the teacher will often be helping individual students, or groups of students, and this may be in a "consolidation mode" or in an "exploratory mode". A more detailed picture of the components of the teacher's approach is shown in Figure 3.

The diagram illustrates that the starting point for the sequence may be concerned with foundation laying but could equally be exploratory. In fact, if we consider these three consecutive lessons as part of a complete sequence covering the concepts of linear equations in two unknowns together with the different possible solution strategies (including a graphical strategy) we see that the whole sequence does indeed start with an exploratory element. Further, according to the teacher's professed approach, the mathematics is often introduced through a situational context. Thus, both the stages of foundation (or consolidation) and exploration may involve a purely mathematical context or may be situational. The analysis of the linear equations lesson also illustrated the importance of a generalization/abstraction stage. This usually comes after an exploratory element but could also come at the end of a foundation element. Clearly, this stage is purely mathematical.

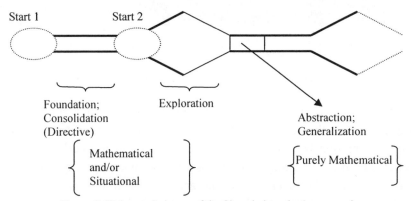

Figure 3. Elaborated picture of the Shanghai teacher's approach

In the analysis, we categorized events in the lesson into exploratory, directive, summarizing, exercises and practice, and assigning homework. (Details of categorizing the events are shown in the appendix). The actual breakdown, in terms of sequences and time, for the first five lessons taught in this topic is shown in Figure 4.

As we can see very clearly, the make-up and distribution of activity varies considerably from lesson to lesson. Once again this confirms very strongly the importance of viewing a teacher's performance over a sequence of lessons rather than a single lesson. We also see that the whole sequence, in terms of time, is dominated by three elements, namely Foundation/Consolidation, Exploration, and Guided Practice. The relative proportions of time for these elements over the five lessons is Foundation/Consolidation (32%), Exploration (19%), and Guided Practice (45%) making up 96% of the total time.

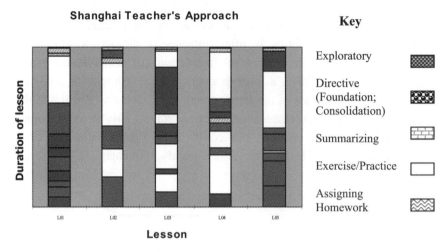

Figure 4. Distribution of the teacher's approach over five lessons

However, we should also highlight another significant element in the sequence, even though it takes a relatively small amount of time. This is the Summarizing element which is in accord with the teacher's expressed beliefs about his teaching. It is striking that a summary is given by the teacher at the end of every lesson (in fact, this was true of *all* the lessons recorded) and in the fourth lesson we see that there was also a summarizing element in the middle of the lesson. This is clearly in accord with the teacher's use of Gu's theory as his guiding principle. We have not attempted to incorporate this element into the diagram in Figure 3, since, in contrast to the Foundation/Consolidation and the Exploratory elements, this *does* occur at rather precise regular intervals (i.e., normally at the end of a lesson). As such, it could be misleading to incorporate it into a diagram that is not meant to represent equal and regular time elements.

7 Concluding Remarks

Our detailed analysis of three of this teacher's lessons has strikingly re-affirmed our initial belief that it is not only unrealistic, but indeed dangerous, to attempt to identify a teacher's "script" for a lesson. Such a characterization carries with it the implicit assumption that a teacher's approach is almost invariable from lesson to lesson. Nevertheless, we have tried to show that by using a different lens on the situation (i.e., a sequence of lessons rather than a "snapshot" lesson), we may still be able to identify a "pattern" of teaching that characterizes a teacher's approach. To be a little more precise, we define a "pattern of teaching" to mean: *The identifiable features of a teacher's classroom practice, occurring in a repeated manner over a period of time, that together constitute the characteristics of the teacher's style.*

We may illustrate the concept and importance of pattern by considering an analogy with a carpet pattern. Suppose we focus on a very small element of the carpet. We may find some very interesting features to study and analyze within this element but we shall certainly not be able to discern the pattern of the carpet. If the pattern is a very simple one, we may begin to see it by zooming back a small distance. However, the more complex the pattern, the more we need to draw back in order to appreciate the overall pattern. The same principle holds with any study of a teacher's pedagogical approach in the classroom. But, of course, we must remember that human behavior is *not* mechanistic, in the way that a well-defined carpet pattern is. Humans are complex beings and teaching, as a human activity, is also necessarily complex. This is why our definition of a pattern of teaching refers to repeated identifiable features but this does not imply precise regularity in a temporal sense.

In this chapter, we have discussed three lessons in detail and also taken a brief overall look at a sequence of five lessons. From this, we have attempted to describe the pattern of teaching, as defined above, that characterizes this particular teacher. Have we "zoomed back" far enough to fully describe his teaching pattern? When we have analyzed a sequence of ten or fifteen of his lessons, will we be able to add other identifiable features to the pattern? Will other teachers in Shanghai conform to a similar pattern and how will this compare to teachers in Hong Kong and in other parts of the world? These and many other exciting questions are inevitably raised by our analysis in this chapter and the rich data we now have at our disposal will ensure that much fruitful follow-up work remains to be done.

References

Clarke, D. (2002). *The Learner's Perspective Study: Methodology as the Enactment of a Theory of Practice*. Paper presented at the interactive symposium 'International Perspectives on Mathematics Classrooms' at the Annual Meeting of the American Educational Research Association, New Orleans, April 1-5, 2002.

Experimenting Group of Teaching Reform in mathematics in Qingpu County, Shanghai. (1991). *Learning to teach* [In Chinese 学会教学]. Beijing: People Education Publishers.

Law, N. (Ed.). (1996). *Science and mathematics achievements at the junior secondary level in Hong Kong: A summary report for Hong Kong in the Third International Mathematics and Science Study (TIMSS)*. Hong Kong: TIMSS Hong Kong Study Centre, University of Hong Kong.

Law, N. (Ed.). (1997). *Science and mathematics achievements at the mid-primary level in Hong Kong: A summary report for Hong Kong in the Third International Mathematics and Science Study (TIMSS)*. Hong Kong: TIMSS Hong Kong Study Centre, The University of Hong Kong.

Lopez-Real, F., & Mok, I. A. C. (2002). Is there a Chinese pedagogy of mathematics teaching. *Perspectives in Education, 18*(2), 125-128.

Mullis, I. V. S., Marin, M. O., Gonzalez, E. J., Gregory, K. D., Garden, R. A., O'Connor, K. M., et al. (2000). *TIMSS 1999 international mathematics report: Findings from IEA's repeat of the Third International Mathematics and Science Study at the eighth grade*. Boston: The International Association for the Evaluation of Education Achievement.

Stigler, J., & Hiebert, J. (1999). *The teaching gap: Best ideas from the world's teachers for improving education in the classroom*. New York: Free Press.

Watkins, D. A., & Biggs, J. B. (Eds.). (1996). *The Chinese learner: Cultural, psychological and contextual influences*. Hong Kong: Comparative Education Research Centre, The University of Hong Kong; Melbourne, Australia: Australian Council for Education Research.

Watkins, D. A., & Biggs, J. B. (Eds.). (2001). *Teaching the Chinese learner: Psychological and pedagogical Perspectives*. Hong Kong: Comparative Education Research Centre.

Appendix

Criteria for Categorizing Events Demonstrating a Teacher's Approach

(B01)   Exploratory
   ♦   The focus is on a relatively open or difficult problem which has more than one possible answer.
   ♦   The teacher gave a signal for pair discussion. (Sometimes this was skipped. The exploration was facilitated directly by the teacher in a whole class discussion.)
   ♦   A whole class discussion with the following features: inviting more than one student to give answers, inviting explanations, inviting peer comments.

(B02)   Directive (Foundation; Consolidation)
   ♦   No comment on the student's answer, no attempt to discuss the answer with the other students, simply stating what should be done (e.g. the conventional notation).
   ♦   Emphasis is purely on following a convention.
   ♦   Insistence on precise language.
   ♦   Repetition of what had been learnt in an earlier lesson or in the earlier part of the lesson in a fast pace, using this as a foundation for establishing further knowledge.
   ♦   Insistence on articulation of procedures.
   ♦   Clear and directive definition of a concept or method after an illustrative example or discussion.
   ♦   Teacher plays the role of directing students to work on problems.
   ♦   Probing for 'expected' answers.
   ♦   Directive explanation by teacher.

(B03)   Summarizing
   ♦   Teacher does summarizing during the lesson, or to conclude the topics or problems discussed.

(B04)   Exercise and Practice (sometimes includes whole class checking exercise)
   ♦   In the situation of doing textbook exercise, there can be teacher talking about/explaining the question, and students having seatwork.
   ♦   Teacher checks exercise with students.

(B06)   Assigning Homework
   ♦   Teacher assigns homework or questions for students to do at home.

Chapter 15

Differences within Communalities: How Is Mathematics Taught in Rural and Urban Regions in Mainland China?

MA Yunpeng   ZHAO Dongchen   TUO Zhongfei

Based on a field study of four schools in rural and urban regions in northeast China, this chapter describes how Chinese primary school teachers teach mathematics and how teachers organize learning activities in the classroom in rural and urban primary schools in Mainland China. The communalities and differences in rural and urban mathematics classrooms were analyzed, which were demonstrated in both preparations of lessons and actual teaching. Inspirations for improvements of mathematics learning and teaching in Mainland China were discussed.

Key words: mathematics teaching, rural and urban, case study, Mainland China

1 Introduction

As is well known, the design and implementation of the curriculum in primary and secondary schools has been traditionally centralized in Mainland China. Not only a national curriculum was laid down, but all students in Mainland China used the same set of textbooks published by an official publisher since the late 1980s. In the 1990s, the central government has attempted to somewhat relax this system. The policies of "one syllabus, many textbooks" (一纲多本) and "many syllabi, many textbooks" (多纲多本) were gradually implemented. Firstly, Zhejiang Province and Shanghai City have been allowed to develop their own curricula that are different from the national ones. Secondly, more publishers have been permitted to publish textbooks. Despite the

413

loosening of central control, the nature of the curriculum development system has remained unchanged. The cases of Shanghai and Zhejiang could be seen as pilot schemes. The publishers who are granted the right to publish textbooks have to base their materials on the national curriculum and their outputs have to go through an official review process (see Wong, Han, & Lee, this volume).

Curriculum theorists have widely discussed the comparative advantages of a centralized curriculum system and a school-based system (Clune, 1993; Morris, 1996; Skilbeck, 1984). A major drawback of a centralized system is the fact that it fails to cater for the needs of students and schools in different settings. Considering China being a large country of approximately 9.60 million square kilometers with notable variations in both terrain and climate across different regions, yet most areas in China still are using the same syllabus and textbooks published by the same publishers. Since September 2001, a reform of the basic education curriculum was under experimentation, which imposed a new approach that was quite contrary to the idea of a unified curriculum (Basic Education Curriculum Material Development Centre, 2001).

Implementation studies in the West over the past three decades have helped educators and teachers gain a great deal of insight into the mechanics and the complexity of the implementation process (Fullan, 1991). Curriculum implementation is affected by a wide range of factors, including the nature, clarity and complexity of change, the support of the local education authority, the quality and involvement of the teaching force, the participation of school principal, the culture of teachers, and the support of the central government etc. (Fullan, 1991; Nias, Southworth, & Campbell, 1992; Snyder, Bolin, & Zmwalt, 1992). Among these factors, the role of teachers, particularly their role in the classroom, is of great importance (B. Clarke, D. Clarke, & Sullivan, 1996; Fullan, 1991).

Teachers seldom implement a curriculum exactly as stated in curriculum documents; rather they tend to make their own adaptations. Studying teachers' decision-making process can therefore help us understand how they make changes. Teachers have been found to adopt a practical stance in deciding what to teach and how to teach (Doyle & Ponder, 1976/77). Their decisions are affected by their knowledge, beliefs and school culture (Calderhead, 1996; B. Clarke et al., 1996; Hargreaves, 1992; Nespor, 1987). Teachers without sound professional knowledge will have difficulty in adapting a curriculum (Lam, 1996). Teachers' attitudes and beliefs are also important. Competent teachers feel that they are capable of shaping students' performance and they have high expectations of their students (Tuckman, 1995).

Despite the new idea of the government's allowing more school/teacher autonomy of the new curriculum, for so many years, the unification of textbook design and management has already affected mathematics teaching in Chinese primary schools extensively and profoundly. It has both theoretical and practical significance to ask how teachers implement the intended curriculum according to the different contexts and constraints they are in. Contrasting the situations in urban and rural schools in China would let us understand how teachers adapt themselves to the centralized curriculum in depth (Lam, Ma, & Wong, 1999). In this connection, how do Chinese mathematics teachers in primary schools understand and implement the curriculum and how do they design and organize their own teaching accordingly? How different are the teachers in the cities and the rural areas in their knowledge of the curriculum and teaching and how do they actually teach in class? How do these primary mathematics teachers make decisions during lesson preparations and actual teaching and what are the factors affecting their decisions? All these important issues in the research of mathematics teaching in primary schools in China will be discussed in this chapter. The researchers attempt to understand teachers' perspectives of teaching and the factors affecting teachers' teaching through the analysis of teachers' preparation and their actually teaching. Furthermore, a comparison between urban teachers and rural teachers is made.

2 Methodology

China has 5.78 million primary school teachers (China Education and Research Network, 2002). Mathematics is one of the main subjects in primary schools. Currently, some urban schools have specialized mathematics teachers, which means that mathematics and language subjects are taught by different teachers. Some other urban schools and most rural schools work under the "class-all-round system", which means that mathematics and language subjects of a class are taught by the same teacher and very often teachers who work in the rural areas are also responsible for moral education and science subjects. Therefore, more than half of the total number of teachers, estimated to be 3.5 million, should be counted as mathematics teachers. According to statistics, the percentage of qualified teachers has reached as high as 97.39% in 2001 (China Education and Research Network, 2002). However, the rise does not necessarily mean a proportional improvement in teaching quality. The discrepancy is more obvious in the rural regions than the urban regions. We took the above factors into account when choosing our samples in order to reflect rural primary teachers' characteristics as accurately as possible.

2.1 *Sampling*

In this research, purposive sampling was used. Two representative sample schools from each area (urban and rural) were selected based on their school size, teacher experience, student demographics, and the proportion of the structure of administrators and teachers. The following is a brief description of the four schools.

"Urban–1"[1], located in Changchun City, Northeast China, is a district[2] school with a relatively high students' academic standard, consisting of 2238 students and 85 teachers.

"Urban–2" is similar to "Urban–1", located in Changchun, with a relatively high academic standard, consisting of 1422 students and 55 teachers.

---

[1] Urban-1 denotes the first school in the urban area. Similar notations are used for the other three schools.
[2] District is one unit level of local government lower than urban region. In the urban region, the district government and the district education department administer the primary schools and middle schools.

"Rural–1"is a village[3] school, located in a mountainous area in the east of Jilin Province[4]. There are six grades, one class in each grade, with 177 students and 9 teachers, including the principal.

"Rural–2"is similar to "Rural–1". There are six grades, one class in each grade, with 133 students and 11 teachers, including the principal.

A total of 28 teachers from the four schools are selected as follows. For the urban schools, all mathematics teachers in a particular grade participated in this study and at least one teacher from each of the other grade levels. In Urban–1, grade three is the focal grade, while in Urban–2, grade four is the focal grade. The choice was made according to school condition and after consultation with the principals.

For each rural school, since there is only one class and one mathematics teacher in each grade, all the teachers were selected to the study.

2.2 *Method*

The research was carried out for more than one month on site in each school through classroom observations and in-depth interviews. It took a total of 14 weeks. 41 lessons were observed and 81 persons were interviewed. In addition, we also attended five lesson preparation sessions and took part in three education research seminars.

The interviews were conducted before and after classes. The following questions were asked:

- Please tell me about your general idea and design of this lesson. (pre-lesson)
- How do you think about this lesson? Have you finished what you had designed ahead? Is there anything special about the class? (post-lesson)
- How do you prepare for your lesson?

---

[3] Village is the lowest level administrative organization in a rural region under the local government. In general, town is above village in the governmental system, while county is above town. One village usually includes some rural areas and village schools are located in the place where the village governing committee is located. Students living in other rural areas must go there to study.

[4] Changchun is the capital of Jilin Province.

- What are included in your mathematics lesson plan generally?
- In general, what is the basic structure of the lesson and how do you allocate your time?
- What kinds of teaching methods do you adopt? And which one do you use most often?
- What factors would you take into account when you are planning and preparing for the lesson?

The observations included in-class observations and after-class observations. In-class observations focused on the activities of the teachers and students in the classroom. After-class observations focused on various activities which took place outside of the classrooms, such as relevant meetings, lesson preparation sessions, and other interactions among the teachers, etc.

3   Lesson Preparation of the Teachers

In this study, by observing the teachers and talking with them, the researchers obtained better understanding of how the teachers prepare for the lessons, in terms of formats, methods, effects, and other relevant factors. It was found that there were prominent differences in the format and method of preparation, and the use of curriculum resources between the urban and rural mathematics teachers.

Preparation is an important component of teaching. In China, primary school teachers are required to prepare for lessons and write up a lesson plan. A properly prepared lesson does not only reflect the teachers' professional accomplishment, but also reflects the achievement of the schools or teaching and research groups[5]. The study found that almost all the schools and teachers conformed to the practice that teachers prepared for lessons before teaching. However, the preparation could be remarkably different in the urban and rural schools, which could be observed in their formats of preparation.

Basically, the formats of preparation include individual preparation

---

[5] There are one or more teaching and research groups (教研组) in most schools in China.

and group preparation. The research reveals that urban schools integrate both methods, while rural schools always adopt the latter.

3.1 *Lesson preparation in urban schools*

In urban schools, there are usually two to four mathematics teachers in one grade and one teacher teaches two classes. In some cases, one teacher teaches only one class. The so-called "group preparation" refers to the meeting where several teachers in the same grade discuss and research on the content of the lesson together, including analyzing the possible difficulties of teaching the lesson and give relevant advices to each other, etc. The following is a record of group-preparation in "Urban–1".

> A: Next, we are going to talk about the division with zero in the middle and at the end of the quotient. It's not very difficult but easy to make mistakes. It's not hard to explain, but it might have problems, especially, with the zero at the end.
> B: It's easy to make mistakes at the end digit, when there're remainders.
> A: Firstly, see how the quotient is like. Judge how many digits are there in the quotient. Secondly, check them again.
> C: I think that under the direction of the teacher, the students can tell the number of digits correctly, but, when they're calculating the problem themselves, they might not do that very well.
> A: Their calculation is a bit slow. They're not skillful enough.
> A: There're three examples in the unit and they should be taught three times. Example 13 should be taught first.
> B: It's easy to miss the zero when the students are calculating.
> A: What should we do? Ask the students to check and judge how many digits there are in the quotient first?
> C: The students can understand what you said when you're teaching, but when they do the calculation by themselves, something would go wrong.
> A: The students work very slowly, because they are not familiar with the calculation method. Ask the students to prepare a piece of paper and ask them to work on the sums at any time.

> Let the more capable students do quiz competitions and reward the quicker students by letting them go out to play.
>
> C: Two days before, we had a small test. The students could not be permitted to go home without finishing the test. The capable students in my class took only 10 minutes to finish it, but I didn't know whether I should really let them go away.
>
> A: I think if they got them all correctly, I will let them go.

The above record shows that the group-preparation centers on next week's topic, "the division with zero in the middle and at the end of the quotient", and briefly explained how to teach the topic and how to improve students' accuracy and speed of calculation. Teaching methods were suggested around the topic and possible difficulties students would encounter in their learning were also brought up and analyzed with suggested solutions, etc. In general, before the preparation meeting, one of the teachers would be responsible for pointing out questions that may arise pertaining to the topic, suggesting relevant advices, and addressing other issues that may occur. The discussion circles around content and technique that students should learn, meanwhile teachers must make sure that they have full knowledge in the content, be aware of the possible issues, and choose efficient methods.

Group-preparation is very popular in China's urban schools, which creates a kind of "school culture" and becomes considerably influential to the quality of teaching. It is usually held once a week, formally or informally. Such activity provides teachers an opportunity to interact among themselves. They can raise their ideas regarding the use of textbooks and classroom teaching, which could improve teachers' professionalism as well, especially for young teachers. However, the study found that teachers paid more attention to the content and technique acquisition of students but no emphasis on other teaching goals, thus such group discussion seemed to involve only a few number of problems.

Besides group-preparation, teachers also do individual-preparation. Teachers are required to get ready for the teaching plan one week ahead of the teaching schedule. The teachers usually prepare for lessons individually by reading textbooks and teachers' reference books. The following interviews show how individual preparation is carried out.

> *"We don't have enough time to read more during preparations but we will consult some reference books before the lessons. We write lesson plans at the very beginning and try to keep doing so during the semester. But the actual lessons are more or less different from the plans. For example, we may come up with new problems during the class, especially when we write the plans one or two weeks ahead of time, but we don't have so much time to write the plans at the end of semester .Although we prepare before the lessons, there would still be changes which couldn't be predicted when writing the plan."* (US1-Interview-F)[6]

Some teachers regard preparing lesson plan as tedious and formalism and some teachers have their own methods and habits. These characteristics can be shown in the following interviews.

> *"We're required to finish the plan one week before the lessons, but I never have such habits. On the one hand, I don't think there is enough time; on the other hand, I used to prepare one day ahead of the lesson. If I prepare long before the lesson, I would forget something in class. It is because writing the plan is not as clear as teaching in class and I can hardly remember anything a week later. So what I usually do is to prepare one day ahead of the teaching."*

> *"Generally, we finish the plan in advance. We all consider it as a burden for teachers, so teachers seldom write the plans or really use the plan for teaching. The plan was like written for inspection only."* (US1-Interview-F)

3.2 *Lesson preparation in rural schools*

Individual-preparation is the main practice in rural schools and group-preparation is very unlikely to happen. There is normally only one class in each grade, especially in the village. One single teacher is

---

[6] "US1-interview-F" refers to interview with teacher F in Urban-1. Similar notations are used for other teachers.

responsible for teaching all the subjects of the class, thus there won't be any other teacher who teaches the same content at the same time and so group-discussion is impossible. Hence, individual-preparation is the only possible way to prepare for lessons in rural schools, which is similar to that in the urban schools, as shown in the following interview:

"Teachers usually prepare lessons according to the textbooks in units, such as reviewing how the word problems (应用题) look like. The first is multiplication and the second is division. Then the teacher will prepare one by one, what questions to ask and how to use the two methods of calculation in the sums; these are the questions that need to be solved during preparations. These preparations also help teachers recognize the goal of this unit according to the reference books, including how to allocate time in the course of teaching." (RS1-interview-C)

The teachers must write the plans beforehand and prepare for lessons according to the Ministry of Education. Teachers follow the teaching schedule and content which are set in the textbooks and reference books and deal with the questions one by one. However, the actual teaching in the classroom may not be exactly the same as planned. The plan is more like a task for inspection. Of course, it is still important for young teachers, as they can get familiar with the textbooks and the design of teaching through preparing lessons. Writing up lesson plans is also the process of learning from other teachers, including the understanding of the teaching methods mentioned in the reference books.

3.3 *Characteristics of the lesson preparation*

Lesson preparation is an important stage in mathematics teaching. It is emphasized both in urban and rural schools. To learn how to prepare for lessons and write up lesson plans are important tasks in teacher education programs, especially during their teaching practice in schools. For new teachers, the basic skill they need to master is how to prepare for lessons and to learn from the more experienced teachers. The administrators (directors and principals) often tell the teachers that "Do not ever enter the classroom without preparations and never teach without the plan". Preparing for lessons has become one of the regulations for teachers. Since the lesson plan is something substantial and also easily accessible, writing plans equated to having prepared for the lessons. However, due to the availability in resources and culture across schools, the differences in lesson planning between urban and rural schools become apparent, according to the above analyses:.

First, the form of the preparation is different. Teachers from urban schools can join the group-preparation organized by the District Teaching and Research Bureau (区教研室) or by the teachers of the same grade in school. They can also prepare the lessons individually. Thus, teachers can understand the textbooks and syllabi through different channels using different forms of preparation. Group-preparation is very common in urban schools, which plays an important role in the improvement of the quality of the preparation. In the interviews, many teachers talked about how the group-preparation can improve their teaching skills, which are especially useful for new teachers.

> *"There are group-preparations every week. We think about the teaching contents in the syllabus and textbook and the prerequisites of learning these contents. We also discuss the knowledge base of the student: the target, knowledge, ability, moral aspects, difficulties, teaching aid …… Schools are strict on the lesson preparations, and we may spend more time on some more complex topics. At the beginning, the teachers were not used to the format, but they could adjust themselves to it gradually, and felt comfortable later."* (US1-interview-G)

However, there are few opportunities for teachers in rural schools to communicate among themselves. Hence, in the rural areas individual-preparation is a common practice. Teachers prepare for lessons merely based on their own understanding of textbooks and reference books.

Second difference is in the effectiveness of the preparations. Teachers in urban schools have opportunities to engage in group discussion and do individual-preparation, therefore they seem to be able to write a more formal and complete lesson plan. While for teachers in rural schools, teachers' reference books are their main, if not only, resources for lesson preparation. Since these teachers mainly depend on their individual knowledge and experience, much more differences in the understanding of content would exist among them. Therefore, the preparation in rural schools is relatively limited and monotonous compared to that in urban schools.

4   Teaching in the Mathematics Classroom

The researchers observed 41 lessons in the four sample schools in the study. The analysis of the lessons provides a better understanding of mathematics classroom teaching in both urban and rural primary schools. The following shows two teaching cases, one from urban school and the other from rural school, followed by an analysis from the perspectives of lesson structure and teaching method.

4.1 *Teaching cases*

In China, each lesson lasts for 40 minutes in primary schools. There are several types of mathematics lessons, including learning new topics, doing exercises, reviewing lessons, and taking tests. The following two teaching cases are about "learning new topics". This type of lessons will take up two-thirds of all lessons. Most preparations are mainly done for this type of lessons, including group- and individual-preparation.

4.1.1 *Teaching case 1*

Teacher: urban school, female, 17 years of teaching experience
Grade: primary three
Topic: division word problems (除法应用题)

Teaching episode:
(a) Introduction (3 minutes and 30 seconds)
T (Teahcer): There are many kinds of quantitative relationships in our daily life. Now we will learn some basic quantitative relationships.
(Writing on the blackboard)

[Question 1]

T: Let's recall yesterday's assignment, to investigate "how much does mother spend on 500 grams of vegetables?"

S (Student): Mother spent 2 *yuan* on 500g of tomatoes.

S: Mother spent 1 *yuan* on 500g of vegetables.

T: How much does one exercise book cost?

S: 5 *jiao*[7].

S: 3 *jiao*.

T: Ok, what do we call the amount of money your mother spent on 500g of vegetables and you spent on your exercise book?

S: It is called "unit price".

T: Good, (writing on the blackboard). Repeat together.

S (altogether): Unit price

[Question 2]

T: How many meters can you walk per minute?

S: 20 meters per minute.

T: That's too slow.

S: 50 meters.

T: OK. So, do you know how many kilometers does the train travel per hour? Did you check it?

S: 60 kilometers.

S: 65 kilometers.

T: Ok, so what do we call the distance you or the train travel per hour?

S: Speed.

T: Good, speed. Repeat together.

S (altogether): Speed.

(b) Teaching new topic (19 minutes and 50 seconds)

T: Look at the blackboard and read out the problem.

S: The price of one tape recorder is 320 *yuan*. How much do four recorders cost?

T: Look for the given condition in the question and the answer needed.

S: There are two known conditions: first is the price of one recorder, 320 *yuan*, and the other is buying 4 recorders. The answer needed is how much is needed altogether.

T: Good, how to solve it?

S: 320×4.

T: Why?

---

[7] Ten cents.

S: Because the price of one recorder is 320 *yuan*. The question is how much do the 4 recorders cost, that is, how much is four "320 *yuan*". The answer is 1280 *yuan*.

T: Good. The price of one recorder is 320 *yuan* and what do we call the price of one product? What do we call the number of products bought? What do we call the amount of money spent on buying the 4 recorders? In this problem, how many quantities are there? Discuss it in groups and we'll see which group is the most enthusiastic.

(Student discussion) (45 seconds)

T: Which group would like to have a presentation?

S: There are three conditions: unit price, total amount, and total price.

T: Does any other group have other opinion?

S: In this problem, there are three conditions: unit price, amount, and total price.

T: Good. What do we mean when we say a recorder costs 320 *yuan*?

S: The cost of one recorder is the "unit price".

T: What is the meaning of "unit price"?

S: The "unit price" is the price of one product.

T: What is the meaning of "quantity"?

S: Amount.

T: What is the meaning of "amount"?

S: The amount is the number of pieces to be bought.

T: Are there other kinds of "quantity"?

S: Total price.

T: What is the meaning of "total price"?

S: The total price is how much the recorders cost together.

T: Good. In this problem, what are the "unit price", "amount", and "total price"?

S: The "unit price" is 320 *yuan*, the "amount" is 4, and the "total price" is 320 ×4 = 1280 *yuan*.

T: Correct or not?

S: Yes.

T: According to the equation, can you tell me the relationship among the "unit price", "amount", and "total price"?

S: unit price × amount = total price.

T: The following is a revision from what we have learnt before, how to rewrite multiplication word problems into division word problems. Now, can you change this word problem into division?

S: Four recorders cost 1280 *yuan*, so how much does one recorder cost?

T: Good, how can we solve it?

S: $1280 \div 4 = 320$, the unit is *"yuan"*. So, one recorder costs 320 *yuan*.

T: Can you summarize the equation from this problem?

S: The total price ÷ the amount = the unit price.

(c) Exercise (16 minutes and 5 seconds)

T: Based on the equation "speed × time = distance", what is "time" equal to? What is "speed" equal to? The first one?

S: time = distance ÷ speed.

S: speed = distance ÷ time.

T: Based on the equation "unit price × amount = total price", what are "unit price" and "amount" equal to, respectively?

S: "unit price" = total price ÷ amount. "amount" = total price ÷ unit price.

T: Based on the equation "efficiency × time = total workload", what is "efficiency" equal to? And what is "time" equal to?

S: "efficiency" = total workload ÷ time. "time" = total workload ÷ efficiency.

(d) Summary (1 minute 25 seconds)

4.1.2 *Teaching case 2*

Teacher: rural school, male, 12 years of teaching experience
Grade: primary six
Topic: division word problems

Teaching episode:

(a) Revision (1 minute and 10 seconds)

T: Let's review how to solve word problems by equation. What are the general steps when we solve word problems?

S: Understand the meaning of the problem, find out the unknown quantity, and then use x to represent it.

T: This is the first step.

S: Sort out the relationship of quantities in the question, write out the equation, solve the equation, double-check, and write the answer.

T: Good, someone else?

S: Understanding the meaning of the problem, find out the unknown quantity, and use x to represent it. Sort out the relationship of quantities in the question, write out the equation, solve the equation, double-check, and write the answer.

(b) Teaching new content (12 minutes and 10 seconds)

T: Now there are two word problems. (The teacher writes the word problem on the blackboard, and the students look at the blackboard); (1 minute and 30 seconds)

T: Now, look at this problem and who would like to read it?

S: The speed of light is 300 thousand kilometers per second. This distance is 7 times and twenty thousand kilometers more than the length of the equator. Then, how long is the equator?

T: Good, sit down please. Look at Example 1. Who can solve it? I hope you could solve it through equations not in the arithmetic way.

S: Let the length of the equator be x thousand kilometers and we can write the equation: $7x + 20 = 300$, $7x = 300 - 20$, $7x = 280$, $x = 40$.

T: Good, sit down please. Let's take a look if he got it right. (Writing out the equation). He said '$7x + 20 = 300$'; is it right?

S: Yes.

T: Of course he is right. But in order to show the given condition, what is the best way to write an equation?

S: $300 - 7x = 20$

T: Good, sit down please. $300 - 7x = 20$, (writing on the blackboard). Is it right or wrong? OK, these two are both right. But the second one matched a particular type of equation word problems — the bigger one subtracts the smaller one equals to the difference. (The teacher writes it on the blackboard and the students repeat after the teacher.)

T: The first one is easier to solve, then, how to solve the second one?

S: $7x = 300 - 20$, $7x = 280$, $x = 40$.

T: Good. Do not miss out the answers.

(The teacher writes the solution on the blackboard)

(c) Exercise (18 minutes)

T: Now, we will do some exercises. Turn your textbook to Page 84. Please use the exercise book. Equations should be used here. Only write the steps but don't calculate.

(d) Checking answers (6 minutes)

4.2   *Analysis of how mathematics lessons are structured*

The study analyzed the form of main class activities of the 41 sampled lessons and qualitative statistics was used to describe the different characteristics of activities between urban and rural mathematics classrooms. The following charts show the amount of time spent on different class activities, which help to understand the whole picture of classroom activities and their characteristics.

The analysis of percentages of teaching time allocated for different activities (see Figure 1) shows that delivering the new topics took up 55% of the whole class time and more than 30% of class time was spent on exercises in both types of schools. Moreover, rural schools spent more time on exercises than urban schools (37% vs. 32%).

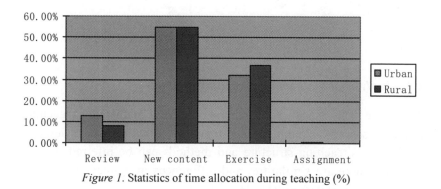

Figure 1. Statistics of time allocation during teaching (%)

The analysis of different activities (see Figure 2) shows that in both urban and rural schools, an average of 15 minutes were spent on general questions in the lessons, and the students' exercises took up about 13 minutes on average. The two activities altogether took 28 minutes, 70% of the whole class time. There is little cultivate questioning, which took only about 2 minutes on average. Rural teachers spent more time on explanation than urban teachers. However, Figure 2 shows that rural teachers did not spent time on discussion and operation, whereas urban teachers did so, although time spent was little (Discussion: 1 minute; Operation: 2 minutes).

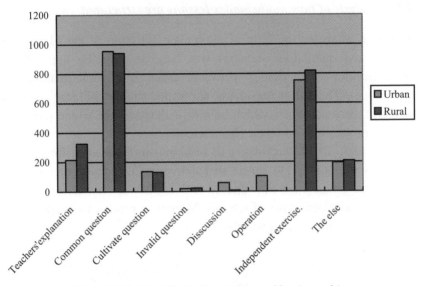

Figure 2. Statistics of activities during teaching (seconds)

4.3 *Analysis of mathematics teaching methods*

The above analysis shows the general context of mathematics teaching in primary schools. Summarizing together with the interviews, the mathematics teaching structure and methods can be inferred. It can be seen that there are similarities and differences in mathematics teaching between urban and rural schools.

4.3.1 *Common characteristics of mathematics teaching*

The analysis of different activities in mathematics lessons reveals the following common characteristics in urban and rural schools.

Firstly, the new topic is mainly delivered through oral communication between teachers and students. The dialogue between teachers and students is the main body of teaching. This kind of dialogue starts mainly from a question asked by the teachers and goes on in the format of "question and answer". Both the questions and the answers are very short. There are few open and inspiring questions that require student's critical thinking. Even in urban schools, simple questions are mostly asked. Dialogues between teachers and students have become a traditional or habitual teaching practice, during the lecturing and doing exercise in primary schools. Since 1950s, this kind of dialogue has become the mainstream in mathematics teaching. Such a teaching method shows that teachers and students are sharing the same experience and activity, but this sharing is only unilateral communication instead of interaction between the two. Students have few opportunities to raise questions and the teachers do most of the asking, which greatly limits the nurturing of student's critical thinking and independent problem solving.

Secondly, the process of teaching and learning centers on examples and exercises in the textbook. It can be inferred that teachers depend highly upon the textbook. The lessons typically begin with teacher-student dialogues following by analyzing in detail one or two examples in the textbook, which intends to help students to be familiar with the examples and the appropriate methods used. Then, teacher lets students do some exercises similar to the examples, giving students opportunities to express their understanding. If there is still some time, students will be given more tasks to do on their own. In case 2 above, the teacher firstly taught Example 1, then questioned the students how to solve the example, after that, the teacher asked the students to do Example 2 and analyzed the solution to the example. This process of teaching centered on these two examples.

Doing examples and exercises form the core of mathematics teaching, therefore many teachers often think and discuss with colleagues about the arrangements of examples and the design of exercises during lesson preparation and actual teaching. Besides the textbooks, workbooks are another main teaching resource, which are also identified as a form of textbooks. This aspect shows that teachers are "loyal" to the textbooks.

During the interview with teachers, many of them talked about their faith in the textbook. For example, one teacher said:

> *"I teach Example 7 first in this lesson and then do some exercises. There is another question, which is the transfiguration of Example 7. I ask the students to do it by themselves, and do exercises afterwards together. I would let students compete with each other and ask one or two students to show their calculation*

on the blackboard. Initially, I thought of teaching Example 6 and Example 7 together when I was preparing for the lessons, but the reference book suggested that this is a three-hour lesson, so I taught Example 6 yesterday followed by Example 7 today and did more exercises afterwards." (RS1-interview-E)

The teachers just followed the suggestions of textbooks and seldom deviated from it. The teaching methods adopted by the teachers are also a kind of imitations of those given in the reference books, especially in rural schools.

Lastly, doing exercise in the classroom occupies a large portion of teaching time. Previous quantitative statistics of classroom activities (see Figure 1) shows that the exercise session takes more than one-third of class time in both urban and rural schools. These exercises include independent and teacher-assisted exercises. The latter is more common in the classroom. In general, teachers would show students a few exercise questions from the textbooks. The whole class will then do some typical questions together with teacher leading them to find the solutions. Some time will also be given for students to complete other exercises on their own. In many classes that we observed, teachers did not let students do independent work due to the time constrain, although it was originally planned. Teachers usually planned a lot of activities during lesson preparations and students' independent exercise is often arranged at the end of the lessons. Whenever any other class activity overruns, students' independent exercise will be shorted or even cancelled. Thus, teachers and students often complete exercises together in classes.

Doing exercises has played an important role in mathematics teaching, which is related to teachers' perceptions of mathematics teaching in primary schools. "Practice makes perfect" (熟能生巧) has long been an important principle in mathematics teaching. Since 1960s, "integration of teaching and exercise" (讲练结合) and "teach only the essential and ensure plenty of practice" (精讲多练) have been dominant in the teaching methods. It is believed that doing more exercises is the key to good grades in mathematics. Mathematics teachers pay too much attention to the role of exercises under the idea that calculation is the core of mathematics teaching. Although the new curriculum reform is trying to change this concept and emphasize the training of students' ability to analyze and solve real life problems, this deep-rooted concept of mathematics teaching lasting for many years has made it difficult for people to change their minds about doing exercises in the near future.

4.3.2 *Difference in mathematics teaching between urban and rural schools*

The first difference is the format of questions asked by teachers in class. Teacher-student dialogue is the main teaching method used; therefore, how a question is posted highly influences the teaching quality. When reviewing the teaching cases, we found that more inspiring questions were asked in urban schools than in rural schools. Questions such as: "How to solve this problem?" "Why do you calculate in this way?" and "Is there another way to solve the problem?" were frequently asked. While in rural schools, these kinds of questions were seldom asked and simple dialogues between teachers and students were more likely to happen. Take the following questions as examples. When urban teachers asked questions like: "Could you tell me why?" and "Let's recall what we have learnt on rewriting multiplication to division and try to do it now", rural teachers would ask questions like: "Who can tell the class how to work out Example 1? It should be solved with equation not in the arithmetic way" and "Two known conditions are available. When we write the equations, the best way is find a given condition directly from the question. What conditions can be found in Example 1?" The difference in forming the questions matters, as inspiring questions can help students to improve their thinking ability and mathematics literacy.

The second difference is the format of activities in class. Urban classrooms make use of various teaching methods and are highly flexible. The interviews with urban teachers show that using various methods has become a regular practice in their daily teaching.

"Generally, the teaching method used depends on the teachers' habits. I usually ask the students to do the problems first and then ask students who can work out the problems to tell the class how to solve it. Students who make mistakes will be required to

analyze the reasons. I call this method "trial teaching".
Sometimes, I would let students talk over the questions, as there
are many issues to discuss. Each student may only have little
time to stand up and talk, but their ability to express themselves
must be trained through these kind of interactions in class."
(US2-interview-A)

The classroom observation shows that besides dialogues, students in urban schools also have many opportunities to engage in other forms of activities, such as discussions, demonstrations with teaching aids, group activities, observations, and practices, etc. In contrast, rural teachers teach in a more monotonous way, mainly through lecturing and asking simple questions, while other methods are seldom used. Teachers from rural schools usually follow a set pattern and use methods suggested by textbooks and reference books. The difference in the forms of class activities between urban and rural schools might be caused by the different approaches used by the teachers, assuming that the teaching contents are the same.

The third difference is the ability to make adjustments during classroom teaching between urban and rural teachers. When students come across difficulties in class, urban teachers usually guide students to think and encourage them to express their own ideas and allow them to come out with a variety of solutions. The teachers in the rural schools are more likely to go on with the pre-designed lesson plans and more concern with teaching schedule. Urban teachers usually handle students' queries through guiding them to understand further; instead, the teachers in the rural schools are more concerned with accomplishing the teaching task but less with students' needs. It seems that urban teachers' "student-oriented" teaching approach and rural teachers' "textbook-oriented" approach might produce different teaching effects. The following are the responses of two teachers in urban and rural schools respectively, which reflect the above connection.

"Normally, the students should be able to answer this question,
but today I don't know why the students did not answer the
questions correctly. Only a few students can answer correctly.
Actually, I did not intend to let students discuss today. However,

students today seemed not to understand the content well, so I asked them to discuss. Normally, if the students can understand the problem easily, I will simply lecture; if students have a clear mind of their own ideas, I would like them to discuss with each other. Sometimes it is beneficial to the students. The students can understand quickly after the discussion." (US1-interview-I)

"These two examples are not simple. I am afraid that the students could not finish them, so I explained to them instead. If there was enough time, I would like to ask the students to summarize and an exercise should be done. In the self-study period today, the students were told to memorize instead of discuss. Today we didn't have enough time, so I did the explanation". (RS1-interview-C)

The above shows that urban teachers are more flexible in adjusting their teaching arrangements: they would deal with students' difficulties at any time when students face problems during teaching. It is especially more evident for the more experienced teachers. Rural teachers pay more attention to finishing the teaching task. They fear that they cannot finish the lesson, so they explain a lot instead of letting students do the thinking and talking. Time constrain is usually the main reason for lack of exercises in rural schools. For rural teachers, keeping the teaching schedule and completing all the teaching tasks are important.

5 Factors that Influence Mathematics Teaching Method

There are many differences between mathematics teaching in rural and urban schools, and these differences are influenced by many factors, which are outlined in the following:

The first is the size of urban and rural schools. Urban and rural schools differ largely in their size, as there are 3-5 classes in each grade in urban schools, while in rural schools, especially the village primary schools, there is only one class in each grade. Urban schoolteachers have more opportunities to interact among colleagues than rural teachers do. Urban schools are able to ensure that constant communication is substantial among the teachers in the system through means like group-preparation. While in the rural schools, as there is only one class in each grade, it is quite impossible for teachers to find suggestions from other teachers, not to mention arranging group-preparation.

The second is the difference in the professionalism of teachers. If the school size is an external factor, the professionalism of teacher is an inherent factor. Rural teachers differ greatly in knowledge and competence from urban teachers. The educational level of rural teachers is usually up to junior high school level and some of them attended education institutes or colleges on the job. The initial education level of urban teachers is usually senior high school or above. The study shows that teachers' understanding about knowledge and the design of teaching methods can reveal the difference in teachers' professionalism. The following tables display the differences in subject knowledge and pedagogical content knowledge between the urban and rural teachers (see Table 1 and Table 2).

Table 1
Comparison of Subject Knowledge between Urban and Rural Teachers[8]

	Understanding of the current content			Mastering the focal points and difficulties			General understanding of the textbooks		
	Accurate	Moderate	Inaccurate	Accurate	Moderate	Inaccurate	Accurate	Moderate	Inaccurate
Urban	93%	7%		86%	14%		97%	7%	14%
Rural	5%	75%	15%	5%	65%	30%	15%	5%	75%

Table 2
Comparison of Pedagogical Content Knowledge between Urban and Rural Teachers

	Understanding of the mistakes students make easily	Understanding of the students' method of study	Clear description of the teaching process
Urban	10	14	15
Rural	4	2	2

The difference in teachers' professionalism reflects the difference in their pedagogical beliefs. Urban and rural teachers both believe that students' computational skills are crucial and put emphasis on the

---

[8] The data in t he tables are from the interviews with the teachers in the four schools.

training of the calculation during classes. They believe that computational skills are very important in the study of mathematics (see Wong, 2001, this volume). "Practice makes perfect", therefore, they ask students to do a lot of exercises, which is apparent in the interviews with the teachers and observations in the classrooms. Urban and rural teachers have different beliefs of their expectations on students. Urban teachers are more demanding and ask students to learn more and work harder. Rural teachers only require the students to learn the content in the textbooks without any other further requirement.

Teachers in the two types of schools also have different attitudes towards low achievers. Urban teachers believe that there are both personal and institutional reasons for low achievers. They affirm that by using appropriate and various ways of teaching can help low achievers' learning. However, rural teachers think that students get poor grades due to their low intelligence and their parents' ignorance, so that they believe that no effective way could be used to improve this kind of students' achievement.

The third difference is teaching culture in schools. School culture is an important factor in lesson preparation and classroom teaching. In the urban schools, faculties pay more attention to the education reform. Some teachers study the reform program and do research on problems that arise through daily teaching from their teaching experience. There are often public teaching activities about educational research or teaching practices. Teachers who do not join in the research can also attend these activities. Through these activities, the teachers can learn more teaching methods and accumulate valuable experiences. Interviews with the teachers and observations in Urban–1 show the relationship between teachers' concepts and researches conducted by the school. For instance, the teaching methods advocated by the research team are often tested by the pilot teachers; school seminars hosted by expert teachers are also incorporated. Obviously, this kind of research-oriented culture has affected day-to-day teaching. In the rural schools, even if there are any research programs, teachers have few opportunities and aspirations to participate. Although the teachers know how to solve the issues occurred during teaching, they seldom consider those as research topics or study on those issues consciously. Day after day, the teachers impart knowledge according to their understanding of the textbooks. This kind of cultural atmosphere is not helpful for teachers to improve their professional knowledge and capability.

In the urban schools, there is a culture of collegial exchange, which has great influence on the curriculum decision. The establishment of open classes (公开课) and seminars held by experienced teachers for young teachers (some schools adopt the apprentice system, where new teachers are led by their more experienced colleagues) are helpful to strengthen the culture. This culture brings more opportunities for teachers to understand each other's teaching design, to share different teaching beliefs, and to learn different teaching methods. The research shows that this kind of culture is helpful for teachers to improve their teaching, especially for the young teachers. The research on Urban–1 and Urban–2 shows that many young teachers believe that their professional growth is enhanced by such schools' class observation activities. They observe others' lessons and also have opportunities to be observed by others. Some teachers even actively requested the researchers to visit their lessons in this study. The teachers believe that their improvement in teaching skills is related to such an interaction and exchange. In contrast, there are few opportunities for teachers to communicate and study each other in rural schools. There was only one activity organized by the county during the two months of the study and only a few teachers attended the activity. To a certain extent, it limits teachers' development and improvement.

The fourth difference is the availability of teaching resources. There are great differences in the resources used in the lesson preparation of urban and rural schools. Besides textbooks and teacher reference books, there are plenty of out-of-school resources for the urban teachers, including a sufficiently sized library. Both the two urban schools in this study have a teachers' reading room, in which there are more than 10 kinds of professional periodicals and reference books. The teachers can refer to the related materials at any time. Moreover, the cities have bookstores and teachers can buy various teacher reference books conveniently, such as workbooks for students and other guidance materials. Whereas rural schools have limited teaching resources, there are no teachers' reading room and library at all in both two rural sample schools and only one or two kinds of professional periodicals are available. Besides teacher reference books, there are no other resources available for teaching. The difference of accessibility to teaching resources greatly influences teaching results.

6 Discussion

Primary mathematics schoolteachers form a big community in China and the analysis above only outlined some characteristics of their lesson preparation and classroom teaching. Due to the variation in the development among the districts, there are great differences between developed and developing areas. Though the cases in this chapter cannot illustrate the whole scene of mathematics teaching in the country, the teachers in the studies are representative in some common situations of mathematics teaching in China. The research does not include excellent teachers who have created and used new teaching methods and formats. This could be a limitation of this study. The new basic education curriculum reform issued in 2001 raised many new ideas and methods and it has been gradually implemented throughout the country. The new beliefs, like "care about the development of students", "everyone learns useful mathematics", "pay more attention to the real life situations", "advocate proactive explorations, communications and co-operations in teaching" and so on, have become the new directions for the teachers' endeavor. With further curriculum reforms, it is hoped that mathematics teaching in Chinese primary classrooms will make a greater progress based on the existing experiences.

Furthermore, the traditional mode of mathematics teaching is still deeply rooted in Chinese teachers' minds. There is a socially common conception among teachers, principals, and parents on the development of mathematics of the students, the value of mathematics, and classroom teaching. High regards on the practice of computational skills, emphasis on basic concepts and skills in teaching, and on lecturing and provision of an abundance of both in-class and out-of-class exercises are some of those. These are all apparent in the above analyses of both urban and rural mathematics classroom teaching. In recent years, some schools began to experiment discovery learning, learning through communications, and cooperative learning. Yet, the process of integrating these new teaching methods could be long and the process would also have vast differences between urban and rural schools. It is hoped that through the years of efforts, there could be great improvement in connecting mathematics with real life situations and the mode of classroom teaching in China, especially in teacher-student interactive learning. Moreover, it is believed that the atmosphere of having discourse among mathematics teachers, including group-preparation and action research, should be maintained and continuously improved. In this way, higher order thinking abilities, such as mathematical thinking, problem solving, and communication can be fully developed on the strong foundation of basic knowledge and basic skills.

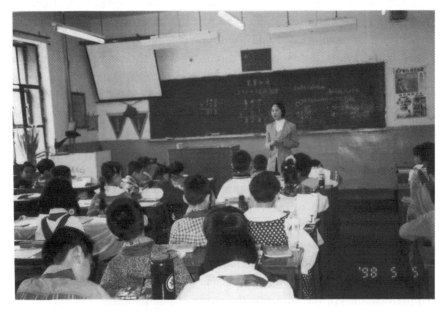

Figure 1. An urban classroom

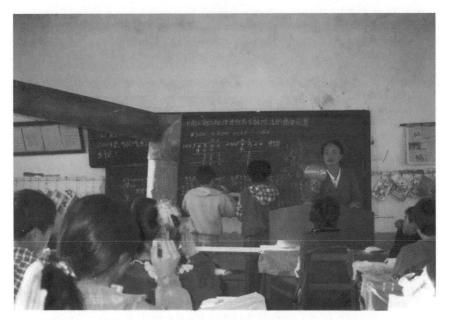

Figure 2. A rural classroom

References

Basic Education Curriculum Material Development Centre. (2001). *National mathematics curriculum standards at the compulsory education level (draft for consultation)* [In Chinese: 义务教育阶段国家数学课程标准(征求意见稿)]. Beijing: Beijing Normal University Press. (Retrieved from http://www.cbe21.com)

Calderhead, J. (1996). Teachers: Beliefs and knowledge. In D. C. Berliner & R. C. Calfee (Eds.), *Handbook of educational psychology* (pp. 709-725). New York: Macmillan.

China Education and Research Network. (2002). *China education development statistics annual report* [In Chinese: 2002 年全国教育事业发展公报]. Beijing: Author.

Clarke, B., Clarke, D., & Sullivan, P. (1996). The mathematics teacher and curriculum development. In A. J. Bishop, K. Clements, C. Keitel, J. Kilpatrick, & C. Laborde (Eds.), *International handbook of mathematics education* (pp. 1207–1233).

Clune, W. H. (1993). The best path to systemic educational policy: Standard/Centralized and differentiated/decentralized? *Educational Evaluation and Policy Analysis, 15*(3), 233–254.

Doyle, W., & Ponder, A. (1976/77). The practicality ethics in teacher decision- making. *Interchange, 8*(3), 1–12.

Fullan, M. G. (1991). *The new meaning of educational change* (2nd ed). New York: Teachers College Press.

Hargreaves, A. (1992). Cultures of teaching: A focus for change. In A. Hargreaves & M. G. Fullan (Eds.), *Understanding teacher development* (pp. 216-240). New York: Teachers College Press.

Lam, C. C. (1996). *Target oriented curriculum: A dream which will never come true?* (Monograph 1) [In Chinese 目标为本课程: 一个遥不可及的理想?]. Hong Kong: Hong Kong Institute of Educational Research, The Chinese University of Hong Kong.

Lam, C. C., Ma, Y., & Wong, N. Y. (1999, March). *How Chinese primary school mathematics teachers adapt the centrally-developed curriculum in their schools: A case study of two primary schools in Northeast China.* Paper presented at AERA annual meeting, Montreal, Canada.

Morris, P. (1996). *The Hong Kong school curriculum: Development, issues and policies* (2nd ed). Hong Kong: Hong Kong University Press.

Nespor, J. (1987). The role of beliefs in the practice of teaching. *Journal of Curriculum Studies, 19*(4), 317-328.

Nias, J., Southworth, G., & Campbell, P. (1992). *Whole school curriculum development in the primary school.* London: The Falmer Press.

Skilbeck, M. (1984). *School-based curriculum development.* London: Harper & Row.

Snyder, J., Bolin, F., & Zmwalt, K. (1992). Curriculum implementation. In P. W. Jackson (Ed.), *Handbook of research on curriculum* (pp. 402-435). New York: Macmillan.

Tuckman, B. W. (1995). The competent teacher. In A. C. Ornstein (Ed.), *Teaching: Theory into practice* (pp. 57–75). Boston, MA: Allyn & Bacon.

Wong, N. Y. (2001). The lived space of mathematics learning: From conception to action. Plenary lecture. In L. Sun (Ed.), *Proceedings of the international Conference on Mathematics Education* (pp. 6–19). Changchun, China: Northeast Normal University.

Chapter 16

Teaching Approach:
Theoretical or Experimental?

LI Jun

Probability is becoming a required part of school mathematics curriculum in China. In order to find an appropriate teaching approach, both theoretical and experimental approaches were examined in this chapter. The results of two studies on the two approaches show that each approach has its limitations. When probability was taught in a theoretical and formal way, students' intuitions could not be modified directly. When probability was taught in a frequentist and experimental way, students' knowledge of classical probability was not improved simultaneously. It is practical to teach both classical and frequentist definitions of probability at school level.

Key words: probability, curriculum development, cognitive framework

1 Introduction

Influenced by the worldwide growing movement to introduce elements of statistics and probability into school curriculum, the Ministry of Education (MOE) of China is pushing a reform to include statistics and probability in its elementary and secondary curriculum. In fact, this is not the first time in Mainland China to try to include them in its school curriculum. In 1980, the MOE once planned to arrange probability as a required part of contents for all senior high school students, but failed. Until 2001, probability was not taught at school level in most areas of China. Only a very few cities, such as Shanghai, have about 8 hours in total for the topic in grade 12, following the topic of permutation and combination.

There are at least three barriers for integrating statistics and probability into the school curriculum in China. First, the role of statistics and probability in solving real world problems was underestimated at that time. There was little use of data, probabilistic arguments, and language in newspapers and other media. For many people, only mathematicians or gamblers need probability. Second, from 1983, the MOE adjusted its innovation plan and set probability as an optional topic. Then probability was eliminated from National University Entrance Examinations. For Shanghai, only four out of 150 marks were allotted to probability in its University Entrance Examinations each year. In China, the National University Entrance Examination for school teachers is described as the baton to a band. With the significance placed on the National University Entrance Examinations, it was not surprising that probability was not taught or taught for a very short time in practice. Third, the teaching approach was highly abstract and formal. Quite a lot of senior high school students had difficulties in solving problems with complicated permutation and combination calculations shown below:

1. There are 8 different books, including 3 mathematics books, 2 foreign language books, and 3 other books. If put these books in a row on a bookshelf randomly, then the probability that all the mathematics books are put together while both foreign language books are also put together is _____. (Shanghai Municipal Educational Examinations Authority, 1996)

2. There are 4 white marbles and 3 black marbles in a bag. Pull out 3 marbles randomly. The probability that you get only one black marble is _____. (Shanghai Municipal Educational Examinations Authority, 1998)

Likely, these tasks are beyond most students' knowledge and abilities as well as teachers.

Before continuing further, let me first explain the meaning of the term "probability". There are three methods for assigning a probability to an event: namely, the classical, frequentist, and subjective definitions of "probability" (Johnson, 1992; Konold, 1991). The classical interpretation, or theoretical interpretation, defines the probability of an event as the ratio of the number of alternatives favorable to that event to the total number of equally likely alternatives. The frequentist interpretation, or experimental interpretation, defines probability in terms of the relative frequency of occurrence of an event in an infinite, or near infinite, number of trials. The subjective interpretation, or intuitive interpretation, is a personal evaluation of the likelihood of chance phenomena. The initial estimation is subject to adjustment according to new information such as the results of actual trials.

Probability was taught in a theoretical and formal way in the Mainland China. The frequentist and experimental definition of probability was despised, since it is posterior and inexact. Chinese students almost had no experiences of being involved in any concrete activities and simulations. Such a situation was also true in some other countries at that time. However, in 1977, Efron independently invented a resampling technique for handling a variety of complex statistical problems (Peterson, 1991). The development and application of that technique, especially in assistance of computer simulations, has elevated the experimental approach. Educators have suggested and implemented some reform projects that could be carried out at school level (Interactive Mathematics Program, 1998; Lovitt & Lowe, 1993; National Council of Teachers of Mathematics [NCTM], 1992; Newman, Obremski, & Scheaffer, 1987; Simon, 1992). A major aim of these projects is to provide opportunities for students to gain experiences in stochastic situations through problem solving or simulations, either manually or by using a computer, before being taught theoretically. Such an approach focuses on students' comprehension and application by the use of real data, activities, and visual simulations. It has attracted more and more attention in teaching. In this chapter, two studies on these two approaches (theoretical and experimental) were reported. Given the limited length of this chapter detailed results of the two studies can be found in Li (2000).

2 Study 1

The question of interest here is whether students' understanding of probability could be improved naturally without any formal instruction on this topic? According to the literature, western students' knowledge of the stability of frequencies was very weak (Fischbein & Gazit, 1984; Green, 1983; Piaget & Inhelder, 1951/1975). But did Chinese students also have poor understanding of the frequentist probability? Compared to students without any formal statistics and probability training, how better could the students who were trained under the theoretical approach behave when answering chance interpretation and chance comparison problems? In 1998, this author conducted a survey in Shanghai.

2.1 *Sample*

The sample was selected to include both students with and without any prior instruction in probability. Half of the classes were selected from ordinary schools (average schools) and the other half from advanced schools (containing about the top 10% of students). A total of 567 students were enrolled in 12 classes, 3 grades in 7 schools. The numbers of students in grades 6, 8, and 12 were 174, 209, and 184 and their average ages were about 11, 13, and 17 years old, respectively. The grade 12 students were the only group who had received prior instruction in probability (about 8 hours using a theoretical non-experimental approach to probability). Four classes were selected at each grade. A subset of 64 out of the 567 students was further interviewed.

Before 1997, high schools in Shanghai were classified into two streams, advanced and ordinary. But from 1997 on, the classification at the junior high level was eliminated. So for the grade 6 students, there was no general streaming examination, but as 1998 was the first year after the change, one advanced school was permitted to select its new grade 6 students from the whole city. One class in grade 6 was selected from this school and it was labeled as an advanced class.

2.2 *Questionnaire*

A total of 83 items (a sample of the items was included in Appendix) were used in each class, but each student was only required to answer one set of questionnaire, about 9 items (see Table 1). The 83 items covered four general categories: Category I – Identification of impossible, possible, and certain events; Category II – Interpretation of chance values; Category III – Chance comparison in one-stage experiments; and Category IV – Chance comparison in two-stage experiments.

Table 1
Overview of the Nine Sets of Questionnaire Used in Study 1

Set	Category I	Category II	Category III	Category IV
A	1(1), 2(2), 4(6)	1(3), 2(4), 3(8)	1(1), (2)	1, 6
B	1(2), 2(1), 4(5)	2(3), 3(4), 1(8)	1(3), (4)	8
C	1(3), 3(5), 4(1)	3(3), 1(4), 2(8)	2(1), (2)	9
D	1(4), 3(6), 4(2)	3(2), 1(6), 2(7)	2(3)	3, 7
E	1(5), 4(3), 3(4)	1(1), 2(5), 3(9)	2(4), 5, 9	
F	1(6), 4(4), 2(3)	2(1), 3(5), 1(9)	3(3), (4), 6, 10	
G	2(5), 3(1)	3(1), 1(5), 2(9)	4(1), (2), 7, 8	
H	2(6), 3(2)	1(2), 2(6), 3(7)	3(1), (2)	2, 10
I	2(4), 3(3)	2(2), 3(6), 1(7)	4(3), (4)	4, 5

Except 9 open-ended items, all the other 74 items were given in multiple-choice form, but students were allowed to give an answer that did not appear in the options. Moreover, students were also asked to provide explanations for their answers.

2.3 *Data coding*

The SOLO (Structure of the Observed Learning Outcome) taxonomy (Biggs & Collis, 1982; Collis & Biggs, 1991) was chosen as a cognitive framework describing students' hierarchical responses in this study. The students' responses to each item were labeled at five levels: prestructural

(P), unistructural (U), multistructural (M), relational (R) and extended abstract (E). The following cognitive framework, Table 2, guided by SOLO taxonomy was generated for coding.

Table 2
A Cognitive Framework Relating to Different Categories of Items Used in This Study

SOLO Level	Summary Description
P	Blank, fully irrelevant, illogical, egotistic answers or inability to become engaged in item answers.
U	Explains that probability just means may or may not happen and believes chance cannot be measured mathematically so chance comparison is impossible.
	Considers an incomplete set of outcomes in solving problem.
M	May consider all possible outcomes for a one-stage and sometimes for a two-stage experiment in qualifying uncertainty or estimating subjective chance value. For example, assigns an equal chance to each possible outcome for fairness.
	Interprets most likely to happen as meaning it should happen or interprets chance by frequency but without fully understanding the role of repetition.
	Uses rudimentary non-proportional reasoning in chance comparison.
R	Groups all possible outcomes in favor of a target event together and uses ratio as a measure of probability.
	Uses proportional reasoning in chance comparison.
	Knows that a larger number of repetitions is a more reliable predictor and expresses the idea of making a few repetitions automatically.
E	Assigns a calculated probability value in complicated situations, for example, involving two bags, two spinners and bases chance comparison on the values.
	Uses a generative strategy to construct sample space in a two- or three-stage experiment to work out probability.
	Suggests collecting data from a series of experiments and finding trends across sampling.

In this study, each student was assigned a descriptive understanding index, formed by a set of SOLO codes for all his or her written responses. All the responses, except for about 4% of them that could not be understood or where students answered another question that could not be coded, were labeled with a SOLO level.

2.4 *Results*

Table 3 shows that, both grade 6 and 8 students in the ordinary schools had the poorest understanding of probability, grade 6 and 8 students in the advanced schools had a slightly better understanding, but not as good as the grade 12 students in the ordinary schools. Grade 12 students in the advanced schools performed the highest among all the students tested.

Table 3
Number of Responses to All the Four Categories' Items by Response Level and by Grade

Number of responses in each level or cannot be coded	Grade 6		Grade 8		Grade 12	
	Adv	Ord	Adv	Ord	Adv	Ord
	463	1142	931	995	896	799
Prestructural	9 (2)*	72 (6)	18 (2)	35 (4)	12(1)	18 (2)
Unistructural	90 (19)	322 (28)	183 (20)	274 (28)	91 (10)	105 (13)
Multistructural	288 (63)	645 (57)	581 (62)	585 (58)	471 (54)	520 (66)
Relational	53 (11)	73 (6)	125 (13)	76 (8)	217 (24)	115 (14)
Extended abstract	5 (1)	0 (0)	8 (1)	2 (0)	83 (9)	32 (4)
Cannot be coded	18 (4)	30 (3)	16 (2)	23 (2)	22 (2)	9 (1)

*Numbers in brackets represent the proportion of the responses.

If we ignore the streams and compare the results for grades 6 and 8, the two grades without any formal probability training are virtually identical. It appears that there is no improvement in developmental level at the two grades.

Table 4 was generated to compare students' understanding in different categories. For all the grades, the lowest percentages of R or E responses were observed in Category I. This was mainly due to the fact that the items in this category (identification of impossible, possible, and certain events) could be answered appropriately without calculating probabilities. Therefore, the majority of responses observed in this category are at U or M level.

Table 4
Percentages of R or E Level Responses to All Categories' Items

Category	Streams	Grade 6		Grade 8		Grade 12	
I	Ordinary	R: 0%	0%	R: 1%	2%	R: 2%	12%
		E: 0%		E: 0%		E: 5%	
	Advanced	R:1%		R: 2%		R: 6%	
		E: 0%		E: 0%		E: 9%	
II	Ordinary	R: 5%	6%	R: 4%	7%	R:15%	21%
		E: 0%		E: 0%		E: 0%	
	Advanced	R:10%		R: 9%		R:25%	
		E: 0%		E: 0%		E: 1%	
III	Ordinary	R:14%	16%	R:17%	22%	R:23%	41%
		E: 0%		E: 0%		E: 6%	
	Advanced	R:20%		R:25%		R:42%	
		E: 3%		E: 2%		E:9%	
IV	Ordinary	R:10%	14%	R:14%	22%	R:23%	44%
		E: 0%		E: 1%		E: 7%	
	Advanced	R:22%		R:28%		R:25%	
		E: 2%		E: 1%		E:33%	

A slightly more but still few R and E responses were observed in Category II, where students' frequentist explanations of probability were investigated. In each grade, the vast majority of the responses were multistructural responses (for grades 6, 8, and 12, the percentages of M responses were 82%, 82%, and 70% respectively). It seems that student age, streams, and backgrounds in probability did not play a significant role in this category.

Does the skewed distribution towards the M level is a result of the ceiling effect? Table 5 shows that the percentages of items with R and E ceiling levels are similar in Categories II and III. However, Table 4 shows that more R level responses were observed in Category III in each grade. This means that the skewed distribution observed in Category II is not a result of the ceiling effect, but the students' limited knowledge of frequentist probability. Chinese students' understanding of frequentist probability was poor compared to their understanding of classic probability.

Table 5
Numbers of Items in Each Category that Have a Ceiling Level of M, R, and E

Ceiling level	M	R	E	SUM
Category 1	14	2	8	24
Category 2		18	9	27
Category 3		16	6	22
Category 4		2	8	10
Total				83

The variation between grade 12 students and the younger students, who have had no exposure to probability, appears to be less pronounced in Category II (interpretation of chance values) and more pronounced in Category IV (chance comparison in two-stage experiments). This result is not surprised, given the limited experience that the grade 12 students had with the frequentist definition of probability and their probability lessons were mainly focused on probability calculations.

3 Study 2

Before 2001, probability was not a part of school mathematics for all Chinese junior high school students. Is it possible to start the teaching of probability earlier if the experimental approach was applied? An activity-based short-term teaching intervention was done in Shanghai in 1999.

3.1 *Sample*

Two ordinary grade 8 classes, one with 23 students and the other with 26 students, participated in the study. The students' ages were 13-14 years, except for one student who was 15 years old.

3.2 *Questionnaire*

Nine parallel items were used in the pre- and post-test. Eight of them were selected directly from the 83 items developed for study 1 and the other one, relating to the frequentist explanation of probability, was new. All the students were interviewed individually before and after the two tests and all of the interviews were audiotaped.

3.3 *Teaching*

Six 40-minute lessons (twice a week) outside regular class time were conducted with the two grade 8 classes. The teaching was activity-based combined with whole class discussion. It focused on the misconceptions related to identification of impossible, possible, and certain events and the frequentist definition of probability observed from Study 1. The two classes were taught slightly differently: one with a computer and the other without a computer. For the class with computer, once all students had finished their trials with dice, coins, and so on, and pooled their data, teacher (this author) would ask the students to look at the big screen and observe what would happen when she made different trials by computer simulations. For another class without visual simulations, the students were asked to read the data from a long series of experiments printed at the end of their workbooks and they were told that the data were computer generated. However, most of the teaching conditions such as activities, workbooks, problems for whole class discussion, and teacher were the same for the two classes.

The structure of each day's lesson is similar, as illustrated below:

1. The meaning of the terms "impossible", "possible", and "certain" were explained by teacher on the first day. On the

other days, the main problem that had been solved in the last class was briefly reviewed by the teacher.

2. The main problem being presented was described.
3. An explanation was given on how to carry out the activity and how to record the data.
4. A presentation outlining some of the wrong conclusions or reasons related to the specific task, such as number 6 is the hardest number to be rolled, was made and the wrong conclusions or reasons printed in their workbooks were briefly discussed.
5. Students did the activity in pairs and recorded the results.
6. The students' data were pooled or they were given the computer-generated data, depending on time.
7. The wrong conclusions were discussed again in light of the results of the experiment they had completed.

3.4 *Results*

Two of the major findings associated with the teaching are included here. First, an activity-based short-term teaching program can help grade 8 students improve their understanding of probability. Table 6 describes the students' performance in terms of the SOLO analysis of responses.

Table 6
Overall Picture of Students' SOLO Levels in Pre-test and Post-test

Percentages of responses in each level	Pre-test		Post-test	
	W/ 26	W/O 23	W/ 26	W/O 23
Prestructural	0%	2%	0%	0%
Unistructural	33%	31%	3%	2%
Multistructural	58%	53%	55%	49%
Relational	8%	14%	29%	30%
Extended abstract	1%	0%	13%	19%

Second, it appears that studying frequentist probability does not necessarily contribute to students' knowledge of classical probability. In the teaching intervention, the frequentist definition of probability was emphasized but the classical definition was not given. After the teaching, it was found that some students could use proportional reasoning in chance comparison but actually they did not know the real chance values.

4 Conclusions and Implications

The following conclusions can be drawn from the two studies: (1) Students' understanding of probability does not improve naturally with age - teaching plays an important role; (2) Students' understanding of probability can be improved after instruction; (3) Introducing probability in the experimental approach or in the theoretical approach cannot replace each other; each has its own role in helping students' understanding of probability; and (4) Students' cognitive development in frequentist probability is slow, if no direct instruction is given.

What didactical implications can be indicated from the two studies? According to the results of Study 2, we can state the first implication, that is, it is possible to introduce probability effectively to Chinese students at an earlier age by an experimental approach.

Compared to the tasks selected from National University Entrance Examination Test Paper, the chance comparison items given by questionnaires are simple. However, about 50% of responses to Category III and IV given by the grade 12 students in Study 1 were at U or M level. Many of these responses revealed that students had misconceptions such as "chance cannot be measured mathematically" and "equiprobability". The percentages of the grade 12 students used these two misconceptions at least once are 19% and 18% respectively (Li & Perira-Mendoza, 2002). Therefore, it is possible to learn some basic probability calculations in a short time, however, this does not mean the students really believe or have confidence in the results of their calculations and abandon their intuitions when they are contrary to the theory. In Study 2, after the teaching intervention, it was found that the misconception "chance cannot be measured mathematically" could be overcome obviously but for some students, misconceptions such as "equiprobability" were remaining. So the second implication here is in order to modify students' intuitions, it's better to spread probability teaching for a few years. Concentrate all the probability teaching in a short term does not help overcoming some stable misconceptions that students have developed from a relatively early age.

The third implication is that both the frequentist and classical definitions of probability should be taught. In Study 1, the grade 12 students had poor understanding of frequentist probability. In Study 2, some of the grade 8 students could use proportional reasoning in chance comparison but actually they did not know how to calculate the chance values. These facts suggested that both classical and frequentist definitions of probability should be taught and both theoretical approach and experimental approach are needed at school level.

Is it now the right time for China to introduce probability into school mathematics again? Are not the three main barriers mentioned above existed any more now? Fortunately, some changes have taken place during the past twenty years. The numerical, experimental approach of teaching probability has been introduced into China. Some researchers (e.g., Garfield & Ahlgren, 1988; Hawkins & Kapadia, 1984; Konold, 1991; Shaughnessy, 1993) have recommended teaching strategies to improve students' understanding in probability, One of the teaching strategies is related to the creation of situations to encourage students to examine, modify, or correct their own beliefs of probability or others' common misuses of probability by the use of real data, activities, and visual simulations. They preferred to base the teaching on authentic situations rather than abstract and irrelevant contexts. Garfield (1995) affirmed these recommendations again but noted the tendency to incorporate technology such as computers, calculators, multimedia, and internet resources in teaching. These recommendations should be helpful and useful for the current curriculum reform in China.

Acknowledgments

This paper is based on the author's doctoral dissertation, which was completed under the supervision of Dr. Lionel Pereira-Mendoza.

References

Biggs, J. B., & Collis, K. F. (1982). *Evaluating the quality of learning: The SOLO taxonomy*. New York: Academic Press.

Collis, K. F., & Biggs, J. B. (1991). Developmental determinants of qualitative aspects of school learning. In G. Evans (Ed.), *Learning and teaching cognitive skills*. (pp. 185-207). Melbourne, Australia: Australian Council for Educational Research.

Fischbein, E., & Gazit, A. (1984). Does the teaching of probability improve probabilistic intuitions? *Educational Studies in Mathematics, 15*, 1-24.

Garfield, J. B. (1995). Reflections on the past 15 years. *Teaching Statistics, 17*(2), 77-78.

Garfield, J. B., & Ahlgren, A. (1988). Difficulties in learning basic concepts in probability and statistics: Implications for research. *Journal for Research in Mathematics Education, 19*, 44-63.

Green, D. R. (1983). School pupils' probability concepts. *Teaching Statistics, 5*(2), 34-42.

Hawkins, A., & Kapadia, R. (1984). Children's conceptions of probability – A psychological and pedagogical review. *Educational Studies in Mathematics, 15*, 349-377.

Interactive Mathematics Program. (1998). *Interactive mathematics program. (Integrated high school mathematics)*. Berkeley, CA: Key Curriculum Press.

Johnson, R. (1992). *Elementary Statistics*. Boston, MA: PWS-KENT Publishing Company.

Konold, C. (1991). Understanding students' beliefs about probability. In E. von Glasersfeld (Ed.), *Radical constructivism in mathematics education* (pp. 139-156). Dordrecht, The Netherlands: Kluwer Academic.

Li, J. (2000). *Chinese students understanding of probability*. Unpublished doctoral dissertation, National Institute of Education, Nanyang Technological University, Singapore.

Li, J., & Pereira-Mendoza, L. (2002). Misconceptions in probability. In B. Phillips (Ed.), *Proceedings of 6th International Congress on Teaching Statistics* [CD-ROM]. Voorburg, the Netherlands: International Statistical Institute.

Lovitt, C., & Lowe, I. (1993). *Chance and data investigations* (Vol. 1 & 2). Carlton, Vic: Curriculum Corporation.

National Council of Teachers of Mathematics. (1992). *Data analysis and statistics across the curriculum*. Reston, VA: Author.

Newman, C. M., Obremski, T. E., & Scheaffer, R. L. (1987). *Exploring probability*. Palo Alto, CA: Dale Seymour.

Peterson, I. (1991). Pick a sample. *Science News, 140*, 56-58. (Also retrieved from http://www.resample.com/content/teaching/texts/picksample.txt)

Piaget, J., & Inhelder, B. (1975). *The origin of the idea of chance in children*. (L. Leake, Jr., P. Burrell, & H. D. Fishbein, Trans.). New York: Norton. (Original work published 1951).

Shanghai Municipal Educational Examinations Authority. (1996). The 1996 National University Entrance Examination Test Paper in Shanghai [In Chinese 1996 年全国普通高等学校招生统一考试上海数学试题（理工农医类）]. *Mathematics Teaching* [In Chinese 数学教学], *146,* 32-35.

Shanghai Municipal Educational Examinations Authority. (1998). The 1998 National University Entrance Examination Test Paper in Shanghai [In Chinese 1998 年全国普通高等学校招生统一考试上海数学试题（理工农医类）]. *Mathematics Teaching* [In Chinese 数学教学], *157,* 36-37.

Shaughnessy, J. M. (1993). Probability and statistics. *The Mathematics Teacher, 86,* 244-248.

Simon, J. L. (1992). *Resampling: The new statistics*. Belmont, CA: Duxbury Press.

Appendix

Sample Items Used in Questionnaires

Category I items:

I1   A six-sided normal die is rolled once. Please indicate whether the following outcome is impossible, possible or certain to happen. Tick where appropriate:

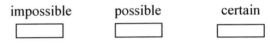

impossible   possible   certain

a) the number rolled is an even number.
b) the number rolled is smaller than 7.
c) the number rolled is bigger than 6.
d) the number rolled is 2.
e) the number rolled is 6.
f) the number rolled is not 6.

Category II items:

II2(1) A mathematician filled a bag with black and white marbles. He didn't really know how many black marbles and white marbles were in the bag. After mixing them thoroughly, he took a look and predicted that "if I pull out a marble from the bag without looking, the chance that it will happen to be white is 80%." Which of the following has the closest meaning to "the chance that it will happen to be white is 80%"?
a) the marble pulled out will certainly be white
b) the marble pulled out will certainly be black
c) suppose that the game is repeated 10 times, white marbles are pulled out around 8 times

  d) suppose that the game is repeated 10 times, white marbles are pulled out exactly 8 times

II2(4) A mathematician filled a bag with black and white marbles. He didn't really know how many black marbles and white marbles were in the bag. After mixing them thoroughly, he took a look and predicted that "if I pull out a marble from the bag without looking, the chance that it will happen to be white is 80%." He pulls out a marble. The marble is white. Do you think the mathematician's prediction is accurate or not?

II2(7) A mathematician filled a bag with black and white marbles. He didn't really know how many black marbles and white marbles were in the bag. After mixing them thoroughly, he took a look and predicted that "if I pull out a marble from the bag without looking, the chance that it will happen to be white is 80%." Here are five situations. Comparatively speaking, in which situation can the mathematician's prediction be considered very accurate?
  a) pulling out a marble and it happens to be a white marble
  b) pulling out a marble and it happens to be a black marble
  c) suppose that the game is repeated 10 times, white marbles are pulled out 10 times
  d) suppose that the game is repeated 10 times, white marbles are pulled out 9 times
  e) suppose that the game is repeated 10 times, white marbles are pulled out 8 times

Category III items:

III1 A class has 20 girls and 22 boys in it. Each pupil's name is written on a piece of paper and all the names are put into a box and mixed thoroughly.

  (1) The teacher picks 1 name out of the box casually without looking. Which statement below is correct?
  a) it is more likely to pick out a boy's than a girl's name

       b) it is less likely to pick out a boy's than a girl's name

       c) it is equally likely to pick out a boy's as a girl's name

       d) it is impossible to compare the likelihood of the two outcomes

(2) Return the name into the box and mix thoroughly again. Now, the teacher picks 6 names out of the box casually without looking. The 6 names are 2 girls and 4 boys. He placed the 6 slips on the table, closes his eyes and does the 7th draw from among the rest of the slips in the box. Which statement below is correct?

    a) it is more likely to pick out a boy's than a girl's name this time

    b) it is less likely to pick out a boy's than a girl's name this time

    c) it is equally likely to pick out a boy's as a girl's name this time

    d) it is impossible to compare the likelihood of the two outcomes

III5   There are 8 red marbles and 16 black marbles in bag A. There are 50 red marbles and 70 black marbles in bag B. Mix the marbles in each bag thoroughly. Close your eyes and suppose you want to pull out a black marble. Which statement below is correct?

    a) the likelihood of pulling out a black marble from bag A is greater than that from bag B

    b) the likelihood of pulling out a black marble from bag A is less than that from bag B

    c) the likelihood of pulling out a black marble from bag A is the same as that from bag B

    d) it is impossible to compare the likelihood of the two outcomes

Category IV items:

IV5   There are 8 red marbles and 16 black marbles in bag A. There
        are 50 red marbles and 70 black marbles in bag B. Mix the
        marbles in each bag thoroughly. Put your hands in two bags and
        pull out a marble from each bag without looking. Which
        statement below is correct?
        a) it is most likely that both marbles are red
        b) it is most likely that both marbles are black
        c) it is most likely that one marble is red and the other
            one is black
        d) it is impossible to indicate which one is the most
            likely among the three outcomes

Chapter 17

Capturing the Chinese Way of Teaching: The Learning-Questioning and Learning-Reviewing Instructional Model

AN Shuhua

This study explores the mythical qualities of learning mathematics in China by addressing the unique characteristics of Chinese mathematics teaching and learning: using the learning-questioning and learning-reviewing instructional model to enhance students' understanding of mathematics concepts and reinforce mathematics proficiency. Furthermore, this study investigates Chinese teachers' beliefs in using the learning-questioning and learning-reviewing instructional model and their impact on teaching and learning mathematics. Four fifth-grade mathematics teachers from four schools in a large city in Jiangsu Province participated in this study. Data were collected via classroom observations and interviews with participating teachers. Findings indicate that Chinese teachers were able to apply various methods to help students learn mathematics, focusing on questioning and reviewing strategies and helping students to understand mathematics concepts and develop mathematics proficiency. Furthermore, Chinese teachers' beliefs have a deep impact on their teaching practices: teachers believe that conceptual understanding and procedural development are equally important in mathematics teaching; teaching mathematics is teaching the thinking method.

Key words: questioning and reviewing, thinking method, teachers' beliefs, prior knowledge, mathematics proficiency

1 Introduction

In the past decades, international perspectives in mathematics education have been broadly growing in various areas. Many studies have focused on teachers' knowledge. Ma (1999) focused on mathematical content knowledge and advocated that elementary teachers should have profound mathematics knowledge, while An (2000) indicated that a connection is needed between content and pedagogical knowledge and called to enhance mathematics teachers' pedagogical content knowledge. Other studies explored students' learning and found that Chinese students were good at computation skills (J. Cai, 2000, 2001). Evidences from international studies, such as the TIMSS and TIMSS-R, indicate that teaching is one of the major factors related to students' achievement. These studies revealed that Asian students, such as students in Singapore, Japan, South Korea, and Hong Kong, scored highest among 41 regions in the Third International Mathematics and Science Study (National Center for Education Statistics, 1999). To understand why Asian students are more proficient in mathematics and to know what vital factor makes Asian students successful in learning mathematics, substantial international study is needed to explore the characteristics of mathematics classroom teaching from an insider's perspective. Furthermore, it is also necessary to investigate the cultural and belief systems in mathematics education and to find out the impact of the culture and beliefs on mathematics learning and teaching. This international study will lead researchers and educators to develop a deep understanding of the various aspects of mathematics teaching and learning and it will lead teachers to question their own traditional teaching practice and bring out better choices in constructing the teaching process (Stigler & Perry, 1988).

The culture and societies in Asian countries, such as China, have different philosophies and beliefs compared to the West, regarding the teaching and learning of mathematics. This results in different approaches to teaching and learning mathematics. Examining these different beliefs and approaches provides opportunities for sharing, discussing, and debating important issues of mathematics education (Robitaille & Travers, 1992) and sparks a light of understanding on how to teach and learn mathematics differently and effectively using common goals.

For many years, mathematics learning in China has been mythlike to the West; questions on how Chinese students learn mathematics effectively and differently have often been inquired into by international studies in recent years. This study attempts to explore the mythlike qualities of learning mathematics in China by addressing the special characteristics of Chinese mathematics teaching: using the learning-questioning and learning-reviewing instructional model to build students' understanding of mathematics concepts and enhance their proficiency in mathematical skills. Furthermore, this study investigates Chinese teachers' beliefs on the learning-questioning and learning-reviewing instructional model and their impact on teaching and learning mathematics in elementary schools.

2   Learning-questioning and Learning-reviewing Instructional Model

2.1   *The influence of Chinese culture on mathematics teaching and learning*

China's five thousand years of civilization is greatly respected and admired all over the world. Whitehead (1925) stated, "The more we know of Chinese art, Chinese literature, and Chinese philosophy of life, the more we admire the heights which that civilization attained" (p. 6). In China, Confucius' philosophy plays an important role in China's civilization and has a deep impact on Chinese education. The successful education systems in China, Japan, and Singapore are all based on their use of Confucianism (Spring, 1998).

Under the influence of Confucian philosophy, the Chinese believe that learning is honorable, which means in order to be at the top of society, one must be a scholar (Ashmore & Cao, 1997). For many centuries, Chinese education was characterized as scholar-nurturing education. One of the distinctive features of scholar-nurturing education was building a solid foundation in education by practicing a rigorous examination system (An, 2000). Mathematics education in China was equated with proficient and fluent skills that could be used to pass rigorous examinations, and ultimately, to apply and solve real world problems.

Traditional mathematics in China was also influenced by the *Nine Chapters on the Mathematical Art* from the Tang Dynasty (581-618 A.C.). The salient feature of this book is a sequence of mathematics questions, answers, and principles. Specifically, the procedure of this model of education is to pose a question, to find the solution to the question, to use the principle to explain the problem, and to apply it in the real world. The center of this instructional model is the use of the questioning strategy, while the emphasis is on the proficiency of computations. The teaching model of the *Nine Chapters on the Mathematical Art* had a great impact on the development of mathematics education in China. It has brought forward a traditional mathematics style that is very useful in application and calculation (Li & Chen, 1995).

2.2 *Inquiry process of learning—questioning and reviewing*

According to Confucianism, to acquire knowledge one needs to not only study for knowledge but also question new learning, which requires thinking while learning; to retain the knowledge and reinforce understanding, one needs to not only learn but also review, which means that the learning should integrate "reviewing" into the learning process. These beliefs in learning are reflected in the construction of the Chinese words for "knowledge" and "learn." The word "knowledge" in Chinese is formed by two verbs: learn (学) and question (问), which address the approach to learning: to learn well, one must ask questions; it also addresses the approach to teaching: to teach for understanding, one must use questions to promote students' thinking. The Chinese word 学习 (learn) is constructed from two verbs: learn and review, which mean that one must consistently review the knowledge that has been learned in order to learn well. These two phases of learning indicate Confucianism's belief that in reviewing prior knowledge, one can always find new knowledge (X. Cai, & Lai, 1994). Together, learning-questioning and learning-reviewing became an important instructional model in Chinese mathematics teaching.

In the process of learning-questioning-learning-reviewing, learning becomes a cycle in a process of inquiry. This inquiry process provides a model for effective teaching and learning. To help students acquire knowledge, teachers need to pose questions to promote students' thinking, in which students review prior knowledge and make a connection to new knowledge and acquire new knowledge; to reinforce understanding of new knowledge, teachers engage students in a review of new learning and also use questions to support students' thinking and to gain new insight from the review (see Figure 1). In this model of learning, teachers ask questions to promote students' active thinking and connect their prior knowledge to the new learning. To achieve proficiency in conceptual understanding and procedural development, students review regularly and constantly by doing extensive and layered practices. Mathematics education in China has followed this pattern for classroom teaching and learning for centuries.

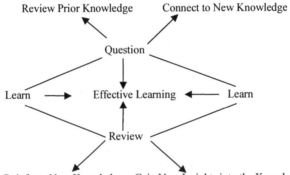

Figure 1. Inquiry process of learning in China

This study investigates how Chinese teachers use the unique inquiry process of the learning-questioning-learning-reviewing instructional model in teaching mathematics in order to enhance students' understanding of mathematics concepts and reinforce students' mathematics proficiency. Moreover, this study examines Chinese teachers' beliefs in this instructional model and their beliefs' impact on teaching in elementary schools in China.

3 Methodology

3.1 *Subjects*

The subjects were four fifth-grade mathematics teachers from four schools in a large city in Jiangsu Province in China. All teachers had a three-year education certificate from Normal Schools after finishing nine years of primary and junior high school education; some of them also had a three-year university diploma. They had an average of 15 credit hours in mathematics courses in college or at a Normal School. Their average length of teaching experience was seven years. The subjects were selected according to the following criteria: (1) currently teaching mathematics in fifth- to sixth- grades, (2) having at least three years of teaching experience at the fifth- to sixth- grade levels, (3) teaching in schools that have typical characteristics of public schools in China, and (4) willing to provide the data relevant to the reliability and validity of this study, including classroom observations and interviews.

3.2 *Procedures*

Data were collected via observations and interviews with participating teachers in four schools in China.

3.2.1 *Classroom observation*

The observations were conducted at a pre-arranged date and time and each teacher was observed once. Field notes and audiotape recordings were conducted during the classroom observations by using an Instructional Criteria Observation Checklist as a guide for observation. The Checklist was constructed using the criteria for analyzing the instructional quality of mathematics textbooks (American Association for the Advancement of Science, 2000). The goals of the observations were to explore how Chinese teachers teach mathematics in classrooms, and to identify some effective strategies in mathematics teaching.

3.2.2 *Interviews*

After each observation, an interview was conducted by using a set of interview questions. The interview was conducted in each teacher's office and it took 30 minutes for each interview. The sample interview questions related to teaching strategies and included the following: What is your primary focus in teaching mathematics? What do you think is the most effective teaching method? What teaching methods do you usually use? How do you know about your students' thinking and understanding? How do you promote students' ability to think? Describe the type of questions you ask. These sample questions have as the objectives of the interviews to examine teachers' beliefs about teaching strategies and the impacts of these beliefs on their teaching practice, and to confirm the learning-questioning and learning-reviewing instructional model as one of the effective teaching approaches in the observed Chinese mathematics classrooms.

3.3 *Data analysis*

Transcriptions were made of the observations and interviews. The responses to the interview questions and the field notes and checklists from the observations were also analyzed through the use of concept mapping to identify teaching strategies and clarify teachers' key beliefs and their impacts on teaching practices. The results of data analysis confirmed that the teachers' responses to the interview questions about the learning-questioning and learning-reviewing instructional model were consistent with their actual classroom practices.

4 Results

A report of classroom observations on the instructional model of the learning-questioning-learning-reviewing process and a discussion of teachers' beliefs and their impacts on mathematics teaching are included below.

4.1 *Observation of classroom teaching*

The duration of observation of classroom teaching was 45 minutes for each class. The following were selected sample segments of classroom teaching in this study. These samples are presented in two planning variations in this study: (1) learning-questioning and learning-reviewing at the beginning of the new lesson and (2) learning-questioning and learning-reviewing during the new lesson.

4.1.1 *Beginning of the lesson – Connection of prior knowledge using question strategies*

In order to help students learn new concepts and skills, all four teachers integrated question strategies into their teaching. They designed layered questions in a logical and sequential order. These questions promoted students' recall of prior knowledge and its relation to new learning. Furthermore, the questions encouraged and supported students' thinking. The following examples addressed how Chinese teachers used the question strategy at the beginning of the new lesson.

Ms. Ren's class. A fifth-grade teacher with 14 years of teaching experience knew the importance of promoting students' thinking. In the lesson on comparison of volumes and surface areas of rectangular prisms, Ms. Ren first related the lesson to prior knowledge on how to find surface area and volume and then posed three questions on the blackboard to introduce the comparison of the volume and the surface area of rectangular prisms:

1. What is the meaning of the surface area of a rectangular prism? What about the volume of the rectangular prism?
2. What is the basic unit of the surface area for a rectangular prism? Of the volume?
3. To calculate the surface area of the rectangular prism, what sides do we need to measure? What about volume?

To help students understand the questions, she had a student read the problem to the class first and grouped the students by four to observe the rectangular prisms they made on paper; they then discussed these three questions.

In order to know students' thinking, Ms. Ren asked two students to report the results of the group discussion. To reinforce students' understanding, Ms. Ren summarized their key points: The differences between the surface area and the volume of a rectangular prism are in meaning, basic units, and methods of calculation; to find the surface area and volume of rectangular prisms, we need to measure the length, width, and height.

In this lesson segment, Ms. Ren posed three questions linked closely to the central point of the new lesson. Question 1 connected students' prior knowledge on finding the surface area with their knowledge on volume; questions 2 and 3 encouraged students to think about the differences of the basic units and of the calculations for surface area and for volume. By having students discuss and answer these questions, Ms. Ren provided a connection for students to learn new knowledge by comparing the volume and the surface area of rectangular prisms.

Ms. Jing's class. Ms. Jing has been teaching for four years, and like Ms. Ren, she also connected students' prior knowledge to the new lesson first. The topic of the lesson was to change fractions into decimals using terminating and non-terminating concepts.

The first introductory activity was to have students solve a set of five fractions orally.

She asked, "How do you change the following fractions to decimals?", and had students change the following fractions to decimals:

$$\frac{3}{10}, \frac{7}{100}, \frac{9}{100}, \frac{35}{100}, \frac{125}{1000}$$

These five fractions with denominators in powers of 10 directed students to recall a simple way of changing fractions into decimals. However, after students answered the questions, Ms. Jing asked, "If fractions do not have denominators like 10, 100, 1000... how can we change these fractions into decimals?" This question encouraged students to think further about changing fractions into decimals and connected students' knowledge to the new lesson.

She showed a second set of fractions with different denominators and asked, "How do you change the following fractions into decimals?" and "How many ways can you solve them?"

$$\frac{3}{4}, \frac{7}{25}, \frac{9}{40}, \frac{3}{14}, \frac{7}{9}$$

These questions promoted students thinking for finding different ways to change fractions into decimals: (1) using division and (2) for some problems, changing denominators to 100.

In the above teaching, Ms. Jing designed two sets of different levels of fractions to connect the new lesson of changing fractions into decimals. By answering questions and solving these problems, students were ready to explore changing fractions using terminating and non-terminating concepts.

4.1.2 *Beginning the new lesson – Connection of prior knowledge using the review process*

All Chinese teachers were able to design a set of problems for students to review at the beginning of the new lesson. All teachers not only had students solve problems but also required students to solve them orally (mentally), so students were always ready for the new lesson.

Ms. Bao's class. As a fifth-grade mathematics teacher for eight years, Ms. Bao likes to provide a set of problems to students and call on them to answer questions orally before starting the new lesson. For example, at the beginning of the lesson on finding simple ways to add or subtract fractions, she asked students to do the following eight problems:

$$\frac{2}{3} + \frac{1}{6}, \qquad \frac{3}{4} + \frac{1}{2}, \qquad \frac{7}{8} + \frac{1}{4}, \qquad 1\frac{7}{10} + \frac{8}{10}$$

$$\frac{5}{9} + \frac{8}{9}, \qquad \frac{3}{4} + \frac{1}{6}, \qquad \frac{5}{12} + \frac{3}{8}, \qquad 1\frac{3}{4} + \frac{3}{5}$$

In two minutes, the students answered the questions one by one and all students got right answers.

After finding out students' prior knowledge, Ms. Bao had students complete a problem orally from the book; whoever finished first stood up until the entire group (row) of students finished. She then told the groups to sit down and asked students in each group to explain how they got their answer. This activity took about five minutes.

Next, she gave two problems for all the students to complete independently in five minutes. She then asked the students who did a problem right to raise their hands and present their reasoning to the whole class. She asked students, "How did you arrive at the answer?" and "Why did you solve it using this method?" She showed two students' work on the projector. By having students compare their strategies of problem solving for these two problems, Ms. Bao provided an opportunity for students to think of different ways to solve problems.

With the above 12-minute review and practice of prior knowledge, Ms. Bao spent about 1/4 of the class time retrieving and aiding in retaining students' prior knowledge. Not only did it enhance students' proficiency in fraction addition and subtraction, but it also created a solid readiness for students to start the new lesson on finding simple ways to add or subtract fractions.

4.1.3   *During the new lesson – Focus on the thinking method using question strategies*

During the lesson, Chinese teachers focused on training the "thinking method" using carefully designed questions to promote students thinking in a critical and logical way. The "thinking method" in mathematics teaching in this study is reflected in how teachers elicited and supported students' thinking by connecting students' understanding of prior knowledge to the new knowledge and directing students to compare and contrast different ways of problem solving.

Ms. Fang's Class. After reviewing prior knowledge and practicing orally, Ms. Fang started the new lesson on mixed operations of fractions and decimals with Example 4 on the pre-prepared small blackboard:

$$3\frac{3}{4} - 0.63 + 1\frac{2}{5}$$

She asked, "If there are fractions and decimals in the problem, how do you solve it?"

Two students shared their answers with procedures from two methods on the blackboard:

$$3\frac{3}{4} - \frac{63}{100} + 1\frac{2}{5} = 3\frac{75}{100} - \frac{63}{100} + \frac{140}{100} = 4\frac{52}{100} = 4\frac{13}{25}$$

$$3.75 - 0.63 + 1.4 = 3.12 + 1.4 = 4.52$$

Then Ms. Fang asked, "Which way is easier? Why?" This question elicited students' thinking in comparing the two methods and identifying the better way to solve the problem. Most students were able to identify the second way as an easier way because in the first way they have to change the mixed numbers and the decimal into fractions and reduce the fraction. Ms. Fang summarized students' responses, "If fractions can be changed to terminating decimals, then mixed operation problems can be solved by changing the fraction into a decimal. It is a simpler way."

To further confirm and reinforce students' understanding, Ms. Fang gave two problems for students to practice using the easy way and asked, "If the fraction cannot be changed to a terminating decimal, how can you get an accurate result?" Ms. Fang provided Example 5:

$$3\frac{5}{6} - 4.5 + 1\frac{3}{4}$$

From doing the problem and comparing it with Example 4, students found that $3\frac{5}{6}$ could not be changed into a terminating decimal to get an accurate result; the fraction way is a good way to do Example 5.

In the above lesson segment, Ms. Fang used various questions to elicit students' thinking and used carefully designed problems to support and extend students' thinking. By comparing Examples 4 and 5, Ms. Fang fostered students' "thinking method" on mixed operations and supported students' thinking at a high level of decision making using the best approach for solving the problem.

4.1.4 *During the new lesson – Reinforce understanding and enhance proficiency by the review process*

To reinforce students' understanding of new learning and enhance their proficiency in mathematics, Chinese teachers liked to provide intensive practice at different levels, immediately followed by new learning.

Ms. Jing's class. To enhance students' proficiency in changing fractions into decimals, Ms. Jing had students do the following 10 fractions in three minutes: 1/2, 1/4, 3/4, 1/5, 2/5, 3/5, 4/5, 1/8, 1/20, and 1/25.

474   *How Chinese Learn mathematics: Perspectives from Insiders*

She required all students to quickly remember these basic facts in one minute. Then she asked the students to give the answers again one by one. All students answered simultaneously.

To reinforce understanding of new learning, Ms. Jing ended the class with a set of problems. She asked students to determine which fraction could be changed into a terminating decimal:

$$2\frac{2}{5}+\frac{14}{15}, \qquad \frac{7}{8}-\frac{1}{2}, \qquad 3\frac{3}{4}-0.67, \qquad 4.5+3\frac{5}{6}$$

By answering orally and simultaneously, students showed their proficiency and understanding. She summarized the key points of the lesson. This practice not only reviewed the new knowledge, but also strengthened students' understanding.

4.2 *Teachers' beliefs*

The above samples of Chinese classroom teaching addressed how Chinese teachers integrated the learning-questioning and learning-reviewing instruction model to enhance students' learning of mathematics, focusing on using oral and layered practice to promote students' thinking, reinforce their understanding, and help students achieve proficiency in mathematics. What are the beliefs about learning-questioning and learning-reviewing strategies of these teachers? The following Chinese teachers' beliefs explained why they used learning-questioning and learning-reviewing strategies to enhance students' learning.

4.2.1 *Primary focus on teaching mathematics*

In responding to the question of the primary focus in mathematics teaching, Chinese teachers believe that both conceptual understanding and procedural development are important. Ms. Jing describes her point of view on the importance of both types of knowledge:

Skills cannot be separated from concepts. Depending on the lesson being taught, I decide to focus on the concepts or the procedure. In today's lesson, I focused on skill development; I had students discover rather than instill knowledge into the students. Usually proficiency relates to skills and the mastery method relates to concepts.

Ms. Jing expects her students to master basic skills and learn thinking methods. In order to develop basic skills in her students, Ms. Jing requires them to have clear concepts and do intensive practice. However, she does not emphasize the result but the thinking process. In order to concentrate on the thinking methods in teaching, she designs and selects good practice problems for her students.

Ms. Fang's primary focus in teaching mathematics is the development of conceptual understanding. She said, "Only if students have conceptual understanding can they answer questions; by answering questions, students develop skills." Therefore, she helps students develop skills through practice with all kinds of problems.

4.2.2 *Thinking method and thinking ability*

Thinking method in mathematics learning is referred to as "approaches of thinking in mathematics" in this study. Thinking method is not just a one-dimensional way of thinking; it includes understanding and analysis of a problem from various angles, comparing and contrasting different strategies, reasoning and justification for the strategies, making a decision for the best approach, and reflecting on problem solving. All Chinese teachers in this study believe that teaching mathematics is teaching a "thinking method." For example, Ms. Ren considers that mathematics teaching is easier than teaching other subjects, because "it teaches methods." She believes that she is teaching a thinking method when she teaches mathematics.

Ms. Bao has no doubts about the belief that teaching mathematics is similar to teaching a method: "Students should learn methods (skills) and enhance their thinking ability" and "When students can solve problems that involve critical thinking, they feel successful". In order to enhance students' thinking methods, she believes that students should "learn basic knowledge points and practice techniques."

With rich knowledge of "thinking methods," students will develop strong thinking ability. Most teachers view "thinking ability" in broad terms. Ms. Jing addresses the importance of thinking ability in students' lives, "I like to teach mathematics because mathematics learning helps students to develop thinking abilities that they can use in all areas of life."

To enhance students' thinking ability, Ms. Fang uses practice and questions. She designs practice problems in layers, from easy to difficult. By working on the problems and answering questions orally, students engage in the thinking process and communicate their opinions. "This training of thinking, using both written and oral practice, will improve students' abilities to think for themselves and extend their thinking to a higher level." To know the character of an individual student's thinking, Ms. Fang likes to "ask several ways of solving one problem and try to find a unique approach from the student."

4.2.3 *Question and review strategies*

In this study, Chinese teachers believe that to teach mathematics effectively, a teacher should design different levels of questions to promote and support students' thinking. To learn new knowledge and reinforce new learning, teachers should guide students in reviewing prior knowledge for readiness of new learning and review the new knowledge to gain new insight.

To promote students' ability to think through question strategies, Ms. Fang likes to design practice problems and questions with layers, from easy to difficult, and have students answer them orally. By answering questions, the students solve problems mentally and express their opinions openly. Ms. Fang believes that this training of thinking, using both written and oral practice, will improve students' ability to think.

To promote students' thinking by answering questions, Ms. Jing encourages students to engage in the learning process actively. She explained, "Mathematics is abstract; if students actively engage in the learning process, students will think about questions and try to answer questions. Understanding how students think is very important to the teacher."

Teachers in this study used a review strategy in various forms to help students review and learn new knowledge in the learning process. To Ms. Fang, new knowledge of mathematics is relatively easy to teach, because the new lesson is only taught for about five to six minutes every day; the rest of the time is spent reviewing prior lessons and with practice problems. She pays much attention to helping students review and reinforcing prior knowledge before starting a new lesson. She believes that if students' prior knowledge reaches a certain level of proficiency and fluency, new knowledge will be mastered easily.

Ms. Bao uses oral practice and oral competition activities as a form of review every day. During morning independent study time, students have 15-20 minutes to practice orally. In mathematics class, before starting a new lesson, she always gives a set of problems for students to do orally. For example, in the observed class in this study, she had students answer eight problems orally before the new lesson. During the lesson, she usually has an oral competition to reinforce conceptual understanding and proficiency in basic skills. Students who got the right answer stood up until the whole group was standing up. This activity increased the students' interest in learning mathematics, gave students a chance to stretch, and promoted fluency in concepts and skills.

Ms. Jing believes in a strong connection between prior and new knowledge. She said, "I hope my students do not say 'new' for every day's lesson; students should be able to connect the prior knowledge to the new."

5 Discussion

The results in this study indicate that the process of learning-questioning-learning-reviewing is an effective learning process for promoting students' mathematics thinking, reinforcing understanding, and enhancing proficiency in mathematics. Moreover, Chinese mathematics teachers' beliefs have a deep impact on their teaching practices.

5.1 *Inquiry process of learning mathematics – learning and questioning*

Asking questions is one of the effective ways to engage students in learning and it promotes students' thinking. Probing questions can guide students in developing a deep conceptual understanding and raise their thinking to a higher order. Probing questions are effective in identifying student errors through engaging students in reasoning and thinking processes (Carroll, 1999). In addition, questions assess learning, promote discussion, and provide direction for teachers in planning. Posing questions in mathematics teaching is one of the features of Chinese education, which reflects the main focus of the *Nine Chapters on the Mathematical Art*. Using these guidelines, Chinese teachers are urged to develop and use sequences of questions during planning and use these questions throughout instruction. In this study, the questioning strategy was displayed extensively in the observations of Chinese teachers' mathematics classrooms. For example, Ms. Ren posed three questions on the blackboard at the beginning of class to connect prior knowledge to new learning and promote students' thinking. During the lesson, Ms. Jing posed the questions, "How can we determine if a fraction is terminating or non-terminating? What factor affects the result?", to guide students in observing the solved problems and engage them in an inquiry learning process. By asking "Why do you do it in this way?", Ms. Bao encouraged students to reason and explain their thinking. Questions, such as "Is there any other way?", encouraged students to think in different ways and expand their knowledge. Furthermore, Chinese teachers not only asked focusing questions to identify each student's thinking, but also understood students' thinking in different ways. For example, Ms. Fang's questions, "Which way is easier? Why?", also directed students toward comparing and contrasting different ways of problem solving and to make a right decision in problem solving and extend their thinking toward a higher level in mathematics.

5.2 *Inquiry process of learning mathematics – learning and reviewing*

The observation of classroom teaching in this study showed that Chinese teachers spent at least one-fourth of their time reviewing prior knowledge at the beginning of class and reinforcing new knowledge during the lesson. The review process not only promotes continuity and helps attain a more comprehensive view of topics previously covered, but also is a diagnostic tool that helps teachers identify students' strengths and weaknesses as well as provide valuable insight for future instruction (Suydam, 1984).

In the introduction of new concepts, all the Chinese teachers were able to connect to students' prior knowledge; it helped students not only understand and reinforce the knowledge being taught but also to picture mathematics as an integrated whole rather than as separate knowledge. The classroom observation with Ms. Bao showed that she understood the importance of prior knowledge in students' learning. She provided a total of 11 problems for students to review and make a connection with prior and new knowledge. To increase students' proficiency level in adding simple fractions, she asked students to answer questions orally and quickly. Ms. Jing also posed two sets of five questions for her students to review at the beginning of the lesson, connecting the new lesson gradually and developing conceptual understanding and skills step by step. To reinforce new knowledge, Ms. Jing had students do 10 basic conceptual and skill problems in three minutes during the new lesson. To help students reach a proficiency level, Ms. Jing again required students to quickly remember basic facts from these 10 problems in one minute. Then she asked the students to give the answers again one by one simultaneously.

Reviewing prior knowledge and connecting it to new learning develops generalizations and helps students solidify what they have learned, and allows them to transfer the knowledge to new situations (Suydam, 1984). Linking the new and prior knowledge in context also helps students know why and how to learn the new topic and grasp new knowledge with better understanding. This strategy is supported by the National Council of Teachers of Mathematics (NCTM, 1989): "Connection among topics will instill in students an expectation that the ideas they learn are useful in solving other problems and exploring other mathematical concepts" (p. 84). Furthermore "Because students learn by connecting new ideas to prior knowledge, teachers must understand what their students already know" (NCTM, 2000, p. 18).

5.3 *The impact of teachers' beliefs*

Educators from many countries agreed that mathematics teachers' beliefs have a powerful impact on their teaching (Ernest, 1989). The results of this study confirmed the impact of Chinese teachers' beliefs on their teaching. However, Chinese historical and cultural development influences teachers' beliefs. In this study, the learning-questioning and learning-reviewing instructional model is identified as one of the characteristics of Chinese mathematics teaching and learning. Chinese teachers believe that conceptual understanding and procedural development are equally important in mathematics teaching; teaching mathematics is to teach thinking methods and enhance thinking abilities. To help students develop conceptual understanding and achieve proficiency, mathematics teachers need to direct students' learning using the inquiry process of the learning-questioning-learning-reviewing model. In this process of inquiry in learning, students learn methods of thinking, make connections, reinforce their understanding, gain insights into new knowledge, and enhance their abilities in problem solving. Importantly, this learning process helps students build a strong and solid foundation of basic concepts and skills, which is a bridge to achieving proficiency in mathematics.

5.4 *Conclusion*

This study examined the influence of Chinese culture and teachers' beliefs on the development of the unique characteristics of Chinese mathematics teaching and learning: using the learning-questioning and learning-reviewing instructional model. The results of this study indicate that the learning-questioning and learning-reviewing process is an effective approach to enhance students' understanding of mathematics concepts and reinforce mathematics proficiency in mathematics classrooms.

There is limitation as to how the results can be applied to teachers in China because the samples of subjects included only four teachers in four schools in one city in China. Therefore, this study cannot be generalized to all mathematics teachers in China. However, the results of this study provided insight on how to use the questioning and reviewing strategies in teaching and learning mathematics and how teachers' beliefs impact their mathematics instruction.

References

American Association for the Advancement of Science. (2000). *Middle grades mathematics textbooks: A benchmarks-based evaluation.* Washington, DC: Author.

An, S. (2000). Globalization of education in China. *International Journal of Education Reform, 9*(2), 128-133

Ashmore, R. A., & Cao, Z. (1997). *Teacher education in the People's Republic of China.* Bloomington, IN: Phi Delta Kappa Educational Foundation.

Cai, J. (2000). Mathematical thinking involved in U.S. and Chinese students' solving of process-constrained and process-open problems. *Mathematical Thinking & Learning, 2*(4), 309-340.

Cai, J. (2001). Improving mathematics learning: Lessons form cross-national studies of Chinese and U.S. students. *Phi Delta Kappan, 82*(5), 400-404.

Cai, X., & Lai, B. (1994). *Analects of Confucius.* Beijing: Sinolingua.

Carroll, W. M. (1999). Using short questions to develop and assess reasoning. In L. V. Stiff & F. R. Curcio (Eds.), *Developing mathematical reasoning in grades K-12, 1999 yearbook* (pp. 247-253). Reston, VA: National Council of Teachers of Mathematics.

Ernest, P. (1989). The impact of beliefs on the teaching of mathematics. In P. Ernest (Ed.), *Mathematics teaching: The state of the art* (pp. 249-254). New York: The Falmer Press.

Li, J., & Chen, C. (1993, October). *Observations on China's mathematics education as influenced by its traditional culture.* Paper presented at the meeting of the China-Japan-U.S. Seminar on Mathematical Education. Weifang, China.

Ma, L. (1999). *Knowing and teaching elementary mathematics.* Mahwah, NJ: Lawrence Erlbaum Associates.

National Center for Education Statistics. (1999). *Highlights from TIMSS: The Third International Mathematics and Science Study, 1999. No. 1999-081.* Washington, DC: U.S. Department of Education.

National Council of Teachers of Mathematics. (1989). *The curriculum and evaluation standards for school mathematics.* Reston, VA: Author.

National Council of Teachers of Mathematics. (2000). *Principles and standards for school mathematics.* Reston, VA: Author.

Robitaille, D. F., & Travers, K. J. (1992). International studies of achievement in mathematics. In D. A. Grouws (Ed.), *Handbook of mathematics teaching and learning* (pp. 689-709). New York: Macmillan Publishing Company.

Spring, J. (1998). *Education and the risk of the global economy.* Mahwah, NJ: Lawrence Erlbaum Associates.

Stigler, J. W., & Perry, M. (1988). Cross-cultural studies of mathematics teaching and learning: Recent finding and new directions. In Grouws, D. A. & Cooney, T. J. (Eds.), *Effective mathematics teaching* (pp. 194-223). Reston, VA: National Council of Teachers of Mathematics.

Suydam, M. N. (1984). *The role of review in mathematics instruction.* ERIC/SMEAC Mathematics Education Digest, 2. (ERIC Document Reproduction Service No. ED260891)

Whitehead, A. (1925). *Science and the modern world.* New York: Free Press.

Chapter 18

The Effects of Different Representations
on Mathematics Learning of Chinese Children

XU Binyan

This chapter reports an experimental program on mathematics learning in one primary school in Shanghai, China. The following research questions were addressed: By means of different representations, could Chinese children exhibit their individual cognitive structures (functional versus predicative)? What effects did the different representations have on children's constructing mathematics concepts? Could the children be facilitated to actively learn and think, and to self reflect on their learning process? In the experimental program, children were encouraged to select partial representation by solving mathematics problems. It was shown that children could think in relation or in function of mathematics objects and learn to reflect on their learning process. They could experience the benefits of external representations and manifest the interest in active learning.

Key words: different representations, mathematics learning, Chinese children

1 Introduction

This research is based upon more than 10-year cooperation with professors and the research group from the University of Osnabrueck in Germany. Since the end of 1988, I have studied as a doctoral graduate student in the University of Osnabrueck, guided by Schwank and Cohor-Fresenborg, who researched for a long time the cognitive structures and strategies in solving mathematics problems and constructing mathematics concepts. In particular, Schwank has put forward the theory about functional versus predicative cognitive structures. Through several experiments, we have found that this theory strongly explain different individual behaviors which would be observed. I have also selected such project as my PhD dissertation, namely, I have studied functional versus predicative cognitive structures of Chinese children by constructing the algorithm concepts. According to the conclusion of my PhD dissertation, we can see that Chinese children are also able to exhibit different cognitive structures. The different cognitive structures are independent from culture context. My research could lead to many discussions in the field of Chinese mathematics education: How can we understand children's mathematics learning process? How can we organize lessons to facilitate effective learning by means of the different representations? After completing my PhD dissertation studies, I returned to my University (East China Normal University). While my advisors Schwank and Cohors-Fresenborg encouraged me to continue my research, my colleagues also encouraged me to continue to study how primary school children learn mathematics. The following research work has showed our efforts in this research field, which informed us how Chinese children construct mathematics concepts by means of different representations and what role do external representations play in learning.

In contrast to the traditional situation of learning mathematics of our Chinese children, through this program, children were able to understand basic ideas by constructing and operating the computer program; children were able to pay more attention to the process of forming mathematics concepts; children were brought up to think actively and initiatively and became good at reflective thinking.

2 Theoretical Background

The cognitive-oriented mathematics education has been more and more valued. From the international point, von Glasersfeld, one of the outrunners, who apply themselves to research the individual difference, wrote in 1983 an article and pointed out: *"we come to see knowledge and competence as products of the individual's conceptual organization of the individual's experience, the teacher's role will no longer be to dispense 'truth' but rather to help and guide the student in the conceptual organization of certain areas of experience."* (von Glasersfeld, 1993, pp. 66-67). He emphasized that we must consider in-depth individual cognitive structure while teaching knowledge and competence, so that learners will acquire knowledge by dint of their special experience.

In addition, Davis (1992) proposed to pay attention to mental representation by studying mathematics education. He mentioned that the focal point of didactic research is to investigate how teachers help students to understand problem, pose and solve the problem, and make use of representations of problem. He pointed out that more cognition science oriented research was needed. Children should be treated as individuals and their mental representation while working with problems should be analyzed.

In such a research field, the theory proposed by Schwank from Germany is also significant and revelatory. As early as 1986, she has already mentioned individual diversity of cognitive structure in her paper "cognitive structures of algorithmic thinking" (Schwank, 1986). Since then, she has been working on the individual diversity both in the theoretical and practical sense with her international research group work. Schwank (1993) differentiates predicative structure from functional cognitive structure, by saying that a preference for a predicative cognitive structure in a given situation means the expression of a static relation or the focusing on the structure and its description, whereas a preference for a functional cognitive structure has a distinctive consciousness for processes and thinking in effects. In the following figure, Schwank expound her theory about different cognitive structures.

In addition, Schwank pointed out that when facing same problem situations, the individual will solve problems according to different cognitive orientations. When the external representation fits a preferred cognitive structure of an individual, a resonance between this external representation and the preferred cognitive structure will be formed (Schwank, 1990a). In such a case, problem solving will be most effective and active. In our project, we intend to construct a similar situation, in which children can have a chance to learn effectively and actively.

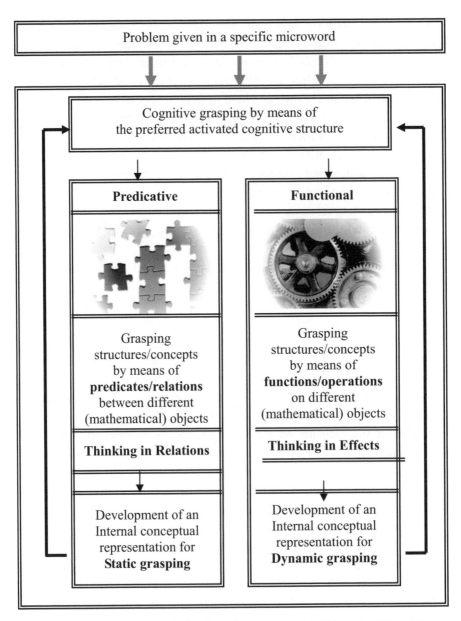

Figure 1. Predicative versus functional cognitive organization (Schwank, 1999, p. 87)

3   Research Question and Hypotheses

In my dissertation (Xu, 1994), I studied the cognitive structures of Chinese children during solving the problems about algorithm, by means of three different external representations (Schwank, 1990b, pp. 18-19, see also the appendix of this chapter). We found that Chinese children manifested their individual cognitive structures: some preferred functional thinking, while some were good at predicative thinking. We observed that different representations played special roles in children's learning process.

In this experimental program, we further analyzed whether Chinese children could exhibit their individual cognitive structures (functional versus predicative) by means of different representations, what effects the different representations had on constructing mathematics concepts, and whether the children could be facilitated to actively learn and think, and to self reflect on their learning process.

After experiencing the three different tools, the children in our project were encouraged to select representations, which they preferred, in solving mathematics problems. It was shown that some children preferred thinking in structures of mathematics objects, while others preferred thinking in function of mathematics objects. In such a learning environment, Chinese children were challenged, they needed to adjust themselves from previous passive learning and teaching strategy, they could learn to reflect on their learning process, they were able to experience the benefits of external representations and show interest in active learning.

4   Method

4.1   *Participants*

The participants in our project included 30 fourth graders, who came from the First Center Primary School in Hongkou District, Shanghai, China. After being briefed about the goals of the elective course, these children volunteered to take part in the course. Most of them were good at or interested in computers.

4.2 *Design*

The experimental program was designed as an elective curriculum in the school, which consisted of 10 sessions. Each session lasted about one hour. During first four sessions, children would learn and experience different representations, while organizing algorithmic activities (e.g., addition or subtraction algorithms). From the fifth to ninth session, children would need to analyze or construct problems and then select representation to solve these complex problems. During these sessions, children worked with computers and observed how computers used algorithms, which they had constructed. In the last session, children would play a game, in which they made use of knowledge, which they had learned.

4.3 *Procedure*

According to the design, we conducted one session per week and each session was screened. After that, all films were analyzed. We tried to understand children's behavior in both verbal and nonverbal activities. After each session was conducted, we discussed with school teachers and our research group to make a adjustment to the instructional design so that children would not be fastened by traditional instructional ideas.

5   Results of the Project

- In this project, we found that there was individual difference in mathematics thinking during problem solving. We concluded that children have their individual cognitive structure (functional or predicative cognitive structure). By means of three different representations, we observed that some children preferred to consider statistic characters, for example, the number of sticks in the box, or the number shown on the switch with rotating number counter. But some children were good at analyzing dynamic process. For example, they considered how and why the number changed and how to control the process.

Situation I: Children studied/acted in the third session. After each group had built one algorithmic machine (circle orbit) with Dynamic Labyrinth (Cohors-Fresenborg, 1976; see the appendix of this chapter), teacher showed the children the orbits built by each group. After which, the children compared and discussed the different orbits and came to recognize how algorithmic problem would be used on each circle orbit. Two children (S1, S2) discussed with the teacher (T):

> *T: Now let us look at the two orbits. Is it built by the third group or the fifth group?*
>
> *S1: Yes, our group made it. Let me show you how we do the addition. [S1 put 2 in the switch 1, put 4 in the switch 2. Now he is shifting the stick in the orbit.]*
>
> *T: Ok, try it.*
>
> *S1: Can you see, now it is 1, here is 5, now it is 0, here is 6. So I have finished it. 2 plus 4 is 6, now here is 6, our orbit is correct.*
>
> *S2: But the way is too long, I think our orbit is better. We can shift the switch 1, then quickly to the switch 2, I am shifting the switch 2, again I am shifting the stick to the switch 1, the number has been changed, go ahead.*
>
> *S1: But we have reached the same outcome.*

Situation II: Children worked in the seventh session. These children had knowledge with addition of two numbers. Here, children would be asked to construct addition algorithms of three numbers. Children could select one of the three different representations, which they have knowledge of. At the end, children should come out with a program of this algorithm. One student (S) wanted to work at first, but she selected the box.

> *S: I will make the addition of 3, 5, and 7. Now, I am putting 3 sticks into the box, 5 sticks into another box, and 7 sticks into this box. 3 plus 5 plus 7. I take one stick, here I put one stick, I take one stick, put one stick, take one stick, put one stick. Now I am looking at another boxes. [S is doing it.]*
>
> *T: Why do you start your work with other boxes?*
>
> *S: There is no sticks.*
>
> *T: How do you know it?*

S: There is only 3 sticks, I have counted it, when I have taken them.

Observation and comment: Now let's analyze the first situation. According to their verbal expressions, we could conclude that the first student (S1) paid more attention to the number status in the switch with the rotating counter, while he shifted sticks in his orbit. That is to say, he didn't consider another position, which also played an important role in using the algorithms. For him, the most crucial was to know whether the solution was correct. We believed that this student was good at thinking in static condition and also good at getting solution, but he didn't consider much about the approach. When we looked at the second situation, we could also conclude that the student (S) preferred to consider static elements, while she used the addition algorithms.

Similarly, we studied the second student in the first situation. This student paid more attention to the change of the number that was reflected on the switch with the rotating counter. Moreover, he could discern which way was essential for using the algorithms. So he judged that his classmate had wasted accessory in building the orbit. We concluded that he was good at thinking in function and approach.

In conclusion, base on the analysis of the above two situation, we argue that there are individual differences in cognitive structure (functional or predicative) in solving mathematics problems.

- The different representations can shape the learn environment in which children could be facilitated to think actively, construct important concepts initiatively, for example, concept of variable, or condition of running algorithms.

Situation I: Children worked in the first session. They acted as a robot and learned basic concepts by using algorithms. In order to control this approach, children tried again and then brought forward several suggestions. Eventually, one student found an activity for controlling algorithmic approach with reasons. The student suggested that robot should touch the box and then judged whether this process could be carried on. Let's look at the following dialogue between two children (S1 and S2) and teacher (T):

> T: *Why did you let the robot stop the operation?*
> S1: *I have counted, the robot has taken 8 sticks. Maybe it must stop.*
> T: *Maybe?*
> S1: *I don't know how many sticks in this box.*
> T: *The robot works automatically, he cannot know how many sticks.*
> S2: *Can the robot touch the box?*
> T: *yes, I have mentioned it.*
> S2: *I think we can order the robot. At first he should touch the box, if there are some sticks.*
> T: *Then?*
> S2: *When there are some, then do it again.*
> S1: *Oh, I know, when he doesn't touch sticks, then he will stop.*
> S2: *Yes, I think so.*
> T: *Good idea.*

Situation II: Children worked in the seventh session. They inputted the algorithmic program into the computer and observed how the computer ran the program (see the appendix of this chapter). One student found something was changing, i.e., on the left of the screen, one scalar, which displayed the number of operational steps the computer took, would be changed, when different input data were used. After a period of observation, the student claimed that the number of operational steps was related to the input data. She expressed the following:

> S: *I think this amount is related to the input data. When we have another input data, then another amount has appeared. When I know input data, then I can count the amount of running operations.*
> T: *Very good.*

Observation and comment: In the first situation, the student (S2) concentrated on constructing addition algorithms. On one hand, he looked into the activity by another children, on the other hand he initiatively manipulated the sticks. Gradually, he realized that the addition algorithms would be conditioned. A crucial idea emerged. He suggested that through the activity 'touch the box', one can control the approach to construct algorithms. This self-constructed concept 'algorithmic condition' was the foundation for analyzing, constructing and understanding algorithms.

The three representations provided children with the opportunities to exhibit their preferred thinking and construct key concepts initiatively. In the second situation, we could see how the student learned the idea of variable and function. While observing the running of algorithms and the changes in elements, the student was inspired to consider the variance of several elements, including output. Then she boldly explained that the number of operational steps depended on the input data. She also pointed out that the relationship between the number of operational steps and input data. It was to show that the elementary idea on variable and function was constructed.

- Through this project, children were be encouraged to reflect on their approach to solve problem in different representation formats, verbal or nonverbal. Children learned to analyze their mistakes or misunderstanding during problem solving. Children's ability in reflection would be facilitated.

Situation I: Children acted in the sixth session. Children and teachers worked interactively. After the children did exercises in the classroom, they were asked to reflect on their work. In particular, children discussed about misunderstandings in the exercises, explored the reasons why they were produced, and how they should be eliminated. About some errors in the exercises, two children (S1, S2) talked to each other as follows:

> *S1: I have forgotten where I should put the symbols. [S1 pointed to the pair of symbols "(,)".] Now I know how I shall use the symbols. I must write this symbol at the end of the program.*
> *S2: No, I don't think so. When we need this operation only once, it means, we don't repeat it, so we don't use of this*

symbol.

S1: Yes, I know the meaning of symbols. It means "repeat". Oh, I only remember the position of symbol, it is not enough. It is "repeat".

S2: Yes, the function of the symbol is "repeat", the stick will shift again. It is easy to know, when we let the computer work, we tell him with this symbol whether it should repeat.

S1: Oh, this symbol means "repeat".

Situation II: Children worked in the eighth session. At first, the addition algorithm about three numbers was reviewed. The Children were asked to write corresponding programs and explain the meaning of the programs. Some children found their errors and modified them, while they listened respectfully to the explanation from other children.

Observation and comment: In some exercise papers, while there were several question marks, children were encouraged to reflect their misunderstanding. Some children analyzed their errors by means of different representations. For example, one student stuck to the structure of symbols, and seldom thought of the function in symbolic form. But another student paid attention to the meanings, which were represented by symbols. We concluded that different representations would motivate children to reflect and evaluate by themselves. Also we observed that while some children reflected on their errors or misunderstandings, other children listened to their explanation. During the process, the latter analyzed their classmates' explanation and then reflected on their own problem solving procedures. We supposed that children had experienced an interactive reflection; reflection made by one child would affect another children' reflection action.

- The different representations provided children with multiple learning situations, in which children choose their preferred thinking structure, meanwhile their learning motivation were strengthened.

Situation: Children acted in the third session. In this session, the learning action taken by the children was to construct a circle orbit to solve an addition problem with the switches from Dynamic Labyrinth. This was new to the children. However, the teacher encouraged the children to make use of those materials to present their ideas bravely. Initially, the children experienced several frustrations, but they gradually finished the task through the cooperation with other children.

Observation and comment: We established an environment in which children experienced the nonverbal actions, which might be ignored during the routine mathematics teaching and learning. In the front of their completed addition orbits, most of the children relaxed and laughed loudly. They vied with each other to test and validate their algorithmic orbits. Spontaneously, several groups marked their solutions as art products (see Figure 2). All these actions made us believe that children were proud of their efforts and achievements. They worked on mathematics problems under internal driven motivation. This learning motivation is like a roll booster, which pushed the participants forward in their learning, so that children experienced interest and challenges of learning mathematics concepts. Such experiences would be more valuable for our Chinese children, because in our traditional instruction, the children worked more on mathematics exercises than did mathematics interactively.

6　Conclusion and Discussion

After analyzing the children's learning processes, we can conclude that the Chinese children exhibited their individual cognitive structures (functional versus predicative) through mathematics problem solving. The different external representations provided the children with opportunities to select such representations to make the resonance between external representation and children' preferred cognitive structures.

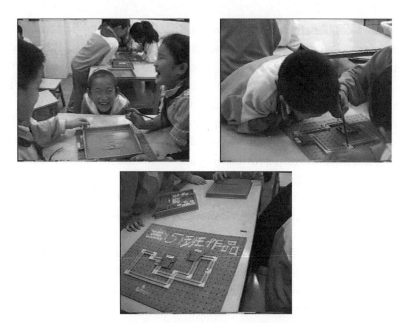

Figure 2. The children were proud of their work

We also realized that using different representations, children would be more actively participating in constructing and analyzing mathematics concepts. They were not only satisfied with the mathematics solutions they have achieved, but also paid attention to the approach of getting the solutions. Gradually, the children gain knowledge about this form of active learning. By going through such an experience, children understood the meaning of mathematics concepts more than just surface learning.

In addition, children reflected their internal motivation during constructing or analyzing concepts with different tools. They were more interested in mathematics learning, which seldom happened in the traditional instructional environment. Children were able to experience the achievements obtained by themselves. These were important factors which facilitated children to learn initiatively.

By investigating and reflecting the projects with the children, we found disadvantages which might be brought on by our traditional instruction. Some of the remarks pointed out by the children in our study were as follows: "in the classroom, sometime classmates spoke so light and that I couldn't hear from them, so that I couldn't understand some exercises."; "sometimes, the teacher explained so few, therefore I couldn't understand it. Please say and explain something more." From the above comments, we can see clearly that those children's learning process heavily relied on their teacher or other children. They were in passive learning status. They were merely waiting for others' input. The reason why they couldn't understand was the knowledge came from others, not themselves. Their learning approach was just memorization.

In conclusion, the study shows that such programs have positive effects on children's learning of mathematics. That is to say, problems given in different external representations activate individual's preferred cognitive structures. The programs provide children with effective environment in which children take the initiative in constructing mathematics concepts. Children experience the effective learning, i.e., learning is to construct knowledge, learning is to negotiate with social interaction, and learning is to actively practice.

In order to design such a learning environment, we have to deal with two kinds of challenges. One is that children must know they are not just recipients of knowledge. They must take initiative in learning and work cooperatively. This will result in maximizing their personality and potential. The other is that teachers must change their conception about learning. Our teachers must understand the new meanings of learning. Teachers must recognize that they are not just initiators, but they must gradually shift their roles as guiders, dialogists, or learners. Teachers must know that individuals have different cognitive structures and recognize the resonance between external and internal representations of knowledge or problems.

Acknowledgements

I am grateful to all the members in the Curriculum and Instruction Development Lab of East China Normal University for contributing their wisdom to the design and implementation of the project; I would like to express my gratitude to the principal, teachers, pupils, and their parents in The First Central Primary School, which was late renamed Chang Qing School, in Hongkou District in Shanghai, China. They have provided us with all necessary support. Thanks go also to the editorial board of this book. They have done the meticulous technical work, but also brought forward vivid suggestions to the writing of this chapter.

References

Cohors-Fresenborg, E. (1976). Dynamische Labyrinthe [Dynamic Labyrinth]. *Didaktik der Mathematik* [Mathematics Education], *1*, 1-21.

Davis, R. B. (1992). *Understanding "understanding"*. *Journal of Mathematical Behavior*, *11*(3), 225-241.

Schwank, I. (1986). Cognitive structures of algorithmic thinking. In L. Burton & C. Hoyles (Eds.), *Proceedings of the tenth International Conference for the Psychology of Mathematics Education* (pp. 195-200). London: Institute of Education.

Schwank, I. (1990a). Zur analyse kognitiver strukturen algorithmischen denkens [On the analysis of cognitive structures of algorithmic thinking]. In K. Haussman & M. Reiss (Eds.), *Mathematische Lehr-Lern-Denkprozesse* [The process of mathematical teaching, learning and thinking] (pp. 31-54). Göttingen: Hogrefe.

Schwank, I. (1990b). *Zur algorithmischen begriffsbildung von Maedchen* [On the construct of algorithmic concepts of schoolgirls]. FMD-Arbeitsbericht 3 [The report of Research Institute of Mathematics Education]. Osnabrück, Germany.

Schwank, I. (1993). On the analysis of cognitive structures in algorithmic thinking. *Journal of Mathematical Behavior, 12*(2), 209-231.

Schwank, I. (1999). On predicative versus functional cognitive structures. In I. Schwank (Ed.), *European Research in Mathematics Education* (Vol. II, pp. 84-90). Osnabrück, Germany: Forschungsinstitut für Matlematikdidatik. (Also retrieved from http://www.fmd.uni-osanbrueck.de/ebooks/erme/cerme1-proeedings/cerme1-proceedings. html)

von Glasersfeld, E. (1983). Learning as a constructive activity. In J. C. Bergeron & N. Herscovics (Eds.), *Proceedings of the fifth annual meeting – North American Chapter of the International Group for the Psychology of Mathematics Education* (Vol. 1, pp. 41-69). Montreal, Canada: University of Montreal.

Xu, B. (1994). *Untersuchung zu praedikativen und funktionalen kognitiven Strukturen chinesischer Kinder bei der Auseinandersetzung mit Grundbegriffen der Programmierung* [Experiment on predicative versus functional cognitive structures of Chinese children while constructing and analyzing basic algorithmic concepts]. Schriftenreihe des Forschungsinstituts fuer Mathematikdidaktik Nr. 25 [The series of Research Institute for Mathematics Education Nr. 25]. Osnabrück, Germany: Forschungsinstitut für Mathematikdidaktik.

Appendix

Three different representations' tools that children used in our project are followings:

- Register box with sticks

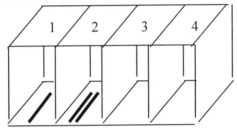

Figure 1. Register box

Register box has a finite number of cases that represent registers. There are sticks, which amounts represent data. In the experiment the cases will be shut out with hanging. Children act as robot and use this representation's tool to do algorithms.

For example, there is a data x_1 in the case 1, and data x_2 in the case 2, the addition (x_1+x_2) will be run by means of this representation as following: Touch the case 1, when there isn't stick, stop the activity, or else take one stick from the case 1, then put one stick into the case 2. The process will be repeated.

- Dynamic Labyrinth

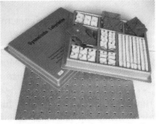

Figure 2. Dynamic Labyrinth

Note. Retrieved from http://www.ikm.uni-osnabrueck.de/aktivitaeten/dl/dynamic_labyrinths/dl-construction-kit.html

Dynamic Labyrinth includes different kits that have special functions. Children use kits (specially, switch with rotating number counter) for building different algorithmic machine. The following is an adding machine.

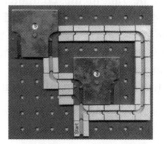

Figure 3. An adding machine

Note. Retrieved from http://www.ikm.uni-osnabrueck.de/akitvitaeten/dl/dynamci_labyrinths/dl-construction-kit.html

The Addition will be run, while children shift a stick through the machine (orbit). It will be observed that the number in the rotating number counter will be greater, while children shift a stick through the right way of the switch. But the number will be smaller, while children shift a stick through the left way of the switch.

- Program language

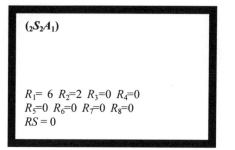

$(_2S_2A_1)$

$R_1 = 6 \quad R_2 = 2 \quad R_3 = 0 \quad R_4 = 0$
$R_5 = 0 \quad R_6 = 0 \quad R_7 = 0 \quad R_8 = 0$
$RS = 0$

Figure 4. The screen of the computer.

By means of this representation children use symbols for programming. There are following symbols that children meet: "S_i" denotes subtract 1 from the register i; "A_i" denotes add 1 in the register i;

"($_i$" indicates judgment: when it is zero in the register i, then algorithm is finished, or else it is going on; ")" indicates repeat. ($_2S_2A_1$) is an adding program. It means: repeat the following procedure, till it is zero in register 2: subtract 1 from the register 2, then add 1 in the register 1.

Such program will be run in the computer. Figure 4 shows, the adding program ($_2S_2A_1$) has been inputted and now the data has also been inputted, 6 in the register 1 ($R_1 = 6$), 2 in the register 2 ($R_2 = 2$). After inputting a special instruction, the computer is running the algorithm and children can observe the data changing in different registers. *RS* records the total amount of running *S* and *A*, while one algorithms is running.

Section 4

INSPIRATION AND FUTURE DIRECTIONS

Chapter 19

The CHC Learner's Phenomenon: Its Implications on Mathematics Education[1]

WONG Ngai-Ying

In the past decades, the outstanding performance of Asian students, especially in the subject of mathematics, had raised the eyebrows of sociologists, educationalists, and psychologists. Many of the studies attributed the success of CHC learners to the ideology of Confucianism itself. At the same time, cautions were made not to "over-Confucianize" in such explanations. The attention has also turned to the identification of good practices (or even just practices) in various regions irrespective of their cultural origins (whether it is "Confucian", "Daoist", "Eastern" or "Western"), aiming at shedding light to contemporary pedagogical practices. In this chapter, after reviewing the trend of CHC studies in the past fifteen years, the author would like to inspect the three Chinese traditions of calligraphy, martial art, and seal carving. We will look into their courses of training and philosophies of pedagogy, especially their view to practices, to see what lessons we can learn from them. The chapter is concluded by the description of the author's perception of the "CHC script".

Key words: Confucian Heritage culture, repetitive learning, practices, memorization, rote learning

For centuries, the Chinese have been fleeing from wars and famines, fighting for survival from North to South, and from East to West. Through it all, they have tried to build a brighter future for their *next generation* through *education*. This mentality has

---

[1] The author wishes to pay tribute to his PhD thesis supervisor, Dr. David Watkins, for initiating the author into the fruitful research field of the CHC (Confucian Heritage Culture) learner's phenomenon.

made the children of the CHC the hardest working learners on earth.

(N. Y. Wong, in press; italics original)

1 The Unfolding of a Myth

In the past decades, the outstanding academic performance of Asian students, especially in the subject of mathematics, had raised the eyebrows of sociologists, educationalists, and psychologists (Bond, 1996a; Lau, 1996; Watkins & Biggs, 1996, 2001; N. Y. Wong, 1998a). "The New Whiz Kids," the cover story appearing in *Time* magazine (Brand, 1987), may have been the first to bring this phenomenon to the notice of the public, as well as sociologists and educationalists. Since then, such a "myth" (as described by scholars like Biggs, 1994, 1996a; Watkins, Regmi, & Astilla, 1991) persisted. CHC regions (including Mainland China, Taiwan, Hong Kong, Singapore, Japan, and South Korea) scored high in international comparisons such as the International Mathematics Olympiads (IMO), International Assessment of Education Progress (IAEP), the Third International Mathematics and Science Study (TIMSS), and Programme for International Student Assessment (PISA).

In the article "The New Whiz Kids", Brand (1987) stated a number of facts that may have been disturbing those who believed in Western superiority to the Oriental system in respect of educational system and who saw the latter relying mostly on drilling and rote learning (Murphy, 1987). The article also deliberately drew a distinction between the Confucian and the Buddhist traditions among various Asian cultures and argued that "immigrants from Asian countries with the strongest Confucian influence — Japan, Korea, China, and Vietnam — perform best. By comparison, ... Laotians and Cambodians, who do somewhat less well, have a gentler, Buddhist approach to life" (p. 45). Thereafter, the CHC learner's phenomenon has become one of the most researched areas worldwide.

In this chapter, we would start off by giving a summary of the discourse in the past decades (which can be conceptualized in Figure 1).[2] With such a background, we would like to report on a recent attempt to bridge between "basic skills" and "higher-order abilities" by the systematic introduction of variations. After that, we would like to offer speculations on the search of the "CHC way" of teaching, if there is anything as such.

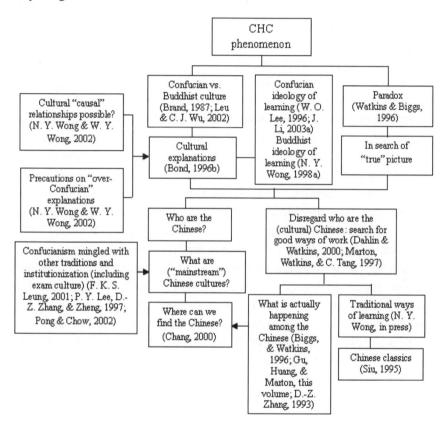

Figure 1. Research on the CHC learner's phenomenon for more than a decade

[2] Earlier versions of some parts of this chapter may appear in the author's previous publications like N. Y. Wong (1998b, 2002, in press) and N. Y. Wong and W. Y. Wong (2002).

2 Common Conceptions and Misconceptions of the CHC Learning Environment

With the brilliant performance of CHC learners, some researchers turned to more in-depth studies on mathematics problem-solving among CHC students (see e.g., Cai, 1995; Stevenson & S. Y. Lee, 1990), while others began to identify features particular to the CHC learning environment. It is generally perceived that the CHC learning environment stresses recitation and memorization, large class with passive learners, teacher-centered, and authoritative teacher. This kind of setting is in sharp contrast to what is found to be conducive to learning (Biggs & Moore, 1993). For instance, an international visiting panel commented in its report to the Hong Kong government that Hong Kong mathematics classroom "has a large size and is crowded, ... with students filling the entire room" (Llewellyn, Hancock, Kirst, & Roeloffs, 1982). In addition, the same report pointed out that the Hong Kong curriculum is examination-driven, putting great emphasis on lecturing, memorization, and preparation for in-school and public examinations (see also Morris, 1985, 1988). Furthermore, disapproval is also a frequently used technique to control social behavior (Winter, 1990). As noted in Biggs (1994), CHC classes are "typically large, usually over 40, and appear to Western observers as highly authoritarian; teaching methods appear as mostly expository, sharply focused on preparation for external examinations. Examinations themselves address low level cognitive goals, are highly competitive, and exert excessive pressure on teachers and exam stress on students" (p. 22; see also Biggs, 1991; D. Y. F. Ho, 1991; Morris, 1985). On top of this, modern Chinese parents place great emphasis on academic achievements of their children (望子成龙) (D. Y. F. Ho, 1986; see also Cai, 2003). Their children, on the other hand, study hard to meet the expectations of their parents (报父母恩); they often attribute their academic success and failure to the efforts they have put into their work (Hau & Salili, 1991, 1996). However, all these could not satisfactorily explain the CHC learner's phenomenon.

3 Revelations from Empirical Studies

On the contrary to the above impressions, it was repeatedly found that CHC students have strong preference to deep approaches to learning, which is the opposite of rote learning, than Western students have (Biggs, 1990, 1991, 1994; G. Y. Chan & Watkins, 1994; Kember & Gow, 1991; Watkins & Ismail, 1994; Watkins et al., 1991). Biggs (1994) made a clear distinction between rote learning and repetitive learning. Other research supported the hypothesis that excellent academic performance of CHC learners may be due to a synthesis of memorizing and understanding which is not commonly found in Western students (Marton, Dall'Alba, & Tse, 1996; Marton, Watkins, et al., 1997; Watkins, 1996). It was also found that recitation was common among CHC learners to bring about sharp focus and better understanding (Dahlin & Watkins, 2000).

Biggs (1994) offered a new perspective on "the teacher as the authority in the classroom" which was often regarded as having a dampening effect on students formerly. He identified the relationship between teacher and students as one of "mentor/mentee relationship." Besides, Hess and Azuma (1991) noted a mixture of authoritarianism and student-centeredness in the CHC classroom. However, regardless of these new insights, the academic success of CHC learners is still largely inexplicable (see also Biggs, 1996a, 1996b). Various empirical research also made similar observations. The CHC teacher was found to bear a moral responsibility of caring for their students and an implicit influence (especially on character cultivation) exists behind the façade of the transmission of knowledge (Gao & Watkins, 2001; I. T. Ho, 2001). In addition, students seem to be passive in the CHC classroom, yet it may be demonstrating a socialization of "listenership" (as opposite to "speakership"). Thus students appear to be silent and passive in class, yet they are attentive and mentally involved (Hatano & Inagaki, 1998; Inagaki, Hatano, & Morita, 1998; J. Li, 2003a, 2003b, this volume).

Series of studies were performed to investigate CHC students' performance in non-routine problems (open-ended problems in particular) and their conception of mathematics. For instance, besides revealing that U.S. students performed in non-routine mathematics problems not much poorer than Chinese students (Cai, 1995), Cai (2000) further discovered that though Chinese students performed better in process-constrained problems than their US counterparts, US students performed much better in process-open problems (see also Cai, Lin, & Fan, this volume).

If CHC learners perform brilliantly in routine problems but not so in non-routine ones, could it be a consequence of how they view mathematics? A series of studies were conducted to investigate students' and teachers' conceptions of mathematics among students in Hong Kong and Mainland China (Figure 2). It was found that CHC learners possess a relatively restricted conception of mathematics In brief, they tend to identify mathematics by its terminologies and perceive it as a subject of "calculables." They consider problem solving in mathematics as being not much more than a process of searching of rules by picking out various clues from the question. Some even do this by identifying the topic (or chapter of the textbook) to which the problems belong. Thus, CHC learners may solve various mathematical problems quickly and with precision, but whether they possess a genuine conceptual understanding of the mathematics concerned is open to conjecture (N. Y. Wong, 2001, 2002).

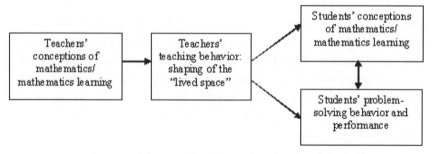

Figure 2. Research framework of conception of mathematics studies

We have similar findings on teachers too. Though CHC teachers possess relatively broader conceptions of mathematics, their conceptions of mathematics basically resemble those of the students (N. Y. Wong, 2001). However, this does not mean that either the CHC learner or CHC learning tradition lacks potential for deep understanding (Siu, 1995, 1999, this volume; Siu & Volkov, 1999; Stevenson & Stigler, 1992; Stigler &

Hiebert, 1999; Watkins & Biggs, 1996, 2001; N. Y. Wong, 1998a). We will return to this point in subsequent sections.

4 The CHC Learner in Prototype

Since the notion of "Confucian heritage" is repeatedly stressed, some scholars turned their attention to the ideology of Confucianism per se. Bond (1996b) integrated classic studies of Hofstede (1983) with the studies of Chinese Culture Connection (1987) and Schwartz (1994), and identified hierarchy, order, discipline, and a strong achievement orientation as the salient values common to such CHC regions as Hong Kong, Singapore, and Taiwan. CHC was often identified as a collective culture too (Kim, Triandis, Kagitcibasi, Choi, & Yoon, 1994). The following are often regarded as salient characteristics of learning in the CHC: social-achievement orientation (as opposed to individual-achievement orientation; see Yu, 1996), emphasizing diligence, attribution of success to effort, a competitive spirit, and a strong belief in the maxim "Practice makes perfect" (熟能生巧) (Bond, 1996b; Bond & Hwang, 1986; Cheng, 1994; Hau & Salili, 1991, 1996; D. Y. F. Ho, 1986; W. O. Lee, 1996). In fact, two sayings demonstrate this belief: first, "diligence could remedy mediocracy" (勤能补拙); second, "familiarity breeds sophistication". In brief, the CHC learner is envisioned as one who works harder instead of one who is smarter.

It has been argued that Confucianism is "congruent with the cultural system of traditional China, basically an agrarian state" (Stover, 1974). This agricultural economy tied the vast majority of the population to the land and peasants can only maintain their livelihood on a subsistence level (Bond & Hwang, 1986, p. 215). The factor contributing to such outstanding performance among CHC students seems to be their orientation toward social achievement, the origin of which could be traced to the Confucian ideology and culture of de-emphasis of individual non-mundane pursuits. When Confucius was asked about life after death, he replied: "We know so little about this life, how can we know about life after death!" (未知生、焉知死?) (*The Analects, 11:12* [论语·先进第十一]) Thus, it was perceived that the CHC philosophy of life is the concentration of one's efforts in achieving secular goals of this life. Moreover, the degree of a person's success in life is judged not only by whether his or her achievement is passed on to the next generation (子嗣), but also by a person's worldly career and his or her contribution to the welfare of society (三不朽); it is believed that though life is perishable, there are "three imperishables": namely, erecting an example of a moral life, contributing to the country or his/her fellow people (or to the welfare of society), and establishing a school of thought. These factors are often seen as the origin of the achievement orientation of CHC societies (Qian, 1945/1976, pp. 7–10). Since it is thought that the target of one's life can be fully achieved by the continuing efforts of one's descendents, parents always have high expectations on their children in respect of academic success. Retrospectively, children try to repay their parents by working hard in school, aiming at honoring them by obtaining good academic results (D.-X. Zhang, 1989). However, some other results of empirical studies are contradictory to this notion. For example, Ray and Jones (1983) discovered that Hong Kong students' achievement motivation was lower than that of Australian students (other studies include Iwawaki & Lynn, 1972; Yang, 1987. For details, see D.-X. Zhang, 1989, pp. 254–269).

Following the above line of thought on the particular concern for mundane success and passing the success to descendents, what is commonly regarded as external motivation could have another meaning. While survival situates at the lowest level in Maslow's (1954) hierarchy, it could represent an intrinsic motivation among those in the CHC since it refers not only to the survival of the self, but also the survival of the community, of the clan, and even of the whole lineage. Though external motivation is often seen as a characteristic of "East Asian" education (F. K. S. Leung, 2001), it is commonly perceived that having high academic achievement (resulting in a high social status) is a means to honor one's ancestors (光宗耀祖), and can even be seen as another form of spiritual pursuit which is in line with the CHC culture of ancestor "worship."

5 Where Is the CHC?

When we try to portray the CHC in this light, we may be subconsciously identifying Asian/Chinese culture with Confucianism and equating Confucianism with what was said by Confucius himself[3].

Though phrases like "the Asian learner," "the Chinese learner," and "the CHC learner" were used interchangeably, it is doubtful what CHC really represents. During an international conference (the First East Asian Regional Conference on Mathematics Education, South Korea, 1998), a participant from Singapore objected the classification of Singapore as a CHC region on the grounds that Singapore was a country of multi-cultures. Hatano and Inagaki (1998) also showed skepticism on whether we can group the Chinese and Japanese mathematics classrooms as "Asian" (p. 94). We can also doubt whether Hong Kong, being greatly influenced by Western culture, could be classified as a CHC city. It is not easy to account for the case of Mainland China when traditional culture was once wiped out by Communism. There are 28 provinces and 56 ethnic groups in China. Geographically, it is not easy to identify central China ("the Central Kingdom") too. It would be difficult to apportion a precise degree of "Chineseness" in this statement: "A girl dressed in *Cheongsam*,[4] playing a Er-hu[5] under a Buddhist pagoda,[6] is sitting on a chair,[7] drinking jasmine tea[8] and watching a lion dance[9]" (see N. Y. Wong & W. Y. Wong, 2002). No wonder was it that Chang (2000) asserted we were all searching the Chinese from the wrong place!

Some scholars even mistakenly equate Confucianism with traditional Chinese culture (J. Tracey, 1983, p. 30). Though it was often asserted that "the unifying intellectual philosophy in the Chinese 'great tradition' was Confucianism" (Yu, 1996, p. 231), it must be remembered that the CHC was also affected by Mohism, Daoism, Buddhism, and other traditions. Chan Buddhism (a school of Buddhist teachings which has flourished in China since the 11th century) received high regard from Western scholars such as Fromm (1960), who took it as a blend of Daoism and Buddhism.

---

[3] Often, just a few sporadic sayings of Confucius are quoted in the literature.
[4] A tribal dress of the Manchus.
[5] A Chinese musical instrument originally from the Northwestern regions.
[6] The Chinese architectural form of "stupa" from India.
[7] Chairs were also brought into the "Central Kingdom" from tribal regions. Ancient "Chinese" knelt on mats while "seated."
[8] Imported originally from Arabia.
[9] Originated from the Tibetan region.

In fact, some later empirical research also found distinctions between Confucian and Buddhist beliefs in teaching and learning. It was found that those teachers influenced by Buddhism stress self-improvement, whereas those influenced by Confucianism stress teachers' modeling (Leu & C. J. Wu, 2002; see also Leu, Y. Y. Wu, & C. J. Wu, 1999).

Even if we confine our understanding of CHC to Confucianism, the Confucian schools at different historical periods[10] held very different ideologies. In some instances, Confucianism was modernized whereas in others, it was blended with other schools of thought such as *Yin-Yang*, the "Five Elements" school of thought, Legalism, Daoism, and Buddhism (see e.g., Lao, 1988). In some cases, Confucianism was simply advocated by the ruling class for governing purposes.

Because it is also fashionable to quote from Confucius (and other philosophers), we must be careful in making interpretations. Ancient Chinese words often carry different levels of connotation. Besides the case of "Practice makes perfect" mentioned above, there are a lot more (for more cases of this kind, see e.g., N. Y. Wong & W. Y. Wong, 2002).

Chang (2000) suggested that the "search" for "Chinese" shall not be targeted at the geographical regions or kinship. Rather, it should be targeted at the "vernacular culture that common people endorse" which includes "the beliefs and values held by ordinary folks who identify themselves as Chinese." This approach no doubt could possibly sidetrack an issue only to find another. Yet, W. O. Lee (1996) did make a brief analysis on the shared beliefs in education (e.g. high regards on education, the educability for all ...) of CHC. This analysis could probably form the basis of further investigation along this line. However, there were counter-arguments to the effect that the above associations could be an "over-Confucianization"; there is also doubt as to whether a "causal relationship" between cultures and phenomena ("Culture $X \rightarrow$ Behavior Y") exists (see N. Y. Wong & W. Y. Wong, 2002).

---

[10] E.g., Zhou Dynasty (770BC–221BC) in which Confucius lived, Han Dynasty (206BC–220AD) when Confucianism was institutionalized, neo-Confucianism in the Song Dynasty (960–1126) and Ming Dynasty (1368–1644), and contemporary Confucianism since the turn of this century.

6 What Counts — Confucianism or Examination?

In CHC, an individual is valued not as an individual but for his or her role (本份) in a vast network of kinship. Thus, it is of utter importance that a person plays precisely the role he or she inherits by birth. In fact, rites (礼) and social norms (cardinal relations, 五伦) are central themes of Confucianism. As a result, one of the major functions of education is to cast youngsters into a certain role that they will take up in society, and act and behave accordingly in the light of their family background and socioeconomic status. This predisposition, however, can be reversed when the examination system comes into play — because this system could bring about social mobility. Social mobility, in turn, sets new rules for a new game. Thus, education, in conjunction with the examination system, has the function of enabling an individual to strive for the best role he or she could attain (力争上游，出人头地). It is understandable, therefore, that the CHC (albeit an adapted one) learner would be strongly motivated toward high academic achievement when it is measured against conventional tests and examinations (N. Y. Wong, 1998a).

Regarding the excellent academic results of CHC students, the "examination culture" (see P. Y. Lee et al., 1997; Pong & Chow, 2002) designed for governance purposes could have a far greater impact on achievement orientation than Confucianism. As remarked in Llewellyn et al. (1982), the curriculum in Hong Kong is "examination driven" and "the examinations are structured so as to dominate style and content of learning in the classroom" (p. 33). Individuals, regardless of their family background, could climb up the social ladder by striving to pass a hierarchy of examinations (see N. Y. Wong, 1998a, 2001, in press). As such, whether CHC students are really more brilliant or just skilful in passing examinations could be another issue worthy of more in-depth investigations (Peterson, 1979; Siu, 1999; Siu & Volkov, 1999).

Rote learning, which is the outcome of an examination-oriented system (of which examinations itself constitute only a part), not only hampers intellectual growth, but may also have a detrimental effect on seeking out new talents since those succeeding in examinations may have passed by means of memorizing standard solutions to stereotyped examination questions. This is obvious if one studies the examination system of the Ming Dynasty (1368–1636) when the "Eight-legged essay-type" (a rigid format of essays comprising eight paragraphs in length) examinations were almost the only channel for the selection of government officials (Peterson, 1979). However, the situation is even more intensified in modern societies since almost all the people who aim at getting a place in the government have to sit for high-stake examinations, whereas in ancient times, the general public (e.g., peasants) are untouched. Besides, the examination system in ancient times did not exert control over curriculum or teaching. In contrast, we see in recent years an expanding scope of educational control through various types of assessment mechanisms (N. Y. Wong, Han, & P. Y. Lee, this volume).

Based on the above, we see that there are no grounds for believing that the examination culture, which is "spoon-feeding" education, is an integral part of the Confucianism. Neither is there any reason to legitimize over-drilling by asserting that CHC learners excel only in rote learning and do not aim for genuine understanding.

7 Looking for Good Ways of Work: Entering the "Way"

Despite the argument of "where is CHC," some turned their attention to the identification of good ways of work in various regions irrespective of their cultural origins (whether it is "Confucian" or "Daoist," "Eastern" or "Western"). By "good ways of work," we only refer to cultural potentials rather than what is actually practiced currently in CHC regions. In fact, despite the conception that CHC education relies on transmission and learning by rote, among all other citations of Confucius, this saying on the process of education is the most oft-quoted: "Enlightenment comes when one is stunned and understanding when one is aroused; if one can't respond with the other three corner if a corner is shown, then one is not in the proper track (of learning)." (不悱不启, 不愤不发; 举一隅不以三隅反者, 则不复也。) (*The Analects*, 7:8 [论语•述而第七]) Confucius talked about experiencing rather than indoctrination, and later Confucians like Zhu Xi stressed on arousing skepticism and reflections of learners in addition. We will have more discussion in the section that follows but we will focus our attention here on the development of "basics," which is seen to be indispensable for further developments. Before that, let us first look at the relationship between "basics" and "higher-order abilities" in the CHC perspective.

Some of the critical aspects in the "middle zone" between the "East" and the "West" have already been identified (Gu, 2000; F. K. S. Leung, 2001; N. Y. Wong, in press; N. Y. Wong, Han, et al., this volume). The two extremes of "product" (content, basic skills, drills, etc.) and "process" (higher-order abilities, creativity, discoveries, etc.) is one such aspect, for which the debate can be dated back at least to the 1960s when there was the "New Math Reform" and the subsequent "Back to Basics" movement (N. Y. Wong, Han, et al., this volume). This may draw a similarity with the notion of *Gei* (art,艺) in Japanese education, which comprises both *Jutsu* (technique, 术) and *Do* (way, 道) (Hirabayashi, 2003). It is clear from the above discussion that CHC pedagogy may recognize the continuum between "content" and "process," not just recognizing that the acquisition of the former is a foundation on which the latter could be developed. Chinese people may believe that the basics are essential for enhancing process ability as it has been pointed out that these abilities cannot be developed out of the mathematics context. The key issue does not lie in striking a balance but in letting the introduction of mathematics knowledge be the foundation of the development of higher-order abilities (N. Y. Wong, 2002). This can be echoed by a common saying in Chinese martial art that "If you only practice combat skills and not develop the inner energy, your efforts will be in vain when you become old; but if you only practice the inner energy and not the combat skills, you would be like a boat that has no rudder." (练拳不练功, 到老一场空; 练功不练拳, 尤如无舵船。) In this regard, repetitive learning by performing a lot of practices becomes an essential part.

As remarked by Biggs (1994), we have to distinguish rote learning from repetitive learning in our discussions. Marton (1997) also pointed out in a public lecture that continuous practice with increasing variations could deepen understanding (see also Watkins, 1996). Confucius' words "Learn the new when revising the old" (温故而知新) (*The Analects*, 2:11 [论语•为政第二]) were also quoted in the lecture. In fact, scholars have pointed out that the first stance of *The Analects* of Confucius on learning — "Learn and practice frequently" (学而时习之) (*The Analects*, 1:1 [论语•学而第一]) — should be interpreted as "Learn and put your knowledge into practice frequently." Confucius did not particularly advocate rote learning and over-drilling (see also W. O. Lee, 1996). Research studies do support the hypothesis that excellent academic performance of Asian learners may be due to a synthesis of memorizing and understanding, a practice that is uncommon among Western students (Marton, Dall'Alba, et al., 1996; Marton, Watkins, et al., 1997; Watkins, 1994). It was also found that recitation is a common practice among CHC learners to bring about sharp focus for better understanding (Dahlin & Watkins, 2000).

One of the central beliefs in Confucianism is that there is always a right way to do anything. The right way is the "rite" that we ought to follow no matter whether the issue is big or small (有子曰:『礼之用……小大由之』。) (*The Analects*, 1:12 [论语•学而第一]). When Confucius entered the great ritual hall, he asked about the details (of the proper way) in each step. Someone called him ignorant but he replied, "This is the rite." ([孔]子入大庙, 每事问。或曰: 孰谓鄹人之子知礼乎? 入大庙, 每事问。子闻之曰: 是礼也。) (*The Analects*, 3:15 [论语•八佾第三]). This is also true in learning. As pointed out in Biggs (1994), "Chinese educators ... believe that art should not only be beautiful but morally good; the idea of one right way pervades teaching" (p. 28). So, there is a standard path, a routine that the learner can and should follow. In mathematics, though there are sometimes different ways to solve a problem, the one posed in the textbook is often the "best" (i.e., most elegant and simplest) way to solve it. Along this line of thought, it may not be advisable for beginners to deliberately create solutions different from the standard ones (H. Wu, 1994).

Following stringently the standard way and practice until one acquires "fluency" could be the first step in learning. N. Y. Wong (2002b) illustrated the case by the example of Chinese calligraphy, a tradition that almost all school pupils have to learn in olden days. The conventional way of learning is to start working with "copy books" (描红). Various basic skills (e.g., the application of brush to effect different kinds of strokes) are also performed during the teaching lesson. Then, the master will choose for the disciple an exemplary calligrapher, say Yan Zhenqing (颜真卿), so that the disciple may imitate (临摹) the calligraphy of Yan to a state that one cannot easily distinguish the calligraphy of Yan from that of the disciple. That is called "entering the Way" (入法). The emphasis is on doing each thing (brush-painting in this case) in the prescribed (or right) way.

Chinese martial art (*kung fu*, 功夫) shares the same approach. Practicing of footwork as well as other kinds of basic physical training like sandbag punching comprise the basics of Chinese martial art. Then there are standard sequences for one to practice. In simple terms, these sequences are "fictitious" courses of fighting. In other words, this is another kind of imitation of the "right" way to attack and defend. Afterwards, there come "paired practices" and other kinds of combat skill training. Of course, the final stage is free fight. In other words, the right way of learning is imitating the "right" way of fighting, accompanied by training of basic skills. These can only be done with a lot of drill and practices.

Certainly, there are other goals of repetition. Automation, which is necessary in some disciplines (for instance, martial art), is one. In mathematics, we often solve problems by applying the "fastest strategies" before going for "backup strategies" (Kerkman & Siegel, 1997). The notion of "techniques", being a bridge between tasks and conceptual reflection, was also put forth; and application of any such techniques should go through the process of naturalization and internalization (Artigue, 2001). We may conclude the role of practices in Figure 3 (for more details, see N. Y. Wong, in press).

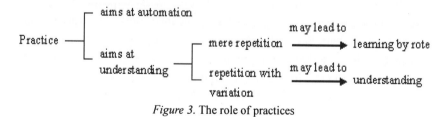

Figure 3. The role of practices

8 Looking for Good Ways of Work: Exiting the Way

However similar the imitation is to the original, even in a state that the imitator's work and the original work are hard to be distinguished, it is still considered as the first step in learning. Using once again the example of calligraphy, one enters the "gate" (i.e., getting to know the basics of a certain specialized knowledge) by way of painting in exactitude the calligraphy style of Yan's. Ultimately, a "personalized Yan-style" should emerge so that people well-versed in calligraphy can see the character of the calligrapher in his or her calligraphy and identify clearly the calligrapher's style originating from the Yan style. This "looking similar but being different" (求其似、求其不似) phenomenon shall be called "exiting the Way" (出法) — transcending the original cast. However, there is no obvious way to tell how a learner can arrive at this stage. Some believe that through incessant practices and a long period of "indulgence" and "hatching," then, mystical though it may sound, insight could be obtained at a certain point. This is clear from the maxim "familiarity breeds sophistication" (commonly translated as "practice makes perfect", 熟能生巧). Familiarity is a necessary but not a sufficient condition for sophistication. The case is similar for martial art. It was said that "when one has practiced for a long time, 'it' [the skills] will naturally be acquired" (习之若恒久, 不期自然至) (Y. Tang, 1986, p. 38). Eventually, the learner might come to a stage where he would exclaim "aha", when the posture comes about naturally without deliberation (技到无心始见奇) (p. 126).

The master's guidance and initiation are of vital importance. It is not easy to show a clear path of instruction, because initiation strategies are situation-dependent. Skilful teachers are able to grasp the right moment to trigger students' "sudden enlightenment" with appropriate means when they know that the disciple is ready. That is why the great Chan (Zen, 禅) master Huang Bo (黄檗) exclaimed, "I did not say that there is no Chan, I only said that we don't have masters!"[11] (for more details, see N. Y. Wong, 1998b, in press)

In brief, reflection forms the core of Confucian and Chan's way of "pedagogy" (bringing about realization). Thus the major task of the master is to arouse a disciple's reflection by generating a state of discomfort and perplexity. To quote from a popular citation of Confucius: "Enlightenment comes when one is stunned and understanding when one is aroused" (不悱不启，不愤不发) (*The Analects*, 7:8 [论语•述而第七]). Doubt and realization form the central theme of learning in Confucianism. Zhu Xi, the central figure of neo-Confucianism in the 12th century, pointed out that "Reading books [learning] is to arouse doubt when one does not doubt and let those in doubt settle in the state of no doubt. This is how one grows" (读书无疑者须教有疑、有疑者却要无疑。到这里方是长进。—朱子语类•卷十一读书法下》) (J. D. Li, 1270/1990, p. 296).

Arousing doubt in a disciple is also a main theme of Chan initiation. As it was said, "It is essential to arouse a sense of doubt in Chan practice. A little doubt leads to small understanding while strong doubt leads to deep understanding." (参禅须是起疑情，小疑小悟，大疑大悟。) (*Progressing through the Chan Gates* [禅关策进]). It was also said, "To make effort, one is only to have great doubt." (明州刚宗软禅师示众：『大凡做工夫，只要起大疑情。』) — 《续指月录》卷十二) (Nie, 1968, p. 759). "Great faith, great doubt and great diligence" are also identified as the "three pillars of Zen (Chan) Buddhism" (Kapleau, 1980). It seems that "doubt – reflection – realization" is a formula for "exiting the Way." This principle can clearly be seen from the words of the Sixth Patriarch of Chan Buddhism, Hui-Neng (慧能). Chapter 10 of his *Platform Sutra* teaches his disciples how to transmit the doctrine:

---

[11] Abbot Huang Bo told the mass, "Do you people know that there is no Chan masters in the entire Tang Empire?" At that time a monk came out from the audience and said, "There are so many masters teaching in so many monasteries, why you said there is no Chan master?" Huang replied, "I did not say that there is no Chan, I only said that there is no master!" (黄檗示众云：『汝等诸人，……还知大唐国里无禅师么？』时有僧出云：『只如诸方匡徒令众，又作么生？』檗云：『不道无禅，只是无师』！— Records of Green Cliff, 碧岩录 (Chinese Buddhist Electronic Text Association, 2001, Vol. 48, p. 1051b)

If someone asks you for the meaning [of something], use "emptiness" in response to questions on "reality"; use "reality" in response to questions on "emptiness"; use "saint" in response to questions on "mundane"; use "mundane" in response to "saint". When two phenomena are contrasted together, the middle way will emerge. So we have questions and answers. All other questioning will follow this method and the truth will not be lost. Suppose someone asks, "What is darkness?" The answer could be, "Brightness is the cause, darkness is the condition; where there is no brightness, there is darkness." We use brightness to illustrate darkness and use darkness to show brightness. Our minds go to and fro between these two notions, and the middle way will emerge. Other questioning will follow this. When you transmit the dharma [doctrine] in the future, you should adopt this kind of teaching so that the spirit of our school will be maintained. (若有人问汝义, 问有将无对, 问无将有对。问凡以圣对, 问圣以凡对。二道相因, 生中道义。如一问一对, 馀问一依此作, 即不失理也。设有人问何名为暗。答曰: 明是因, 暗是缘, 明没则暗。以明显暗, 以暗显明。来去相因, 成中道义。馀问悉皆如此。汝等于后传法, 依此转相教授, 勿失宗旨。—《六祖法宝坛经·咐嘱品》) (see N. Y. Wong, 1998b)

9. Variations: A Bridge over "Basic Skills" and "Process Abilities"?

Repetition until internalizing understanding could be a general strategy employed to bring about reflection and hence deeper understanding. This is well explained in the following words of Zhu Xi:

Generally speaking, in reading, we must first become intimately familiar with the text so that its words seem to come from our own mouths. We should then continue to reflect on it so that its ideas seem to come from our own minds. Only then can there be real understanding. Still, once our intimate reading of it and careful reflection on it have led to a clear understanding of it, we must continue to question. Then there might be further progress. If we cease questioning, in the end there'll be no more progress. (大抵观书先须熟读, 使其言皆若出于吾之口。继而精思, 使其意皆

若出于吾之心。然后可以有得而。然熟读精思既晓得后, 又须
疑不止如此。庶几有进。若以为止如此矣, 则不复有进也。——
《朱子语类·卷十读书法上》) (see also W. O. Lee, 1996)

In addition, recitation, when undertaken with reflection, is a means of bringing about repetitive learning. The following words of Zhu Xi give a clear explanation: "The method of reading books is, read once then reflect once; reflect once then read once again. Recitation is a means of enhancing reflection … if reading is just done in the mouth and not reflected in the mind, you cannot remember the passage well" (读书之法, 读一遍又思量一遍; 思量一遍又读一遍。读诵者, 所以助其思量…… 若只是口里读、心里不思量, 看如何也記不仔细。——《朱子语类·卷十 读书法上》) (see J. D. Li, 1270/1990, p. 170).

In fact, reinterpreting earlier findings in phenomenography (e.g., Bowden & Marton, 1998; Marton & Booth, 1997) leads to the conclusion that one way of experiencing a phenomenon can be characterized in terms of those aspects of the phenomenon that are discerned and kept in focal awareness by the learner (see also Runesson, 1999). Since discernment is an essential element in learning and variation is crucial in bringing about discernment, repetition by systematically introducing variations could be the key to bringing about learning and understanding.

In this light, repetition and practices of basic skills (entering the "Way") form the basis for developing process abilities (exiting the "Way") and thus should not be overlooked. The heart of the matter seems to lie in the quality rather than quantity of these practices, including the systematic introduction of variations.

N. Y. Wong (in press) projected the case to mathematics and looked into the example of introducing the formula for factorizing quadratic polynomials. After students have learned how to factorize quadratic polynomials for completing squares, a series of related problems could be set to let students experience the generalization of the completing square method into the quadratic polynomial formula. For a first trial, one can easily factorize polynomials like $x^2 + 4x + 4$ and $x^2 + 6x - 7$ by completing square. Gradually, we can introduce some variations like $2x^2 + 8x - 8$, $2x^2 + 4x - 7$ and $3x^2 + 5x - 4$. Later on, some parameters can be further introduced, such as $x^2 + 4x + k$, $x^2 + 2bx + 4$, $x^2 + 2px + q$, and $x^2 + px + q$. Finally, the factorization of $ax^2 + bx +$ would come about naturally. Huang (2002) also concluded that learning through exercises with variations is one of the characteristics of Chinese mathematics teaching (p. 236; see also Huang & F. K. S. Leung, 2002). Gu et al., (this volume) further distinguish two theories of variation, originated independently from Marton and Gu. In brief, despite the great communality between the two, Marton's focuses more on concept formation whereas in Gu's theory, skill acquisition is the central part.

Hence, less variation is associated with narrower ways of experiencing a phenomenon and more variation with wider ways of experiencing that phenomenon. Such a restricted conception may be the outcome of a "lived space" shaped by their teachers. In simple terms, we may say that CHC learning is strong in the "basics" but not so strong in the enhancement of "process abilities." This is a notion derived from the studies on teachers. There is a similarity in students' and teachers' conceptions of mathematics. In particular, both students and teachers perceived mathematics as, by and large, a set of rules. Though teachers' conception is not as restrictive (for instance, some appreciated the esthetic aspect of mathematics), this is not realized when setting up students' lived space. The mathematics problems given to the students are found to be closed-ended and stereotyped and required only low-level skills (N. Y. Wong, Lam, & C. S. Chan, 2002). This may be due to the acute examination orientation of CHC, coupled with the cultural expectations of parents. The systematic introduction of non-routine problems should help in widening the "lived space" of mathematics learning; students could acquire broader conceptions of mathematics and become more capable mathematical problem solvers (N. Y. Wong, Marton, K. M. Wong, & Lam, 2002; see also Watkins, 1996). Such an attempt was just made in 2001–2002, arriving at meaningful results (N. Y. Wong, Lam, K. M. Wong, & Chiu, 2003).

One class from each of ten schools in Hong Kong were involved in the project. After establishing shared views about the pedagogy of variation in the group through joint study activities and discussions, the mathematics tasks to be used in the ten classrooms during a school year were designed. To begin with, exemplars of non-routine mathematics problems were given to teachers, and they started designing more problems of the same type afterwards. Here "non-routine" mathematics problems mean those problems that are not frequently met by students or are not usually found in standard textbooks (see Figures 4 and 5). These problems include open-ended problems, problems found in overseas textbooks, problems found in the Internet, and even problems found in local textbooks that appear very different from those used in individual schools. Such non-routine tasks may include mathematics problems that: (1) appear in unfamiliar formats, (2) have more than one answer, (3) allow openness in the solving process, (4) contain missing or irrelevant data, (5) can be solved by a variety of means (for instance, by algebraic means, geometric means, graphical methods, concrete objects, calculators and micro-computers), or (6) involve problem posing (S. S. Leung, 1997). Problem posing here refers to the formulation of new problems or the conversion of existing problems into new ones.

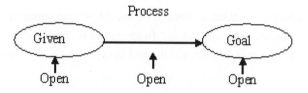

Figure 4. Definition of Open-ended Problems

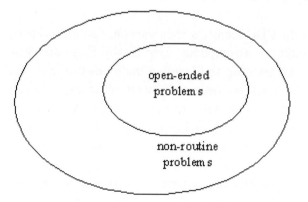

Figure 5. Relationship between non-routine and open-ended problems

The idea was that: at least half of all the tasks used in each classroom were taken from a common pool of tasks. These were constructed by more teachers, including more variations and a greater number of open-ended problems than was usually the case. In sum, variation in the students' learning experience would be introduced through the open-endedness of each task. The variation between such tasks came from: (1) the design of more open-ended tasks by individual teachers, (2) shared tasks developed by different teachers, (3) reflection in sharing session within the teacher groups, or (4) student sharing and discussion of different solutions offered by others in the classroom. In other words, students would encounter not only different tasks authored by other teachers, but also different solutions to the same problem offered by other students. In such a way, the lived space of variation of the students' mathematical experience was widened, and so did the live space of the teachers. In general, it was found that the exposure to non-routine tasks improves students' performances in solving open-ended problems, but the appropriate amount of tasks depends on the academic standards of the students. In brief, students from schools with higher academic standards benefit from high and medium doses of non-routine tasks whereas those from schools with lower academic standards only benefit from medium and low doses (N. Y. Wong, Lam, et al., 2003).

10 In Search of the "CHC" Script

Obviously the CHC learner's phenomenon, like most other phenomena, rests on "cultural" assumptions. That is why Biggs and Watkins (2001) alerted us that teaching and learning traditions that may work well in a certain culture may not necessarily work in another: "adopting Chinese teaching tactics will not solve this one.[12] Rather, Western educators need to develop their own script, using things that work in Western culture and that will engage students socialized the Western way in productive learning" (p. 291). The (classroom-) learning environment ("cultural" setting) is shaped by cultural beliefs, social assumptions, and beliefs on students and student learning. Huang (2002) tried to portray a scene of a Chinese mathematics lesson as follows:

---

[12] The paradox of the Western class having a smaller size but with low performance.

There are teacher, students and mathematics. The teacher presents mathematics and help students engage in the process of exploring the mathematics by providing proper scaffoldings and asking a series of heuristic questions. The students are eager to listen and engage themselves in the process of learning. (p. 237)

Huang (2002) continued to comment that "according to Western concepts such as teacher-centered or student-centered, this description is difficult to understand. However, it seems to be quite understandable and practical in the Chinese cultural setting, which may be due to cultural differences" (p. 237).

Biggs and Watkins (2001) also noted the components of "concentrated learning," "vicarious learning," "careful planning, timed questioning, and associated activity," and "learner-trained learning" in a "good" "CHC learning environment" which is seen to be repetitive, teacher-dominated in the "Western eye" (p. 285). From the discussions of the above sections, we may identify general descriptions of the CHC classroom environments such as:

- obedient and attentive students sitting properly listening to the teacher
- teachers with their lessons well-prepared and structured
- students seldom interrupting the flow of the teaching by asking questions
- teachers checking whether students follow through by asking questions
- teachers not attempting to cater for individual differences in class yet
- students having a lot of guided after-class learning (including homework and tutorial classes)
- teachers giving individual guidance after class
- teachers seeing the moral responsibility of providing individual care, including those not directly related to learning (e.g., personal growth and transmission of cultural values such as listenership)

Research on Hong Kong students repeatedly revealed that a good mathematics teacher as perceived by the students is one who explains clearly, shows concern toward them, treats them as friends, makes sure that they understand, teaches in a lively way, is conscientious and well-prepared, and answers students' queries (after class). A good mathematics teacher should also provide more exercises and generate a lively atmosphere but keep good order; and a good learning environment is one which is not boring, but is quiet, with classmates engaged in learning, where order is observed but discussion with classmates after lesson is possible (N. Y. Wong, 1993, 1996; N. Y. Wong, Lam, K. M. Wong, F. K. S. Leung, & Mok, 2001).

The above picture of the CHC classroom may be in accord with the learning environment that is "both teacher led and student centered" as advocated by Ausubel (1961, 1963, 1988a, 1968b), who argued that his notion of meaningful verbal learning is different from learning by rote (in fact empirical research revealed that "transmission" and "child-centeredness" are distinct dimensions; see Perry, D. Tracey, & Howard, 1998). In such kind of learning environment, the basics of knowledge are transmitted with high efficiency and in large scale in class, so that students are led to "enter the Way." Individual guidance is provided after class, hoping that "exiting the Way" could happen (that may only need to happen occasionally). In order to actualize such a scenario, one can envisage that attention and discipline (in class) is of first priority. By "discipline", it is much more than obedience. Besides as an ends in itself, students should be acquired and accustomed to the various routines in flow of classroom teaching: when to talk, when to do seat work, when to open one's book, when to look at the chalk-board (or computer projection), and so on. Without such a cultural assumption (that students know what should be done in every moment of the class), the above "teacher led and student centered" script cannot be put onto show. These "trainings" are developed through reinforcement, social contracts, conformities, and social negotiations which are so common in the CHC classroom and CHC teacher education programs (e.g., students at a very young age have already known that one should put up one's hand and being called by the name before one can stand up and speak).

The establishment of classroom discipline has dual purposes. It is also a part of moral education. In fact, Gao and Watkins (2001) pointed out that

CHC teachers believe that individual guidance should be handled outside rather than inside the classroom. Furthermore, CHC teachers were found to bear a moral responsibility of caring for their students and an implicit influence (especially on character cultivation) exists behind the façade of knowledge transmission (Gao & Watkins, 2001; I. T. Ho, 2001). It has long been a tradition that teachers should not only "teach books" (which can be done by "lecturing") but "teach the person" (经师易得, 人师难求—《北史》) (which can be done by modeling [言教、身教]). The relationships between "entering the way", "exiting the way" can be conceptualized, in broad strokes, in the "script" depicted in Figure 6.

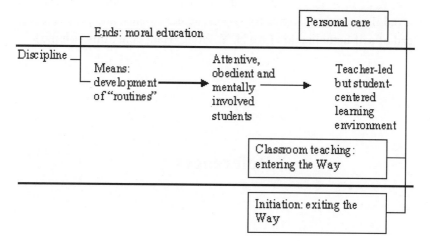

Figure 6. A possible "CHC script"

As remarked by Biggs and Watkins (2001), the West should find their own script, and the CHC regions should find their script too. One should not be satisfied merely with the superficial success in international comparisons since good achievements in international studies should not be the central aim of mathematics education (see N. Y. Wong, Han, et al., this volume). Siu and Volkov (1999) remind us that placing too much focus on practical aspect of (mathematics) education may hamper the development of those talented in mathematics. Likewise, letting high-stake assessments remain the driving force of learning may result in rote memorization. While there is a general misconception that examination is the built-in component of CHC, the above analyses precisely show the opposite. CHC contains full cultural potential for deep understanding. Ideologies of Confucianism and other Chinese philosophies possess nurturing goals far beyond crossing examination hurdles and getting a place in the official hierarchy. In many points in history, it was precisely the aim of those who advocated these philosophies to counteract governments' educational control mechanism. As said by Confucius himself, "the purpose of learning in ancient time is for (enriching) oneself and the purpose of learning nowadays is for (pleasing) others" (古之学者为己, 今之学者为人。) (*The Analects, 14:24* [论语•宪问第十四]). The "soul" of CHC education can never be retrieved if one only searches for scores, achievements, and performances instead of self-actualization (see N. Y. Wong, Han, et al., this volume).

References

Artigue, M. (2001, July). *Learning mathematics in a CAS environment: The genesis of a reflection about instrumentation and the dialectics between technical and conceptual work*. Paper presented at the CAME meeting, Utrecht, The Netherlands.

Ausubel, D. P. (1961). In defense of verbal learning. *Educational Theory, XI*, 15–25.

Ausubel, D. P. (1963). *The psychology of meaningful verbal learning*. New York: Grune & Stratton.

Ausubel, D. P. (1968a). *Educational psychology, a cognitive view*. New York: Holt, Rinehart & Winston.

Ausubel, D. P. (1968b). Facilitating meaningful verbal learning in the classroom. *The Arithmetic Teacher, 15*, 126–132.

Biggs, J. B. (1990). Asian students' approaches to learning: Implication for teaching overseas students. In M. Kratzing (Ed.), *Eighth Australasian learning and language conference* (pp. 1–51). Australia: Queensland University of Technology Counseling Services.

Biggs, J. B. (1991). Approaches to learning in secondary and tertiary students in Hong Kong: Some comparative studies. *Educational Research Journal, 6*, 27–39.

Biggs, J. B. (1994). What are effective schools? Lessons from East and West [The Radford Memorial Lecture]. *Australian Educational Researcher, 21*, 19–39.

Biggs, J. B. (1996a). Learning, schooling, and socialization: A Chinese solution to a Western problem. In S. Lau (Ed.), *Growing up the Chinese way* (pp. 147–167). Hong Kong: The Chinese University Press.

Biggs, J. B. (1996b). Western misconceptions of the Confucian-heritage learning culture. In D. A. Watkins & J. B. Biggs (Eds.), *The Chinese learner: Cultural, psychological and contextual influences* (pp. 45–67). Hong Kong: Comparative Education Research Centre, The University of Hong Kong; Melbourne, Australia: The Australian Council for Educational Research.

Biggs, J. B., & Moore, P. J. (1993). *The process of learning*. New York: Prentice Hall.

Biggs, J. B., & Watkins, D. A. (2001). Insights into teaching the Chinese learner. In D. A. Watkins & J. B. Biggs (Eds.), *Teaching the Chinese learner: Psychological and pedagogical perspectives* (pp. 277–300). Hong Kong: Comparative Education Research Centre, The University of Hong Kong.

Bond, M. H. (Ed.). (1996a). *The handbook of Chinese psychology*. Hong Kong: Oxford University Press.

Bond, M. H. (1996b). Chinese values. In M. H. Bond (Ed.), *The handbook of Chinese psychology* (pp. 208–226). Hong Kong: Oxford University Press.

Bond, M. H., & Hwang, K. K. (1986). The social psychology of Chinese people. In M. H. Bond (Ed.), *The psychology of the Chinese people* (pp. 213–266). Hong Kong: Oxford University Press.

Bowden, J., & Marton, F. (1998). *The university of learning*. London: Kogan Page.

Brand, D. (1987, August 31). The new whiz kids: Why Asian Americans are doing well, and what it costs them [cover story]. *Time, 9*, 42–50.

Cai, J. (1995). A cognitive analysis of U.S. and Chinese students' mathematical performance on tasks involving computation, simple problem solving, and complex problem solving. *Journal for Research in Mathematics Education Monograph series 7*. Reston, VA: National Council of Teachers of Mathematics.

Cai, J. (2000). Mathematical thinking involved in US and Chinese students' solving of process-constrained and process-open problems. *Mathematical Thinking and Learning, 2*, 309–340.

Cai, J. (2003). Investigating parental roles in students' learning of mathematics from a cross-national perspective. *Mathematics Education Research Journal, 15*(2), 87-106.

Chan, G. Y., & Watkins, D. A. (1994). Classroom environment and approaches to learning: An investigation of the actual and preferred perceptions of Hong Kong secondary school students. *Instructional Science, 22*, 233–246.

Chang, W. C. (2000). In search of the Chinese in all the wrong places! *Journal of Psychology in Chinese Societies, 1*(1), 125–142.

Cheng, K. M. (1994). Quality of education as perceived in the Chinese culture. In T. Takala (Ed.), *Quality of education in the context of culture in developing countries* (pp. 67–84). Tampere, Finland: Tampere University Press.

Chinese Buddhist Electronic Text Association. (2001). *Chinese electronic tripitaka series* (Vol. 48) [In Chinese 电子佛典系列] [CD ROM]. Taipei: Author.

Chinese Culture Connection. (1987). Chinese value and the search for culture-free dimensions of culture. *Journal of Cross-Cultural Psychology, 18*, 143–164.

Dahlin, B., & Watkins, D. A. (2000). The role of repetition in the processes of memorising and understanding: A comparison of the views of Western and Chinese school students in Hong Kong. *British Journal of Educational Psychology, 70*, 65–84.

Fromm, E. (1960). *Psychoanalysis and Zen Buddhism*. London: George Allen & Unwin.

Gao, L., & Watkins, D. A. (2001). Towards a model of teaching conceptions of Chinese secondary school teachers of physics. In D. A. Watkins & J. B. Biggs (Eds.), *Teaching the Chinese learner: Psychological and pedagogical perspectives* (pp. 27–45). Hong Kong: Comparative Education Research Centre, The University of Hong Kong.

Gu, L. (2000, July–August). *Exploring the middle zone*. Paper presented at the 9th International Congress of Mathematics Education (Gathering of Chinese scholars), Tokyo/Makuhari, Japan.

Hatano, G., & Inagaki, K. (1998). Cultural contexts of schooling revisited: A review of *The Learning Gap* from a cultural psychology perspective. In S. G. Paris & H. M. Wellman (Eds.), *Global prospects for education: Development, culture, and schooling* (pp. 79–104). Washington, DC: American Psychological Association.

Hau, K. T., & Salili, F. (1991). Structure and semantic differential placement of specific causes: Academic causal attributions by Chinese students in Hong Kong. *International Journal of Psychology, 26*, 175–193.

Hau, K. T., & Salili, F. (1996). Achievement goals and causal attributions of Chinese students. In S. Lau (Ed.), *Growing up the Chinese way* (pp. 121–145). Hong Kong: The Chinese University Press.

Hess, R. D., & Azuma, M. (1991). Cultural support for schooling: Contrasts between Japan and the United States. *Educational Researcher, 20*(9), 2–8.

Hirabayashi, I. (2003). A traditional aspect of mathematics education in Japan: Mathematics as *Gei* (art), its *Jutsu* (technique) and *Do* (way). In F. Lopez-Real (Ed.), *Pre-conference Proceedings of ICMI comparative study conference* (pp. 133–141). Hong Kong: Faculty of Education, The University of Hong Kong.

Ho, D. Y. F. (1986). Chinese patterns of socialization: A critical review. In M. H. Bond (Ed.), *The psychology of the Chinese people* (pp. 1–37). Hong Kong: Oxford University Press.

Ho, D. Y. F. (1991). *Cognitive socialization in Confucian heritage cultures*. Paper presented at the Workshop on Continuities and Discontinuities in the Cognitive Socialization of Minority Children, U.S. Department of Health and Human Services, Washington, DC.

Ho, I. T. (2001). Are Chinese teachers authoritarian? In D. A. Watkins & J. B. Biggs (Eds.), *Teaching the Chinese learner: Psychological and pedagogical perspectives* (pp. 99–114). Hong Kong: Comparative Education Research Centre, The University of Hong Kong.

Hofstede, G. H. (1983). Dimensions of national cultures in fifty countries and three regions. In J. B. Deregowski, S. Dziurawiec, & R. C. Annis (Eds.), *Expiscations in cross-cultural psychology* (pp. 335–355). Lisse, The Netherlands: Swets and Zeitlinger.

Huang, R. (2002). *Mathematics teaching in Hong Kong and Shanghai — A classroom analysis from the perspective of variation*. Unpublished doctoral dissertation, The University of Hong Kong, Hong Kong.

Huang, R., & Leung, F. K. S. (2002). Is there a Chinese approach? — A comparison on the ways of teaching the Pythagoras theorem among Australia, Czech Republic, Hong Kong and Shanghai. In D. Edge & B. H. Yeap (Eds.), *Proceedings of second East Asia regional conference on mathematics education and ninth Southeast Asian conference on mathematics education* (Vol. 2, pp. 247–252). Singapore: Association of

Mathematics Educators & National Institute of Education, NTU.

Inagaki, K., Hatano, G., & Morita, E. (1998). Construction of mathematical knowledge through whole-class discussion. *Learning and Instruction, 8,* 503–526.

Iwawaki, S., & Lynn, R. (1972). Measuring achievement motivation in Japan and Great Britain. *Journal of Cross-Cultural Psychology, 3*(2), 219–220.

Kapleau, P. (1980). *The three pillars of Zen: Teachings, practice, enlightenment.* Garden City, NY: Anchor Books.

Kember, D., & Gow, L. (1991). A challenge to the anecdotal stereotype of the Asian students. *Studies in Higher Education, 161,* 117–128.

Kerkman, D. D., & Siegel, R. S. (1997). Measuring individual differences in children's addition strategy choices. *Learning and Individual Differences, 9*(1), 1–18.

Kim, U., Triandis, H. C., Kagitcibasi, C., Choi, S. C., & Yoon, G. (Eds.). (1994). Individualism and collectivism: Theory, method and application. Thousand Oaks, CA: Sage.

Lao, S. K. (1988). Philosophical thought and education [In Chinese 哲学思想与教育]. In J. Y. To & S. H. Liu (Eds.), *Philosophy, civilisation, and education* [In Chinese 哲学、文化与教育] (pp. 3–62). Hong Kong: The Chinese University Press.

Lau, S. (Ed.). (1996). *Growing up the Chinese way.* Hong Kong: The Chinese University Press.

Lee, P. Y., Zhang, D.-Z., & Zheng, Z. (1997). Examination culture and the teaching of mathematics [In Chinese 考试文化与数学教学]. *EduMath* [In Chinese 数学教育], *4,* 96–103.

Lee, W. O. (1996). The cultural context for Chinese learners: Conceptions of learning in the Confucian tradition. In D. A. Watkins & J. B. Biggs (Eds.), *The Chinese learner: Cultural, psychological and contextual influences* (pp. 25–41). Hong Kong: Comparative Education Research Centre, The University of Hong Kong; Melbourne, Australia: The Australian Council for Educational Research.

Leu, Y. C., & Wu, C. J. (2002). The origins of pupils' awareness of teachers' mathematics pedagogical values: Confucianism and Buddhism-driven. In F. Lopez-Real (Ed.), *Pre-conference proceedings of ICMI Comparative Study Conference* (pp. 49–58). Hong Kong: Faculty of Education, The University of Hong Kong.

Leu, Y. C., Wu, Y. Y., & Wu, C. J. (1999). A Buddhistic value in an elementary mathematics classroom. In O. Zaslavsky (Ed.), *Proceedings of the 23rd international conference of the psychology of mathematics education* (Vol. 3, pp. 233–240). Haifa, Israel: Israel Institute of Technology.

Leung, F. K. S. (2001). In search of an East Asian identity in mathematics education. *Educational Studies in Mathematics, 47,* 35–51.

Leung, S. S. (1997). On the open-ended nature in mathematical problem posing. In E. Pehkonen (Ed.), *Use of open-ended problems in mathematics classroom* (Research Report 176, pp. 26–33). Helsinki, Finland: Department of Education, University of Helsinki.

Li, J. (2003a). The core of Confucian learning. *American Psychologist, 58,* 146–147.

Li, J. (2003b). U.S. and Chinese cultural beliefs about learning. *Journal of Educational Psychology, 95*(2), 258-267.

Li, J. D. (1990). *Selections from the conversations of Master Zhu, arranged topically* (D. K. Gardner, Trans.). Berkeley, CA: University of California Press. (Original work published 1270)

Llewellyn, J., Hancock, G., Kirst, M., & Roeloffs, K. (1982). *A perspective on education in*

Hong Kong: Report by a visiting panel. Hong Kong: Government Printer.

Marton, F. (1997, March). *Student learning: East and West.* Public lecture presented at The Chinese University of Hong Kong, Shatin, Hong Kong.

Marton, F., & Booth, S. (1997). *Learning and awareness.* Mahwah, NJ: Lawrence Erlbaum Associates.

Marton, F., Dall'Alba, G, & Tse, L. K. (1996). Memorizing and understanding: The keys to the paradox? In D. A. Watkins & J. B. Biggs (Eds.), *The Chinese learner: Cultural, psychological and contextual influences* (pp. 69–83). Hong Kong: Comparative Education Research Centre, The University of Hong Kong; Melbourne, Australia: The Australian Council for Educational Research.

Marton, F., Watkins, D. A., & Tang, C. (1997). Discontinuities and continuities in the experience of learning: An interview study of high-school students in Hong Kong. *Learning and Instruction, 7,* 21–48.

Maslow, A, H. (1954). *Motivation and personality.* New York: Viking.

Morris, P. (1985). Teachers' perceptions of the barriers to the implementation of a pedagogic innovation: A South East Asian case study. *International Review of Education, 31,* 3–18.

Morris, P. (1988). Teachers' attitudes towards a curriculum innovation: An East Asian study. *Research in Education, 40,* 75–87.

Murphy, D. (1987). Offshore education: A Hong Kong perspective. *Australian Universities Review, 30*(2), 43–44.

Nie, X. (1968). *Records of moon-pointing (continued).* Taipei: Zheng Shan Mei Publishers.

Perry, B., Tracey, D., & Howard, P. (1998). Elementary school teacher beliefs about the learning and teaching of mathematics. In H. S. Park, Y. H. Choe, H. Shin, & S. H. Kim (Eds.), *Proceedings of the ICMI-East Asia Regional Conference on Mathematical Education* (Vol. 2, pp. 485–497). Seoul, Korea: Korean Sub-Commission of ICMI; Korea Society of Mathematical Education; Korea National University of Education.

Peterson, W. (1979). *Bitter gourd, Chapter 3: Examination man* (pp. 44–63). Yale: Yale University Press.

Pong, W. Y., & Chow, J. C. S. (2002). On the pedagogy of examinations in Hong Kong. *Teaching and Teacher Education, 18,* 139-149.

Qian, M. (1976). Soul and mind [In Chinese 灵魂与心]. In M. Qian (Ed.), *Soul and mind* [In Chinese 灵魂与心]. Taipei: Lian Jing Publications. (Original work published 1945)

Ray, J., & Jones, J. (1983). Occupational and educational achievement motivation in Australian and Hong Kong school children. *The Journal of Social Psychology, 120,* 281–282.

Runesson, U. (1999). *Variationens pedagogic: Skilda sätt att behandla ett matematiskt innehåll* [The pedagogy of variation: Different ways of handling a mathematics topic]. Unpublished doctoral dissertation, University of Göteborg, Sweden. English summary retrieved December 1, 1997, from http://www.ped.gu.se/biorn/phgraph/civial/graphica/diss.su/runesson.html

Schwartz, S. H. (1994). Cultural dimensions of value: Toward an understanding of national differences. In U. Kim, H. C. Triandis, C. Kagitcibasi, S. C. Choi, & G. Yoon (Eds.), *Individualism and collectivism: Theory, method and application* (pp. 85–119). Thousand Oaks, CA: Sage.

Siu, M. K. (1995). Mathematics education in ancient China: What lesson do we learn from it? *Historia Scientiarum, 4,* 223–232.

Siu, M. K. (1999, July). *How did candidates pass the state examination in mathematics in the Tang Dynasty (618–907)? — Myth of the "Confucian-heritage-culture" classroom*. Paper presented at the Third European Summer University in History and Epistemology in Mathematics Education, Louvain-la-Neuve/Leuven, Belgium.

Siu, M. K., & Volkov, A. (1999). Official curriculum in traditional Chinese mathematics: How did candidates pass the examinations? *Historia Scientiarum, 9*, 85–99.

Stevenson, H. W., & Lee, S. Y. (1990). *Contexts of achievement: A study of American, Chinese, and Japanese children*. Chicago, IL: The University of Chicago Press.

Stevenson, H. W., & Stigler, J. W. (1992). *The learning gap: Why our schools are failing and what we can learn from Japanese and Chinese education*. New York: Summit Books.

Stigler, J., & Hiebert, J. (1999). *The teaching gap: Best ideas from the world's teachers for improving education in the classroom*. New York: Free Press.

Stover, L. E. (1974). *The cultural ecology of Chinese civilization*. New York: New American Library.

Tang, Y. (1986). *Brief introduction to Form-and-Will style Chinese martial art* [In Chinese 意拳浅释]. Hong Kong: Form-and-Will Study Group.

Tracey, J. (1983). *Patriarchy and social revolution in Chinese*. Berkeley, CA: University of California Press.

Watkins, D. A. (1994, July). *Memorising and understanding: The keys to solving the mysteries of the Chinese learner?* Paper presented at the 23rd Congress of the International Association of Applied Psychology, Madrid, Spain.

Watkins, D. A. (1996). Hong Kong secondary school learners: A developmental perspective. In D. A. Watkins & J. B. Biggs (Eds.), *The Chinese learner: Cultural, psychological and contextual influences* (pp. 107–119). Hong Kong: Comparative Education Research Centre, The University of Hong Kong; Melbourne, Australia: The Australian Council for Educational Research.

Watkins, D. A., & Biggs, J. B. (Eds.). (1996). *The Chinese learner: Cultural, psychological and contextual influences*. Hong Kong: Comparative Education Research Centre, The University of Hong Kong; Victoria, Australia: The Australian Council for Educational Research.

Watkins, D. A., & Biggs, J. B. (Eds.). (2001). *Teaching the Chinese learner: Psychological and pedagogical perspectives*. Hong Kong: Comparative Education Research Centre, The University of Hong Kong.

Watkins, D. A., & Ismail, M. (1994). Is the Asian learner a rote learner? A Malaysian perspective. *Contemporary Educational Psychology, 19*, 483–488.

Watkins, D. A., Regmi, M., & Astilla, E. (1991). The Asian-learner-as-a-rote-learner stereotype: Myth or reality? *Educational Psychology, 11*, 21–34.

Winter, S. (1990). Teacher approval and disapproval in Hong Kong secondary school classrooms. *British Journal of Educational Psychology, 60*, 88–92.

Wong, N. Y. (1993). The psychosocial environment in the Hong Kong mathematics classroom. *The Journal of Mathematical Behavior, 12*, 303–309.

Wong, N. Y. (1996). Students' perceptions of their mathematics classroom. *Hiroshima Journal of Mathematics Education, 4*, 89–107.

Wong, N. Y. (1998a). In search of the "CHC" learner: Smarter, works harder or something more? [Plenary lecture]. In H. S. Park, Y. H. Choe, H. Shin, & S. H. Kim (Eds.). *Proceedings of ICMI — East Asia regional conference on mathematical education* (Vol. 1, pp. 85–98). Seoul, Korea: Korean Sub-Commission of ICMI; Korea Society of Mathematical Education; Korea National University of Education.

Wong, N. Y. (1998b). The gradual and sudden paths of Tibetan and Chan Buddhism: A pedagogical perspective. *Journal of Thought, 33*(2), 9–23.

Wong, N. Y. (2001). The lived space of mathematics learning: From conception to action. (Plenary Lecture). In L. Sun (Ed.), *Proceedings of the international conference on mathematics education* (pp. 6–19). Changchun, China: Northeast Normal University.

Wong, N. Y. (2002). Conceptions of doing and learning mathematics among Chinese. *Journal of Intercultural Studies, 23*(2), 211–229.

Wong, N. Y. (in press). From "entering the way" to "exiting the way": In search of a bridge over "basic skills" and "process abilities." In F. K. S. Leung, K. D. Graf, & F. Lopez-Real (Eds.), *Mathematics education in different cultural traditions: A comparative study of East Asia and the West, new ICMI study series*. Dordrecht, The Netherlands: Kluwer Academic Press.

Wong, N. Y., Lam, C. C., & Chan, C. S. (2002). The current state of the "lived space" of mathematics learning. *Hiroshima Journal of Mathematics Education, 10*, 27–52.

Wong, N.Y., Lam C. C., Wong, K. M., Leung, F. K. S., Mok, I. A. C. (2001). Students; views of mathematics learning: A cross-sectional survey in Hong Kong. *Education Journal, 29*(2), 37-59.

Wong, N. Y., Lam, C. C., Wong, K. M., & Chiu, M. M. (2003). *The lived space of mathematics learning: An attempt for change*. Manuscript submitted for publication.

Wong, N. Y., Marton, F., Wong, K. M., & Lam, C. C. (2002). The lived space of mathematics learning. *Journal of Mathematical Behavior, 21*, 25-47.

Wong, N. Y., & Wong, W. Y. (2002). The "Confucian Heritage Culture" learner's phenomenon. *Asian Psychologist, 3*(1), 78–82.

Wu, H. (1994). The role of open-ended problems in mathematics education. *Journal of Mathematical Behavior, 13*(1), 115–128.

Yang, J. (1987). Confucian ethics, Weber's propositions and ideology [In Chinese 儒家伦理, 韦伯命题与意识形态]. In J. Yang & N. Tao (Eds.), *Confucian ethics and economic development* [In Chinese 儒家伦理与经济发展] (pp. 227–261). Taipei: Yuen Zhen Civilization.

Yu, A. B. (1996). Ultimate life concerns, self and Chinese achievement motivation. In M. H. Bond (Ed.), *The handbook of Chinese psychology* (pp. 227–246). Hong Kong: Oxford University Press.

Zhang, D.-X. (1989). *Confucian ethics and the order complex* [In Chinese 儒家伦理与秩序情结]. Taipei: Great Current Publications.

Zhang, D.-Z. (1993). Success and inadequacies of mathematics education in Chinese communities [In Chinese 华人地区数学教育的成功与不足]. In C. C. Lam, H. W. Wong, & Y. W. Fung (Eds.), *Proceedings of the international symposium on curriculum changes for Chinese communities in Southeast Asia: Challenges of the 21st century* [In Chinese 东南亚华人社会的课程改革: 二十一世纪的挑战国际研讨会论文集] (pp. 93–95). Hong Kong: The Chinese University of Hong Kong.

Chapter 20

How Do Chinese Learn Mathematics? Some Evidence-Based Insights and Needed Directions

CAI Jinfa   LIN Fou-Lai   FAN Lianghuo

This chapter summarizes some research-based evidence that characterizes how Chinese learn mathematics, and then points out needed directions to understand Chinese learners and their learning of mathematics. The discussion is situated in a comparative context by focusing on the following four important issues: (1) Are Chinese learners really higher achievers in mathematics? (2) Does the teaching of Chinese learners necessarily lead to rote learning? (3) How is the intended curriculum structured to support teaching and learning? and (4) How do Chinese families support students' learning? Available research evidence that addresses each issue is first reviewed, and then research needed to further address the issue is suggested.

Key words: Chinese learners, conceptual development, rote learning, family support, curriculum features, instructional practice

1 Why Do We Care How Chinese Learn Mathematics?

How Chinese learn mathematics is the theme of this volume. This chapter aims at summarizing some research-based evidence for characterizing how Chinese learn mathematics, and then pointing out needed directions to understand Chinese learners and their learning of mathematics. But why should we and readers care about how Chinese learn mathematics? As an attempt to answer this question, we start with a true story about Howard Gardner, a distinguished professor and scholar from Harvard University. In the spring of 1987, Gardner was visiting China studying arts education in kindergartens and elementary schools. During the visit, he, his wife, and son (Benjamin) stayed in the Jinling

Hotel in Nanjing. The key to their hotel room was attached to a large plastic block, which made noise when it was shaken. His son, Benjamin loved to carry the key chain around, shaking it vigorously. He also liked to try to place the key into the slot. Because Benjamin was one and a half years old, it was a challenge to correctly orient the key into the slot. However, Benjamin seemed to enjoy the sound it made when the key banged against the slot, and he also loved this exploratory activity. Since Gardner and his wife were not in a hurry at the time, they allowed Benjamin to have a good time. But they soon observed an intriguing phenomenon. Any Chinese attendant nearby would come to watch Benjamin. At one point, an attendant noticed Benjamin's lack of initial success in placing the key into the slot, so she would hold onto Benjamin's hand and directly help Benjamin insert the key. Then she smiled at Gardner or his wife, as if having done a favor for them and awaiting for "thank you." Interestingly, neither Gardner nor his wife appreciated the intervention of the attendant since what mattered to them was that Benjamin was having a good time exploring. Later Gardner realized that this incident pointed to important differences in the educational and artistic practices between the US and China. After studying Chinese education in general and arts education in particular, the world renown scholar wrote: "Some of my most entrenched beliefs about education and human development had been challenged by my observations in Chinese classrooms." (Gardner, 1989, p. vi)

The above story sheds some light on why we should care how Chinese learn mathematics. Like arts education, the teaching and learning of mathematics is also a cultural activity. Clearly, there are cultural differences in both the views and practices of the teaching and learning of mathematics among different countries. In particular, there are at least three compelling reasons for studying how Chinese learn mathematics.

First, studying how Chinese learn mathematics would broaden our experience and provide different perspectives for addressing practical issues related to the teaching and learning of mathematics. For example, it is widely accepted that to achieve the goal of "algebra for all," students in the early grades should have experiences that prepare them for more sophisticated work in algebra in the middle and high school (National

Council of Teachers of Mathematics [NCTM], 2000). However, curriculum developers, educational researchers, teachers, and policy makers are just beginning to think about and explore the kinds of mathematical experiences elementary school students need in order to prepare them for the formal study of algebra in the later grades. The Chinese elementary school mathematics curriculum includes a variety of activities and ideas to provide students with rich experiences of algebraic thinking in earlier grades. The overarching goal of learning algebra in the Chinese elementary curriculum is to better represent and understand quantitative relationships, with a focus on equations and equation solving. Students in elementary school are consistently encouraged and provided with opportunities to represent a quantitative relationship both arithmetically and algebraically. Furthermore, students are asked to make comparisons between arithmetical and algebraic ways of representing a quantitative relationship. The first-describing-and-then-calculating is one of the key features that make algebra different from arithmetic. The comparisons of arithmetic and algebraic approaches can highlight this unique feature of algebra. Throughout the Chinese elementary school curriculum, there are numerous examples and problems in which students need to identify quantitative relationships and represent them in multiple ways. The Chinese experience in developing students' algebraic thinking in earlier grades may increase teachers' ability to address the issues and challenges they face in other countries (Cai, 2004).

Second, studying how Chinese learn mathematics may provide a unique opportunity for people to reflect on theories and conceptions of teaching and learning mathematics in their own culture. For example, in Western countries, memorization and rote learning are generally considered the same (Marton, Dall'Alba, & Tse, 1996). Western scholars also believe that memorization does not lead to understanding. However, through extensive interviews with 20 Chinese teacher educators, Marton et al. (1996) provided a new way of seeing the relationship between memorization and understanding. For Chinese teacher educators, memorization can be used to deepen and develop understanding. In addition, studying how Chinese learn mathematics may provide a unique opportunity for generating new knowledge and theories. Through examining a group of Chinese teachers' mathematical knowledge, for example, L. Ma (1999) proposed that in order to teach mathematics effectively, teachers should have a profound understanding of fundamental mathematics. Her study not only contributes to our understanding of teachers' subject matter knowledge but also challenges the current practices of teacher preparation around the world.

Third, studying how Chinese learn mathematics can foster Chinese "insiders" to reflect on and systematically synthesize the current practices for the purpose of building theories about the teaching and learning of mathematics. There is no doubt that Confucianism has an impact on the conceptions and practice of mathematics teaching and learning among Chinese. Wong (this volume) has indicated that it is very helpful to use the Confucian Heritage Culture (CHC) to understand and explain some phenomena of Chinese learners. However, we lack empirical data to systematically document and describe Chinese learners. In addition, Chinese teachers and educators have accumulated ample experience about curriculum development and instructional practices. There is an urgent need to systematically synthesize these experiences and generate theories about how Chinese learn mathematics.

In this chapter, we situate our discussion in a comparative context. However, our comparative perspective is limited to comparing Chinese learners with learners in Western countries. Moreover, to characterize Chinese learners, we decided to focus on four important issues: (1) Are Chinese learners really higher achievers in mathematics? (2) Does the teaching of Chinese learners necessarily lead to rote learning? (3) How is the curriculum structured to support teaching and learning? and (4) How do Chinese families support students' learning? In the discussion of each issue, available research evidence that addresses each issue is first reviewed, and then research needed to further address the issue is suggested.

2 Are Chinese Learners Really Higher Achievers in Mathematics?

In the past several decades, a number of cross-national studies have consistently showed that Chinese students outperformed their Western counterparts on tasks routinely learned in schools [See Cai (1995), Fan and Zhu (this volume), and Robitaille and Travers (1992) for reviews]. In fact, a general finding across almost all existing cross-national studies in mathematics was that Chinese students consistently outperformed their Western counterparts across grade levels and mathematical topics. For example, Geary, Bow-Thomas, Liu, and Siegler (1996) examined the development of arithmetical competencies of US and Chinese children in kindergarten, and first, second, and third grades. They found that Chinese children have higher success rates than do US children at each grade level. Stevenson and Lee (1990) used samples of first- and fifth-grade students from Chicago (US) and Beijing (China) to compare their achievements in mathematical topic areas including word problems, number concepts, mathematical operations, measurement and scaling, graphs and tables, spatial relations, visualization, estimation, and speed tests. They found that there were almost no areas in which the children in Chicago performed as well as children in Beijing.

Since recent studies have shown the relative performance between US and Chinese students on various tasks (see Cai & Cifarelli, this volume), however, we may not be able to simply claim that Chinese students are higher achievers in mathematics. Nevertheless, cross-national studies did provide sufficient evidence showing that Chinese students are higher achievers on tasks measuring basic mathematical knowledge and skills in mathematics.

While a number of studies examined Chinese students' achievement in the wider comparative contexts, there are at least three unanswered questions for future exploration. The first unanswered question is related to mastering basic knowledge and skills and the development of higher-order thinking skills. Research has shown that having routine problem-solving skills does not imply having creative, nonroutine problem solving skills (Cai, 2000; Hatano, 1988; Steen, 1999; Sternberg, 1999). As indicated before, Chinese students clearly outperform US students on tasks measuring basic knowledge and skills, but not necessarily on complex, open-ended tasks measuring creativity and nonroutine problem solving. In a recent study, C. Chen et al. (2002) examined whether European Americans and Chinese differ in their creation and evaluation of drawing of geometric shapes. They found high consensus between 50 European Americans and 48 Chinese college students and great similarity in the creativity of drawings generated by the two samples. Cai (2000) found that Chinese students outperformed US students on process-constrained tasks, but on process-open tasks, US students outperformed Chinese students. Therefore, the question is: Does the development of Chinese students' basic skills come at the expense of the development of higher-order thinking skills?

The second unanswered question is related to instructional practice. Given the fact that Chinese students have strong basic skills, a natural question is to explore possible factors contributing to Chinese students' mastering of basic skills and knowledge. How do Chinese students develop basic mathematical skills and knowledge? It is clear that Chinese students in Mainland China, Hong Kong, and Taiwan spend more time in schools than do US students, and many Chinese students also attend cram schools (H. M. E. Huang, this volume). Both in and out of schools, Chinese students are required to do a great deal of practice and memorization. In fact, according to Chinese teachers in Taiwan, cram schools mainly focus on basic skills rather than higher-order thinking skills. Would it be possible that the Chinese students' mastery of basic knowledge and skills necessary resulted from the practice and memorization? As Marton et al. (1996) pointed out, such practice and memorization may lead to rote learning, but it may also lead to understanding (also see Wong, this volume). Under what conditions would the practice and memorization lead to rote learning? Similarly, it is important to explore what kind of practice and memorization would lead to conceptual understanding.

The third unanswered question is related to the interpretation of the achievement results from some of the cross-national studies. Using national representative samples, the TIMSS Video Study (Stigler & Hiebert, 1999) showed that — when compared to German and Japanese teachers' teaching — US teachers focused more on mathematical procedures and techniques and practice of routine problem solving, and less on mathematical exploration and conceptual understanding. If that is the case, why did US students perform so poorly on computation and routine problem-solving tasks requiring procedural knowledge, in contrast to Chinese students and students from other countries? One may argue that since US teachers focused more on procedures, US students might not understand the principles behind the procedures (Hiebert, 1986); thus, they performed poorly on computation and routine problem solving. However, if US teachers focused less on mathematical exploration and conceptual understanding, according to Stigler and Hiebert (1999), and Chinese teachers had a better understanding of elementary mathematics than their US counterparts, according to L. Ma (1999), then why did the US students perform better than the Chinese students on the process-open, non-routine problems? Furthermore, why did US students in Cai's study (2000) perform better on the process-open problems than on the process-constrained problems and vice versa for the Chinese students?

3 Does the Teaching of Chinese Learners Necessarily Lead to Rote Learning?

This is a commonly asked question for those who are interested in knowing how Chinese learners learn mathematics in their schools. Many scholars and observers found that mathematics teaching in Chinese classroom is very traditional, content-based, examination-driven, and teacher-centered. Classroom instruction is usually conducted in a whole classroom setting, with a large class size of 40-50 students, and with little interaction between teachers and students (Leung, 2002). These external characteristics of classroom organization and structures are likely to give people impression that the teaching of Chinese learners may lead to rote learning. In fact, a number of authors in this volume consistently identified these characteristics of instruction in Chinese classroom and suggested the potential link with the rote learning (e.g., see An, this volume; Y. Ma, Zhao, & Tuo, this volume).

However, other researchers found that underlying these external features of classroom instruction, students might engage in deep thinking of important mathematics (see Wong, this volume). For example, R. Huang and Leung (this volume) provided an in-depth analysis of lessons from Shanghai and Hong Kong on the topic of Pythagoras's theorem. Their findings suggest that even though students were not actively involved in the classroom discussion in the setting with a large class size, teachers used well-developed instructional activities and guided students to exploring activities, justification, and exercises with variations. While there was no external observable discourse between students and teachers, it is quite possible that teachers did pay attention to helping students engage in the learning process through these well-structured activities. In fact, one important feature of the mathematics teaching in Chinese classroom can be described as "teaching with variations" (Gu, R. Huang, & Marton, this volume). According to Gu et al. (this volume), in the setting of teaching with variations, even with a large class size, students still can actively involve themselves in the process of learning, make connections, and understand the critical features of mathematical concepts and relationships.

Apparently, there is no simple answer to the question: does the teaching of Chinese learners necessarily lead to rote learning? However, it is clear that the vast majority of the Chinese lessons analyzed are all well structured, even though teachers may have different teaching styles, and teaching in urban and rural areas might be different. Some researchers (e.g., Mok, Cai, & Fung, 2004) have started to explore the advantages and disadvantages of well-structured lessons. One of the desirable future directions is not just to explore, in a superficial sense, if the teaching in Chinese classroom does lead to rote learning; instead, the emphasis should be on understanding underlying circumstances and conditions in which the teaching in Chinese mathematics classrooms leads to rote learning, and how we can avoid the rote learning in classroom. Wong (this volume) proposed that mere repetition of practice may lead to rote learning, but repetition with variations may lead to understanding. This proposal appears to have incredible merit, but empirical studies are needed to reveal what is actually happening in classrooms. The findings from empirical studies can not only provide evidence to verify Wong's proposal, but also provide insightful information in an effort to improve mathematics learning in both Chinese and international societies.

Perhaps a more fundamental question is: After all, what is effective teaching for Chinese teachers? This question is fundamental because answers to this question can not only help researchers and educators to understand what teachers do in classroom, but also help them to interpret why they teach the way they do. We take a position that teaching is a cultural activity (Bruner, 1996; Stigler & Hiebert, 1999). Although there is no universal agreement about what effective mathematics teaching should look like, no one questions the idea that the teachers' instructional practices are influenced by their cultural conceptions of effective teaching. In fact, cultural beliefs about teaching do not directly dictate what teachers do, but teachers do draw upon their cultural beliefs as a normative framework of values and goals to guide their teaching (Bruner, 1996). Limited evidence revealed significant differences in US and Chinese teachers' beliefs about the desirable methods for teaching mathematics (e.g., Stigler & Perry, 1988). US teachers tend to believe that young children need concrete experiences in order to understand mathematics, at times asserting that concrete experiences will automatically lead to understanding. Chinese teachers, however, apparently believe that even young children can understand abstraction and that concrete experience only serves to mediate an understanding of abstract mathematics. Chinese teachers also believe that the more a student struggles, the more the student can learn; therefore, teachers in China usually pose difficult problems to challenge students. US teachers, in contrast, tend to pose problems that will reinforce the idea that mathematics problems should be solvable in a single, insightful motion (Stigler & Perry, 1988). Furthermore, US teachers reported that mathematics was rather easy to teach, whereas Chinese teachers stated that it was difficult to teach. Systematic efforts are needed to understand how Chinese teachers view and practice effective mathematics teaching.

There are two other related and unanswered questions: What are the characteristics of effective mathematics teachers? How do Chinese teachers learn to be effective teachers? It is suggested that effective teachers should know and understand mathematics, students as learners, and pedagogical strategies (NCTM, 2000). Such understanding can be characterized as "profound understanding of fundamental mathematics" (L. Ma, 1999). Teaching is a profession requiring continuous learning and development (Darling-Hammond & Sykes, 1999). It is well-documented that teachers' university preservice experience (including course work and student teaching) sometimes has little direct impact on their subsequent teaching (e.g., Eisenhart et al., 1993; Grossman,

Valencia, & Hamel, 1997; Kennedy, 1998). After a series of studies of elementary and secondary preservice teachers, Ball (1990) concluded that requiring teachers to study more traditional mathematics would not improve their understanding of school mathematics. Instead, teachers need learning opportunities to analyze mathematical ideas and make connections. Teachers learn to become effective teachers through the practice of teaching: not only do they better understand the topics they are teaching, but they also learn the pedagogy for teaching these topics (also see Fan, 1998).

In China, for example, teachers engage in continuous school-based, collegial professional development through "lesson study" or "teaching research groups" (L. Ma, 1999; Paine & L. Ma, 1993). It is possible that they not only engage in situational learning in their process of induction into teaching, but they also actively use a large repertoire of cultural knowledge of teaching shared by experienced teachers. Besides lesson studies or teaching research groups, Chinese teachers also get involved in district-wide "teaching-research activities" that lead to long-term and short-term plans, as well as lesson plans. Despite the wide agreement about the importance of teachers' continuous learning and development, we know little about what Chinese teachers actually learn through lesson study or teaching research groups or how what they learn impacts on their teaching and consequently on students' learning.

One of the unique features of Chinese teachers is their use of the teaching reference books. Besides student textbooks, each Chinese teacher has a set of corresponding teaching reference books. The teaching reference books used by Chinese teachers are quite unique in the sense that they are very different from the teacher's edition of textbooks in the United States. Li Jianhua (this volume) made an attempt to describe the features of Chinese teaching reference books. The teaching reference books provide not only an overall analysis of the treatments of mathematical topics in students' textbooks, but also detailed instructional guidance for teaching these topics. More work is needed to systematically analyze teaching reference books and to understand how teachers use the reference books to teach and learn to teach in classrooms.

4 How Is the Intended Curriculum for Chinese Learners Structured to Support the Teaching and Learning?

A curriculum is an operational plan for instruction that details what mathematics students need to know and what teachers are to do to help students develop their mathematical knowledge (NCTM, 1989). Cross-cultural studies showed a relatively wide consensus that the observed performance differences among students in different countries could be attributed to, at least in part, the variations in mathematical curricula (e.g., Westbury, 1992). For example, the Third International Mathematics and Science Study (TIMSS) clearly showed that across countries, students' learning is highly correlated with curricular treatment of related topics (Schmidt et al., 2002). As revealed in the study of the textbook use in Chinese classrooms, Fan, J. Chen, Zhu, Qiu, and Hu (this volume) found that intended and implemented curricula in Chinese classroom settings are quite consistent. Thus, to understand Chinese learners, it is quite natural and important to look into the intended curriculum.

Analyses of intended curriculum showed that for Chinese learners, curriculum generally supports effectively their acquisition of basic knowledge and basic skills, including pre-identified mathematics concepts, facts, algorithms, procedures, and formulas. Such acquisition is planned in the curriculum structure to be achieved through providing students with experience and exposure so they can gain more memorization of, more familiarity with, and more practice on the so-called basic knowledge and skills. The evidence is consistently shown that mathematics curricula across Mainland China, Taiwan, and Hong Kong promote students' acquisition of basic knowledge and skills (Cai, Lo, & Watanabe, 2002; H. M. E. Huang, this volume; Wong, this volume; Zhang, S. Li, & Tang, this volume). For example, in a recent study, Cai et al. (2002) analyzed the intended treatment of arithmetic average in US and Asian school mathematics. Two US *Standards*-based and two Chinese curricula were included in the analysis (Division of Elementary Mathematics, 1996; Elementary School Teacher Training Center in Taiwan, 1997; Lappan, Fey, Fitzgerald, Friel, & Phillips, 1998; National Center for Research in Mathematical Sciences Education and

Freudenthal Institute, 1997-1998). It was revealed that the Chinese curricula focus more on understanding the concept of arithmetic average as a computational algorithm than on understanding the concept of arithmetic average as a representative of a data set; however, the two US *Standards*-based curricula focus more on the latter exposition of the concept.

In addition, a number of curriculum and textbook analyses conducted in this area have consistently found that Chinese curricula placed more emphasis on applying basic knowledge and routine procedures, on abstract reasoning, and on solving non-contextualized and conventional problems, but less on investigation, on intuitive thinking and visual representation, and on solving contextualized and non-traditional tasks (Bao, 2002; Fan, 1999; Y. Li, 1999; Zhu, 2003). In solving traditional types of tasks, the Chinese curricula provide more challenge for learners (Zhu, 2003). In addition, Chinese mathematics curricula offer a relatively narrow scope of content, but the coverage is often deeper. A larger percentage of content is repeated in US curricula than in Chinese curricula. Flanders (1987) examined the percentage of new content introduced at each grade level (K-8) in three US mathematics textbook series. He reported that the average percentage of new content in the three series ranged from about 40% to 65% at each grade level and much of the new content is introduced at the end of the year. Using the Flanders' coding method, however, Cai (1995) reported that over 95% of the content is new at each grade level (grades 1-6) in the Chinese textbook series published by the People's Education Press and the old content is primarily found in the review section at the end of each textbook.

The curricula in China are usually designed to support individual learning, but not for cooperative learning. For example, Zhu (2003) examined two seventh and eighth grade mathematics textbooks widely used in China and revealed that almost all problems provided in the textbooks are those that support individual learning, whereas many problems in the US books are designed for group work, which supports cooperative learning. Less opportunity is provided in the Chinese textbooks for students to write and present their ideas.

In summary, available evidence from curriculum analyses showed that the intended curricula in Mainland China, Taiwan, and Hong Kong are well structured and support students' acquisition of basic knowledge and skills well. However, it seems to us that few, if any, empirical studies have been conducted to actually document how well these curricula support both students' acquisition of basic knowledge and skills and conceptual development of mathematical knowledge. In the past several years, education reforms in general and mathematics education in particular have been advocated in these regions. For example, in Mainland China, there has been a movement of systematic mathematics curriculum reform. One of the major focuses of reforming school mathematics curriculum is to not only foster students' acquisition of basic knowledge and skills, but also to foster conceptual development of students' learning. Future studies may focus on investigating what students know and are able to do when they use the "reform-oriented" mathematics programs in China.

Classroom teachers are at the heart of the implementation of mathematics education reform. Their interpretation and implementation will determine the ultimate success of the systematic reform initiative. In fact, the effectiveness of the reform-oriented mathematics programs is critically dependent on how they are understood and handled by teachers. Studies are needed not only to empirically document the effectiveness of school mathematics programs, but also to examine the roles teachers play in implementing reform ideas in Chinese educational systems.

5 How Do Chinese Families Support Students' Learning?

Recognition of the importance of family support in students' learning is not new. In fact, in 1897, Hauschmann indicated that "[a]ll are looking for reform in education. ... If [the] building is not to be solid, we must look to the foundations — the home" (as cited in White, Taylor, & Moss, 1992, p. 91). A strong relationship between home background variables and student performance is well-documented (Robitaille & Garden, 1989; Wang, Haertel, & Walberg, 1993). For example, researchers have known that the involvement of parents contributes to both their children's higher academic achievement and their positive behaviors and emotional development.

Previous cross-national studies have surveyed the educational and occupational status of the parents, parental help, the study environment at home, time spent on homework, parents' expectations of their children, and parents' beliefs about their children's future happiness and the way to achieve success. The educational and occupational status of the parents and the study environment at home were not found to contribute to performance differences in mathematics (e.g., Robitaille & Garden, 1989; Stevenson & Lee, 1990). However, time spent on homework, parental help, parents' expectations of their children, and parents' beliefs about their children's future happiness and the way to achieve success do seem to be related to children's school work (e.g., Cai, 2003; Lapointe, Mead, & Askew, 1992; Robitaille & Garden, 1989; Stevenson & Lee, 1990).

Compared to US students, Chinese students not only have longer school year, but also spend more time on homework in all subjects. As far as the time spent particularly on mathematics homework is concerned, data from the second International Assessment of Educational Progress (IAEP) showed that students from Mainland China and Taiwan spent more hours on mathematics homework each week than did US students (Lapointe et al., 1992). In particular, 72% of the students from Mainland China reported that they spent two hours or more on mathematics homework each week, but only 37% of the US students reported doing so. In addition, not only did Chinese students spend longer time on homework, but also the majority of them attended cram schools according to a survey of teachers in Taiwan (H. M. E. Huang, this volume). The time spent on homework is one kind of measures for students' learning in home setting. It is quite possible that for doing the same number and types of homework problems, one group of students may take much longer than the other. Future studies should focus on actually documenting the kinds of homework Chinese students have and the kinds of mathematics-related cram schools they attend. Studies are also needed to investigate the actual impact of the homework and cram schools on students' learning of mathematics.

Regarding parents' involvement in their students' learning, US parents were more likely to help their children with homework than to ask them about their mathematics classes. In contrast, Chinese parents were more likely to ask their children about their mathematics classes than to help them with their homework (Lapointe et al., 1992). US mothers appeared to be less interested in their children's specific academic achievement than in their children's general cognitive development, so they attempted to provide experiences for fostering cognitive growth rather than academic excellence. While both Chinese and US mothers emphasized diligence as a way to achieve success, US mothers stressed independence, innate ability, and acceptance of diversity. Chinese mothers held higher standards for their children's achievement than did US mothers, and they gave more realistic evaluations of their children's academic, cognitive, and personality characteristics. Chinese mothers appeared to believe that the route to future happiness is through hard working and high academic success, while US mothers gave greater emphasis on innate ability (Stevenson & Lee, 1990).

Recently, Cai (2003) conducted a cross-national study to examine parental roles in students' learning of mathematics in the home setting. A Parental Involvement Questionnaire (PIQ) was developed and used to examine five parental roles: motivators, resource providers, monitors, mathematics content advisors, and mathematics learning counsellors. There are several differences and similarities between US and Chinese parents. For example, Chinese parents had a significantly higher mean score than did the US parents on the variable of parents as monitors, while US parents had significantly higher mean scores on the variables of parents as resource providers and content advisers. The findings from the study suggest that Chinese parents are less directly involved in students' learning of mathematics. Instead, Chinese parents tend to support students' learning through monitoring and motivating them (Cai, 2003). The finding of the study supports the argument that the Chinese parenting style is more monitoring and organizational in nature (Chao & Sue, 1996).

US and Chinese parents realized the importance of having a nice learning environment for their children at home. However, there were statistically significant differences between the two samples regarding the mathematics-related books and availability of mathematics tools such as calculators. For example, nearly 90% of the Chinese parents agreed or strongly agreed that they often buy mathematics-related books for their children, but only about 30% of the US parents said so. US parents may buy fewer mathematics-related books for their children because many US parents purchase computer software for their children's learning of mathematics. Over 95% of the US parents said that they had mathematics tools such as calculators available at home, but only about 25% of the Chinese homes had such mathematics tools available. Over 70% of the Chinese parents tried to monitor the amount of time their children spent on mathematics at home while about 50% of the US parents tried to do so. It should be noted that the vast majority of both US and Chinese parents realized the importance of motivating their children to learn mathematics. However, a considerable number of US and Chinese parents stated that sometimes they did not know how to motivate their children to do a good job on mathematics assignments (Cai, 2003).

Cai (2003) also found that parental involvement measured by the PIQ is closely related to students' mathematical achievement. The contribution of the five parental roles together for both US and Chinese students' performance was statistically significant. Although this study has show the important roles US and Chinese parents play in their children's learning in the home setting, how specifically these parents play their roles at home is not documented. One direction for future studies is to systematically document how parents motivate and monitor their children's learning at home, as well as to explore ways to help parents motivate and monitor their children's learning.

6 Final Remarks

How do Chinese learn mathematics? This chapter clearly shows that Chinese students have some unique characteristics in their mathematical performance. This chapter also describes in and out of school contexts in which Chinese learners are nurtured. Chinese students have strong basic knowledge and skills in mathematics. Chinese teachers usually deliver well-structured lessons following the alignment of curriculum. Although Chinese parents are less likely to be directly involved in their children's learning, they seem to be one of the major driving forces behind their children's success in education.

While we believe the contribution of studying how Chinese learn mathematics in the wider educational context, we also realize that it is still too early to paint a clear picture of Chinese learners in mathematics. As we indicated in this chapter, it may not be fruitful by just focusing on cultural explanations (e.g., Confucianism) to characterize Chinese learners, but to clearly characterize Chinese learners, much more effort, research, and development must take place. In this chapter, we have pointed out a number of research issues for empirical investigations. There is a need for researchers in this area to more systematically explore these issues in order to understand Chinese learners better.

It should be indicated that this chapter has a limitation in that we were not able to include a large body of mathematics education literature in Chinese in our review. Otherwise, we might have had an even better picture about how Chinese learn mathematics. In this sense, our work on exploring how Chinese learn mathematics from insiders' perspective is just the first step of a long and exciting journey.

References

Ball, D. L. (1990). Prospective elementary and secondary teachers' understanding of division. *Journal for Research in Mathematics Education, 21*(2), 132-144.

Bao, J. (2002). *Comparative study on composite difficulty of Chinese and British school mathematics curricula.* Unpublished doctoral dissertation, East China Normal University, Shanghai.

Bruner, J. S. (1996). *The culture of education.* Cambridge, MA: Harvard University Press.

Cai, J. (1995). A cognitive analysis of U.S. and Chinese students' mathematical performance on tasks involving computation, simple problem solving, and complex problem solving. *Journal for Research in Mathematics Education monograph series 7*. Reston, VA: National Council of Teachers of Mathematics.

Cai, J. (2000). Mathematical thinking involved in U.S. and Chinese students' solving process-constrained and process-open problems. *Mathematical Thinking and Learning: An International Journal, 2*(4), 309-340.

Cai, J. (2003). Investigating parental roles in students' learning of mathematics from a cross-national perspective. *Mathematics Education Research Journal, 15*(2), 87-106.

Cai, J. (2004). Developing algebraic thinking in the earlier grades: A case study of the Chinese elementary school curriculum. *The Mathematics Educator, 8*(1), 107-130. Singapore.

Cai, J., Lo, J. J., & Watanabe, T. (2002). Intended treatments of arithmetic average in U.S. and Asian school mathematics. *School Science and Mathematics. 102*(8), 391-404.

Chao, R. K., & Sue, S. (1996). Chinese parental influence and their children's school success: A paradox in the literature on parenting styles. In S. Lau (Ed.), *Growing up the Chinese way: Chinese child and adolescent development* (pp. 93-120). Hong Kong: The Chinese University Press.

Chen, C., Kasof, J., Himsel, A. J., Greenberger, E., Dong, Q., & Xue, G. (2002). Creativity in drawings of geometric shapes: A cross-cultural examination with the consensual assessment technique. *Journal of Cross-Cultural Psychology, 33*(2), 171-187.

Darling-Hammond, L., & Sykes, G. (Eds.) (1999). *Teaching as the learning profession: Handbook of policy and practice*. San Francisco, CA: Jossey-Bass.

Division of Elementary Mathematics. (1996). *National unified mathematics textbooks in elementary school* [In Chinese 全国通编小学数学教材]. Beijing: People's Education Press.

Eisenhart, M., Borko, H., Underhill, R., Brown, C., Jones, D., & Agard, P. (1993). Conceptual knowledge falls through the cracks: Complexities of learning to teach mathematics through understanding. *Journal for Research in Mathematics Education, 24*(1), 8-40.

Elementary School Teacher Training Center in Taiwan. (1997). *Experimental mathematics* [In Chinese 数学国民小学实验课程]. Taipei: Author.

Fan, L. (1998). *The development of teachers' pedagogical knowledge: An investigation of mathematics teachers in three high-performing high schools*. Doctoral dissertation, University of Chicago. (UMI No. AAT 9841511)

Fan, L. (1999). Applications of arithmetic in US and Chinese textbooks: A comparative study. In G. Kaiser, E. Luna, & I. Huntley (Eds.), *Studies in mathematics education series II: International comparisons in mathematics education* (pp. 151-162). London: Falmer Press.

Flanders, J. R. (1987). How much of the content in mathematics textbooks is new? *Arithmetic Teacher, 35*(1), 18-23.

Gardner, H. (1989). *To open minds*. New York: Basic Books.

Geary, D. C., Bow-Thomas, C. C., Liu, F., & Siegler, R. S. (1996). Development of arithmetic competencies in Chinese and American children: Influence of age, language, and schooling. *Child Development, 67*(5), 2022-2044.

Grossman, P. L., Valencia, S. W., & Hamel, F. (1997). Preparing language arts teachers in a time of reform. In J. Flood, S. B. Heath, & D. Lapp (Eds.), *A handbook for research on teaching literacy through the communicative and visual arts* (pp. 407-416). New York: MacMillan.

Hatano, G. (1988). Social and motivational bases for mathematical understanding. In G. B. Saxe & M. Gearhart (Eds.), *Children's mathematics* (pp. 55-70). San Francisco, CA: Jossey Bass.

Hiebert, J. (Eds.) (1986). *Conceptual and procedural knowledge: The case of mathematics*. Hillsdale, NJ: Lawrence Erlbaum Associates.

Kennedy, M. M. (1998). *Learning to teach writing: Does teacher education make a difference?* New York: Teachers College Press.

Lapointe, A. E., Mead, N. A., & Askew, J. M. (1992). *Learning mathematics*. Princeton, NJ: Educational Testing Service.

Lappan, G., Fey, J. T., Fitzgerald, W. M., Friel, S. N., & Phillips, E. D. (1998). *Connected mathematics*. Menlo Park, CA: Dale Seymour Publications.

Leung, F. K. S. (2002, October). *Mathematics education in East Asian and the West: Does culture matter?* Paper presented at the International Congress of Mathematics Instruction's Comparative Study Conference. Hong Kong: The University of Hong Kong.

Li, Y. (1999). *An analysis of algebra content, content organization and presentation, and to-be-solved problems in eighth-grade mathematics textbooks from Hong Kong, Mainland China, Singapore, and the United States*. Doctoral dissertation, University of Pittsburgh. (UMI No. AAT 9957757)

Ma, L. (1999). *Knowing and teaching elementary mathematics: Teachers' understanding of fundamental mathematics in China and the United States*. Hillsdale, NJ: Erlbaum.

Marton, F., Dall'Alba, G., & Tse, L. K. (1996). Memorizing and understanding: The keys to the paradox? In D. A. Watkins & J. B. Biggs (Eds.), *Cultural, psychological and contextual influences* (pp. 69–83). Hong Kong: Comparative Education Research Centre, The University of Hong Kong; Melbourne, Australia: The Australian Council for the Educational Research.

Mok, I. A. C., Cai, J., & Fung, A. T. F. (2004, July). *Two sides of a coin: An analysis of a lesson on comparing fractions*. Paper presented at the 10th International Congress of Mathematics Education. Copenhagen, Denmark.

National Center for Research in Mathematical Sciences Education and Freudenthal Institute. (1997-1998). *Mathematics in context*. Chicago, IL: Encyclopedia Britannica.

National Council of Teachers of Mathematics. (1989). *Curriculum and evaluation standards for school mathematics*. Reston, VA: Author.

National Council of Teacher of Mathematics. (2000). *Principles and Standards for School Mathematics*. Reston, VA: Author.

Paine, L. W., & Ma, L. (1993). Teachers working together: A dialogue on organizational and cultural perspectives of Chinese teachers. *International Journal of Educational Research, 19*(8), 675-697.

Robitaille, D. F., & Garden, R. A. (1989). *The IEA study of mathematics II: Contexts and outcomes of school mathematics*. New York: Pergamon.

Robitaille, D. F., & Travers, K. J. (1992). International studies of achievement in mathematics. In D. A. Grouws (Ed.), *Handbook of research on mathematics teaching and learning* (pp. 687-709). New York: Macmillan.

Schmidt, W. H., McKnight, C. C., Houang, R. T., Wang, H., Wiley, D. E., Cogan, L. S., et al. (2002). *Why schools matter: A cross-national comparison of curriculum and learning.* San Francisco, CA: Jossey-Bass.

Steen, L. A. (1999). Twenty questions about mathematical reasoning. In L. V. Stiff & F. R. Curcio (Eds.), *Developing mathematical reasoning in grades K – 12* (pp. 270-285). Reston, VA: National Council of Teachers of Mathematics.

Sternberg, R. J. (1999). The nature of mathematical reasoning. In L. V. Stiff & F. R. Curcio (Eds.), *Developing mathematical reasoning in grades K–12* (pp. 37-44). Reston, VA: National Council of Teachers of Mathematics.

Stevenson, H. W., & Lee, S. Y. (1990). *Contexts of achievement: A study of American, Chinese, and Japanese children.* Chicago, IL: University of Chicago Press.

Stigler, J. W., & Hiebert, J. (1999). *The teaching gap: Best ideas from the world's teachers for improving education in the classroom.* New York: The Free Press.

Stigler, J. W. & Perry, M. (1988). Cross cultural studies of mathematics teaching and learning: Recent findings and new directions. In D. A. Grouws, T. J. Cooney, & D. Jones (Eds.), *Effective mathematics teaching* (pp. 104-223). Reston, VA: National Council of Teachers of Mathematics.

Wang, M. C., Haertel, G. D., & Walberg, H. J. (1993). Toward a knowledge base for school learning. *Review of Educational Research, 63*(3), 249-294.

Westbury, I. (1992). Comparing American and Japanese achievement: Is the United States really a low achiever? *Educational Researcher, 21*(5), 18-24.

White, K. R., Taylor, M. J., & Moss, V. D. (1993). Does research support claims about the benefits of involving parents in early intervention programs? *Review of Educational Research, 62*(1), 91-125.

Zhu, Y. (2003). *Representations of problem solving in China, Singapore and US mathematics textbooks: A comparative study.* Unpublished doctoral dissertation, National Institute of Education, Singapore.

About the Contributors

AN Shuhua is an assistant professor of mathematics education in the College of Education, California State University, Long Beach. She taught mathematics for nine years at college level in China and six years at high school level in Texas, USA. She earned her PhD in mathematics education from Texas A&M University in 2000. Her research interest fields include comparative study, teachers' pedagogical content knowledge, knowledge of students' thinking, and technology integration in mathematics teaching.

BAO Jiansheng is an associate professor of mathematics education and deputy director of Lesson Study Video-case Lab at Soochow University in China. He was a high school mathematics teacher for about 6 years and a visiting research fellow at the University of Exeter for one year. He earned his PhD in mathematics education at East China Normal University in 2002. His research interests embrace teacher education, international comparisons in mathematics education, problem solving, and assessment in mathematics.

CAI Jinfa is a professor and director of Secondary Mathematics Teacher Education at the Department of Mathematical Sciences, the University of Delaware. His research interest is related to students learning and mathematical problem solving. In particular, He is interested in how students learn mathematics and solve problems, and how teachers and teaching impact on students learning and their mathematical thinking. He has explored these questions in various educational contexts, both within and across nations. His work has been published in various research journals and books. He received the 1994 Outstanding Dissertation Award from the Doctoral Association of Educators at Pittsburgh and was a 1996 U.S. National Academy of Education Spencer Fellow. In 2002, he received the International Research Award from the University of Delaware as well as a teaching excellence award from the Delaware Chapter of Kappa Delta Pi. He has been a visiting professor in various institutions, including Harvard University in 2000-2001. He has been serving on the Editorial Panels/Advisory Boards of *Journal for Research in Mathematics Education, Mathematics Education Research Journal*, and *Zentralblatt fuer Didaktik der Mathematik*.

CHEN Jingan is an associate professor in the Department of Mathematics, Yunnan Normal University, China. She graduated from Yunnan University in mathematics in 1982 and completed a graduate program in mathematics education in 1998. Her research areas include mathematics education and teacher education.

CIFARELLI Victor is an associate professor of mathematics and the coordinator of mathematics education in the Department of Mathematics, University of North Carolina at Charlotte. His doctoral research focused on the role of reflective abstraction as a learning process in mathematical problem solving. His current research examines how solvers reflect on and test the viability of their evolving intuitions, and transform their initial hypotheses and conjectures into actual solution activity. Dr. Cifarelli has presented his research at AERA, PME, and PME-NA. His articles have appeared in the *Journal of Mathematical Behavior* and the Proceedings of PME and PME-NA. He has taught a variety of undergraduate and graduate mathematics and mathematics education courses including mathematics for elementary education majors, mathematics education for elementary and middle school education majors, and graduate mathematics courses for secondary mathematics teachers. He has co-directed a pair of projects for elementary, middle, and secondary grades mathematics teachers under the Eisenhower Professional Development Program and also has conducted numerous in-service workshops for middle grades and secondary mathematics teachers.

FAN Lianghuo received his MSc in 1989 from East China Normal University, China, where he has also taught at both school and university levels for about 10 years. He completed his PhD in 1998 at the University of Chicago, USA, where he also worked for the University of Chicago School Mathematics Project. Since then he has been working at the National Institute of Education (NIE), Nanyang Technological University, Singapore. His research interests include assessment and alternative assessment, curriculum studies and textbook development, teacher knowledge development, and algorithmic algebra for polynomials, and he has published in all of these areas. He presided over the Forum for All Chinese Mathematics Educators of the 9th International Congress on Mathematics Education (ICME-9) held in Tokyo, 2000. He is currently leading a research team for a mathematics assessment project under the Center for Research in Pedagogy and Practice (CRPP) of NIE. He is also the chief editor of secondary mathematics textbooks being published by Zhejiang Education Publishing House in China.

GU Lingyuan is a professor of mathematics education at East China Normal University and Shanghai Academy of Educational Sciences, where he is also deputy president. He obtained his BSc from Fudan University and his PhD from East China Normal University. He is well-known for his 20-year long *Qinpu Experiment* catering for effective mathematics teaching since the early 1980s. His research interests are teacher education, school-based development research, and mathematics education.

HAN Jiwei, BA, MPhil (Northeast Normal University, China), PhD Candidate (the Chinese University of Hong Kong); Lecturer, Department of Mathematics, Northeast Normal University. Research area includes mathematics teacher knowledge.

HUANG Hsin Mei, Edith, is a professor of the Graduate School of Curriculum and Instruction, and the Department of Elementary Education, Taipei Municipal Teachers College, Taipei, Taiwan. Her research interests are learning and teaching of mathematics, children's thinking in problem-solving, preservice and inservice development for elementary school teachers. In addition to teaching and research, she has also been involved in elementary school mathematics curriculum and teaching practice through cooperative projects with inservice teachers for empowering teachers professional development purpose.

HUNAG Rongjin is an assistant professor at the University of Macau and East China Normal University. He obtained his PhD from the University of Hong Kong. He is interested in mathematics classroom study, and mathematics education comparative study.

LEE Peng Yee was past vice president of the International Commission on Mathematical Instruction (ICMI) for two terms from 1987 to 1994. He was also head of the Department of Mathematics at the National Institute of Education, Singapore. He has spent 40 years in the educational service, and traveled extensively in Asia, in particular, Southeast Asia, during which he held lecturing positions in Africa and New Zealand. He published most of his papers on Henstock integration and authored the book Lanzhou *Lectures on Henstock Integration* (1989), and jointly with Rudolf Výborný the book *Integral: An Easy Approach after Kurzweil and Henstock* (2000). He has supervised PhD students from Singapore, the Philippines, Indonesia, China, and India. His other research interests are sequence spaces and teaching of analysis at the university level.

LEUNG Frederick is a mathematics educator in the Faculty of Education of the University of Hong Kong, and was dean of the Faculty between 1996 and 2002. Born and raised in Hong Kong, Dr. Leung obtained his BSc, CertEd and MEd from the University of Hong Kong, and subsequently his PhD from the University of London. His major research interests are in the comparison of mathematics education in different countries, and in the influence of different cultures on teaching and learning. He is the principal investigator of a number of major research projects, including the Hong Kong component of the Third International Mathematics and Science Study (TIMSS) and the TIMSS 1999 Video Study. Dr. Leung is co-editor of the *Second International Handbook on Mathematics Education,* and is also author of a series of local secondary mathematics textbooks which is most widely used in the territory. He served as a consultant for a number of educational projects for UNESCO and the World Bank, and he is a member of the Executive Committee of the International Commission on Mathematical Instruction (ICMI). Dr. Leung was awarded the Fulbright Scholarship for the year 2002-2003, and he is also an honorary professor of Beijing Normal University, China.

LI Jianhua joined the People's Education Press in Beijing, where he was involved in the development of elementary mathematics teaching and learning materials both as author and editor, after he graduated from Beijing Normal University in mathematics. Currently, he is finishing his PhD program in math education at the University of Chicago from which he also got his master's degree in mathematics education. He is interested in various issues of learning and teaching of mathematics from Kindergarten to 10th grade, particularly of middle grades.

LI Jin is an associate professor at Brown University. She studies how children in different cultures develop ideas and related affects about knowledge and learning and how their understanding of learning influences their actual learning behavior and academic achievement. Related topics include children's conceptions of knowledge, the relationship between their life goals and the process of learning, the role of affect in learning, and socialization for developing beliefs about learning.

LI Jun is an associate professor of the Department of Mathematics at the East China Normal University. She has special interest in studying students' understanding of mathematics, especially in the field of statistics and probability. She is also interested in some other topics, such as curriculum study, teacher training, using technology in classroom and culture's influence on mathematics education. She is a member of the writing group of The Standards of Mathematics Curriculum for Senior High Schools issued by the Ministry of Education of China in 2003. She is also one of the authors of a textbook being used in junior high schools in China.

LI Shiqi is a professor of Mathematics Education at the Department of Mathematics and the deputy director of the Research Institute of Mathematics Education at East China Normal University. His research areas include mathematics learning and teaching, and teacher education. He has published many papers and books in these areas. He is currently the President of China Association of Mathematics Education Research of Higher Institutions of Teacher Education, an External Examiner of Hong Kong Institute of Education, a member of the editorial board of Korea Journal of *Research in Mathematics Education*, and a member of the International Program Committee for ICMI Study 15.

LIN Fou-Lai is professor of the Department of Mathematics at National Taiwan Normal University, where he also served as the department chair for many years. He holds a PhD and an MA from Fordham University, USA and an MPhil from Cambridge University, UK. He is currently the president of Taiwan Association for Mathematics Education, and the chief editor of *International Journal of Science and Mathematics Education*. He is also co-editor of the book *Making Sense of Mathematics Teacher Education* by Kluwer. His research interests include mathematics education, teacher education, and psychology in mathematics teaching and learning.

LOPEZ-REAL Francis is an associate professor in the Faculty of Education at the University of Hong Kong. He has worked as a school teacher, education advisor, curriculum consultant and university lecturer in England, Kenya, Cyprus, Cameroon, Brunei and Hong Kong. He has published widely in international journals, both in mathematics education and more generally in teacher education. His current research interests include comparative studies of classroom teaching in mathematics, the impact of dynamic geometry software on learning mathematics, and understanding communities of practice in teacher education.

MA Yunpeng is a professor in the School of Educational Science, Northeast Normal University. He earned his PhD from the Chinese University of Hong Kong in 1999. He currently directs two national projects: *Elementary Mathematics Curriculum for Distance Learning* and *Study of Assessment Models and Methods for Basic Educational Quality*. His research interests include curriculum studies, teaching methods, and mathematics education at the primary and secondary level.

MARTON Ference is a professor of education in Gothenburg University since 1977, Distinguished Visiting Professor (1998-2001) and Honorary Professor at the University of Hong Kong (2001), Honorary Doctor at Edinburgh University (2000) and at the University of Helsinki (2003). His special areas of interest are learning, Chinese pedagogy, mathematics education, Phenomenography, Variation theory.

MOK Ah Chee Ida is an associate professor in the Faculty of Education at the University of Hong Kong. Since 1990, she has worked in teacher education, specializing in mathematics education. She has been active in mathematics education in both local community and research. She has a broad research interest which includes mathematics education, learning and teaching of mathematics, learning of algebra, investigation in mathematics classrooms, qualitative research, pedagogy of variations and comparative studies. Her current active project is an international video study comparing the mathematics teaching at eighth grade.

MURPHY John, MA, is a recent graduate of the Department of Child Study at Tufts University. His thesis compared socialization beliefs of Chinese and Euro-American parents. He is now working on a study of how parents make decisions. His long-term interests have been in the study of Chinese language and culture.

QIU Xiaolan is an associate professor of mathematics at Fujian Normal University. She has conducted researches on the education of middle school mathematics for more than 20 years and has authored or coauthored nearly 20 publications.

SIU Man Keung obtained his BSc in mathematics/physics from the University of Hong Kong and his PhD in mathematics from Columbia University, writing a thesis on algebraic *K*-theory in 1972 under the supervision of Hyman Bass. He is now a professor of mathematics at the University of Hong Kong. He has published in the fields of algebra, combinatorics, applied probability, mathematics education and history of mathematics. In 1991, the Chinese Mathematical Society selected his book *Mathematical Proofs* (1990, in Chinese) as one of the seven outstanding books in mathematical exposition.

TANG Ruifen is a professor of the Department of Mathematics at East China Normal University. Before she started to be involved in the research of mathematics education, she had taught geometry and topology for about 30 years. She has wide interests in international comparative study, mathematics didactics theory, mathematics teacher training, and information technology in mathematics education. She has authored and translated several books in these areas. She is currently advisor and examiner of mathematics teaching materials being used in schools of China.

TUO Zhongfei is a master's degree student at Northeast Normal University. She is currently involved in three research projects: the Research of Evaluation of the Quality of Elementary Education, the Network of Mathematics Education of Elementary Education, and the Case Study of the Rural Elementary Education. Her research interests include curriculum implementation, curriculum evaluation, and teaching in mathematic of elementary school.

WANG Tao is currently a doctoral candidate in the Graduate School of Education at Harvard University. He has taught in primary school and university level in Shanghai for eight years before he joined Harvard in 1999. He got his MEd in 2001 from Harvard Graduate School of Education majoring in Human Development and Psychology. His research interests are in language and culture, teacher training, and mathematics education.

WONG Ngai-Ying, BA, MPhil, PhD, PostGrad CertEd (the University of Hong Kong), MA(Ed) (the Chinese University of Hong Kong), FIMA., C.Math, F.S.S., C.Stat.; Professor, Department of Curriculum and Instruction, the Chinese University of Hong Kong; member of various subject committees (mathematics) in Curriculum Development Council, and the Examinations Authority in Hong Kong; Founding President of the Hong Kong Association for Mathematics Education, chief editor of *EduMath*. Research areas include conception of mathematics, affect and Confucian Heritage Culture learner's phenomena.

XU Binyan holds a PhD in Science, with a major in Mathematics Education from the University of Osnabrueck, Germany (1994), and is currently a professor of curriculum and instruction at East China Normal University (ECNU). Her research specialties are curriculum and instruction from the perspective of learning science, mathematics learning and teaching for primary school and junior high school, teacher development. She was the associate dean of the School of Educational Sciences of ECNU. She directs or co-directs five key national research projects and also serves as chief advisers for several school projects. She is author or co-author of 8 books and more than 50 articles, has made over 60 presentations around the country, and has obtained the grants of Excellent Young Teacher of Chinese Ministry of Education. She is currently a research fellow of the Alexander von Humboldt Foundation.

ZHANG Dianzhou is a professor of mathematics and the director of the Research Institute of Mathematics Education at East China Normal University. His main research areas include spectral theory of operator, mathematics history, and mathematics education, and he has a wide range of publications in all of these fields. He is co-chair of a committee responsible for the new national senior high school mathematics curriculum standards in China. He was an executive committee member of the International Commission on Mathematical Instruction (ICMI) during 1995-1998. In 1999, he was elected as Academician of the International Eurasian Academy of Sciences.

ZHAO Dongchen is a master's degree student in the School of Educational Science of Northeast Normal University. His research areas include curriculum and instructional theory, and school educational theory.

ZHU Yan is a research associate in the Centre for Research in Pedagogy and Practice, National Institute of Education, Singapore. She earned her PhD in mathematics education from the National Institute of Education, Nanyang Technological University, Singapore, in 2003. Her research interests include curriculum studies, problem solving, comparative studies, and mathematics assessment.

Name Index

Subject Index